Anesthesia STAT! Acute Pediatric Emergencies in PACU

Susan T. Verghese
Editor

Anesthesia STAT! Acute Pediatric Emergencies in PACU

A Clinical Casebook

Springer

Editor
Susan T. Verghese
Department of Anesthesiology, Pain and Perioperative Medicine
Children's National Hospital
Washington, DC, USA

ISBN 978-3-031-24395-0 ISBN 978-3-031-24396-7 (eBook)
https://doi.org/10.1007/978-3-031-24396-7

This Springer imprint is published by the registered company Springer Nature Switzerland AG
The registered company address is: Gewerbestrasse 11, 6330 Cham, Switzerland

This book is dedicated to all the pediatric perioperative caregivers worldwide, who run the race each day for the safety and well-being of the patients entrusted to them!

Preface

The art and science of pediatric anesthesia has evolved over the years to enable the pediatric surgical team to perform complex surgeries in children of all ages and sizes.

The improvement in continuous intra-operative hemodynamic monitoring, minimally invasive approach to surgical sites, use of short-acting muscle relaxants, hypnotics, narcotics, and of regional blocks have enabled the anesthesiologist to awaken the patient breathing spontaneously with minimal pain after complex surgeries.

The continuation of optimal postoperative clinical safety and care in the immediate postoperative period of these surgical patients is a topic that should interest every pediatric anesthesiologist.

Hitherto, there has not been a single textbook published that has described urgent postoperative complications that occur in a pediatric PACU.

A year ago, two of our PACU nurses, Ms. Kathleen Curtis and Ms. Susan Joslyn asked me this question: "Why is it that no one has written a book about anesthesia stat calls and emergency situations in a pediatric PACU and how to minimize these?"

Since we have collectively managed multiple emergency clinical situations post-operatively in children, I realized that it was time to put down on paper, different urgent clinical scenarios we have managed successfully.

As a pediatric anesthesiologist, blessed with the privilege to work at Children's hospital for more than 4 decades, I thank God for this opportunity to raise awareness among the readers to anticipate these complications in children and perhaps learn to decrease potential anesthesia stat calls.

The goal of this endeavor would be to teach members of the perioperative teams around the globe, how we do things at Children's hospital to keep anesthesia stat calls to a minimum. The authors will first focus on how clinical monitoring and safety of our post-op patients can and must continue after we hand off their care to the PACU team and then describe 24 interesting clinical scenarios that needed urgent intervention in PACU.

The task is undertaken by authors who are friends and colleagues, who describe these clinical scenarios from their experience of caring for children who developed these complications.

Chapter 1 is an introduction to this book—about nuts and bolts of post-op hand-off and why the transfer of information of surgical patient is important for post-op care in pediatric anesthesia. It is titled "Passing the Baton" as in a relay race scenario and is about the transfer of patient's medical and surgical information or the "Baton" between members of the relay team.

The focus of the first half is on how checklists became an important part of handoffs historically and why an ideal complete handoff is necessary for continuation of the patient's safety. The specific focus on lateral or recovery positioning of patients postoperatively and the scientific reason why an emerging patient should be in lateral position is described with studies to support the importance of this positioning. This is one simple effective technique used by the author **Dr. Susan T. Verghese** to maintain airway patency of all patients during transport from OR to PACU. The second half is authored by two experienced nurses at Children's PACU team: **Ms. Kathleen Curtis BSN, RN, and Ms. Susan P. Joslyn BSN, RN.** They highlight the physical PACU setup, the flow of cases from Phase 1 to Phase 2 and the clinical problems seen in pediatric patients from the PACU nursing perspective.

The first clinical scenario by **Giuliana Geng-Ramos,** is about a young child developing anaphylaxis after administration of antibiotic in PACU.

The next clinical scenario titled somnolence in an infant after VP shunt revision is by **Dr. Nina Deutsch** who discusses the etiology of lethargy in a child after placement of a ventriculo-peritoneal shunt.

Dr. Chaitanya Challa takes on the task of detailing an undesirable post-op problem in PACU by describing the scenario of emergence delirium in a toddler after surgery.

An unusual complication of cardiac arrest after central line placement in a child in PACU is described by **Dr. Chinwe Unegbu**.

A 7-year-old young child who has a loose tooth pre-operatively seems to have lost it on arrival to PACU! **Dr. Jonathan Maxwell Teets** takes the reader through a hide and seek game where the tooth was there before but not now! Where is it? Who saw it last?

It is unusual to anticipate problems after a bone marrow biopsy in a child with leukemia. **Dr. Andrew Matisoff** describes a sudden clinical deterioration in a young child who develops intractable cardiac arrythmias after anesthesia for a brief surgical procedure.

Dr. Cassie Rim describes another rare but clinically fascinating scenario where an obese teenager develops shoulder pain and tachycardia after a liver biopsy performed by the interventional radiologist under fluoroscopic guidance.

In a scenario of acute oxygen desaturation in a healthy teen on arrival to PACU after hardware removal, **Dr. Dan Vuong Thoai** describes a classic clinical picture of negative pressure pulmonary edema developing from airway obstruction.

Establishing Latex-free OR environment has made allergic reactions to latex, a rare occurrence. **Dr. Mingfei Wang** takes the reader through an unanticipated case scenario of a child with Spina Bifida developing latex allergy in PACU.

In another interesting clinical scenario, Dr. **David Rico Mora,** describes acute O_2 desaturation developing in a teenager in PACU after esophagoscopy and esophageal dilatation.

Although the lateral positioning of patient is the most beneficial position in patients with OSA, this position may not be possible for the patient to assume in some cases. **Dr. Daniela Perez Velasco** describes the problem of respiratory arrest occurring in a teen with obesity and OSA after a cardiac catheterization procedure.

Caudal anesthesia is an easily performed regional technique used in children to provide intra-operative and postoperative analgesia for urological surgery. **Dr. Elisha Peterson** describes the complication of weakness and the inability to walk in a toddler in PACU after a caudal block.

Dr. Pooja Gupta draws an informative clinical picture of the acute complication of post-extubation croupy cough and desaturation in ex-premature toddler. She highlights important techniques to minimize the development of croup and the ways to treat it in PACU.

Dr. Philip Dela Merced describes the genesis of apnea in an ex-premature infant undergoing hernia repair under spinal anesthesia and describes the current treatment available for this complication.

Dr. Nina Rawtani gives the reader a comprehensive clinical picture of a child with persistent vomiting after eye muscle surgery. She describes the pathophysiology and effective preventable methods to lessen this retching problem in the PACU.

Dr. Gregory Lessans describes an unusual scenario of a healthy young boy developing blindness after undergoing bone marrow harvest in the prone position.

In another dynamic case scenario, **Dr. Claude Abdallah** invites the readers to watch in awe as a clinical storm unfolds in PACU in a teenager who develops tachycardia and hypertension after thyroidectomy.

Dr. Marjorie Brennan describes a clinical scenario of prolonged apnea after laryngospasm treatment in a child with hiccups and coughing in PACU after Botox injection for limb spasticity. Etiology?

What could cause seizures in a child after a caudal block performed after anesthetic induction for circumcision**?** **Dr. Andrew Waberski** invites the reader to take a comprehensive look at this critical problem which can occur after a seemingly successful caudal block.

Dr. Jerry D. Santos takes the readers through a maze of causes for sudden fever after dental rehabilitation in a child. Wait, but could this be malignant hyperthermia?

Dr. Angela Lee details an urgent scenario of a young child vomiting blood in PACU after T&A and enumerates steps to treat this perilous complication promptly to decrease morbidity.

Dr. Phayon Lee describes the scenario of a morbidly obese teenager developing acute oxygen desaturation shortly after arrival to PACU. What went wrong?

Children with sickle cell disease (SCD) require general anesthesia for cholecystectomy for gall stones. **Robert Scott Dingeman** describes an uncommon but alarming vascular complication in an SCD patient who develops sudden onset of confusion and left-sided weakness in PACU.

Managing children with autism can be challenging to the entire perioperative team. **Dr. Alberto Rivera Cintron and Dr. Susan T. Verghese** tackle the problem of profound bradycardia when dexmedetomidine was used for treating agitation on induction and emergence. To Treat or not to Treat this problem—is a dilemma!

Finally, the authors of this book sincerely hope that reading these case series will succeed in helping the reader to anticipate postoperative problems that can potentially occur in children after surgery and attempt to minimize them by early preventive interventions.

For this allegorical relay race from OR to PACU to succeed, the following steps are vital:

***First**, know your patient well by detailed history and thorough physical examination, to plan and provide the safest and best anesthetic for the scheduled surgery.*

Anticipate and prevent possible complications from occurring during transport and in PACU by careful patient positioning and focus on continuous monitoring of vital signs.

***Next**, communicate effectively to the PACU team EVERYTHING necessary regarding the post-op patient, to spur them to continue the same vigilance in monitoring, to provide care and comfort in a seamless fashion.*

It is important to remember that the prize is only won if the race is run for the ultimate safety and comfort of our pediatric patients!

Washington, DC Susan T. Verghese

Contents

Contributors

Claude Abdallah Division of Anesthesiology, Children's National Hospital, Washington, DC, USA

Marjorie P. Brennan Children's National Hospital, Washington, DC, USA

Chaitanya Challa Children's National Medical Center, Washington, DC, USA

Kathleen Curtis Children's National Medical Center, Washington, DC, USA

Nina Deutsch Children's National Hospital, Washington, DC, USA

Robert Scott Dingeman The George Washington University School of Medicine and Health Sciences, Washington, DC, USA

Department of Anesthesiology, Pain and Perioperative Medicine, Children's National Hospital, Washington, DC, USA

Giuliana Geng-Ramos Children's National Hospital, The George Washington University School of Medicine, Washington, DC, USA

Pooja Gupta Children's National Hospital, George Washington University, Washington, DC, USA

Susan P. Joslyn Children's National Medical Center, Washington, DC, USA

Angela C. Lee Division of Anesthesiology, Pain and Perioperative Medicine, Children's National Hospital, Washington, DC, USA

Phayon U. Lee Children's National Hospital, The George Washington University School of Medicine, Washington, DC, USA

Gregory Lessans Department of Anesthesiology, Pain and Perioperative Medicine, Children's National Hospital, Washington, DC, USA

Andrew Matisoff Division of Cardiac Anesthesia, Children's National Hospital, Washington, DC, USA

Philip dela Merced Department of Anesthesia, Pain, and Perioperative Medicine, Children's National Hospital, Washington, DC, USA

Daniela Perez-Velasco Division of Pediatric Cardiac Anesthesiology, George Washington University, Washington, DC, USA

Division Anesthesiology, Pain and Perioperative Medicine, Children's National Hospital, Washington, DC, USA

Elisha Peterson Children's National Medical Center, Washington, DC, USA

Nina Rawtani Division of Anesthesiology, Sedation and Perioperative Medicine, Children's National Hospital—George Washington University, Washington, DC, USA

David A. Rico Mora Department of Anesthesiology, Pain, and Perioperative Medicine, Children's National Medical Center, Washington, DC, USA

Catherine Rim Division of Anesthesiology, Pain and Pediatric Medicine, Children's National Hospital and George Washington University Hospital, Washington, DC, USA

Alberto A. Rivera Cintron Children's National Medical Center, Washington, DC, USA

Domiciano Jerry Santos Children's National Medical Center, Washington, DC, USA

Jonathan Maxwell Teets Department of Anesthesiology, Pain and Perioperative Medicine, Children's National Hospital, Washington, DC, USA

Chinwe Unegbu Division of Cardiac Anesthesiology, Children's National Hospital, Washington, DC, USA

Susan T. Verghese Children's National Medical Center, Washington, DC, USA

Thoai An Vuong Division of Anesthesiology, Pain and Perioperative Medicine, Children's National Hospital, George Washington University SMHS, Washington, DC, USA

Andrew T. Waberski George Washington University School of Medicine, Washington, DC, USA

Mingfei Wang Children's National Medical Center, Washington, DC, USA

Passing the Baton: Check List/PACU Handoff: What Is Best?

Susan T. Verghese, Kathleen Curtis, and Susan P. Joslyn

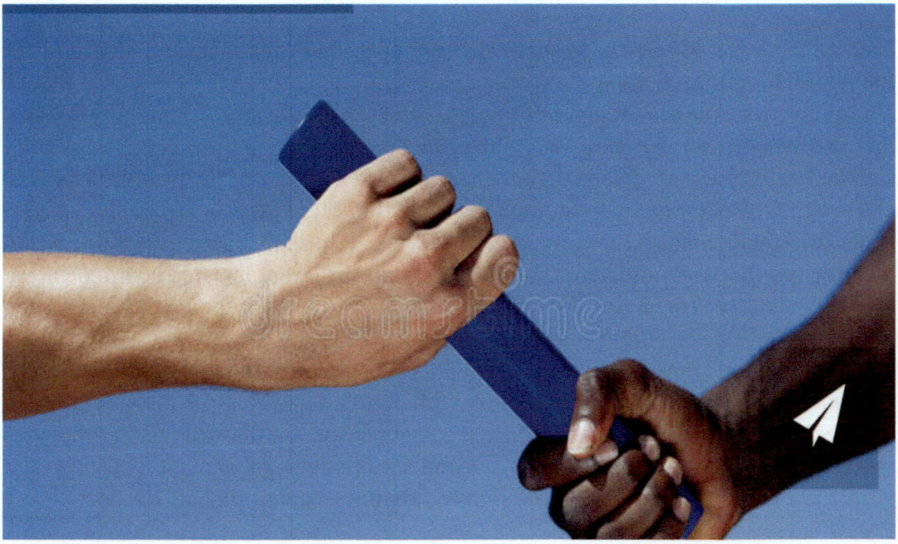

Handing Patient Information as a Baton in a Relay Race. *Illustration of a baton handoff in a relay race*. Need for a structured Handoff—History and Evidence -OR team Handoff to PACU—*as seen from the anesthesiologist view point.* Author: Susan Verghese MD. PACU setup and PACU Nursing Concerns in PACU: OR team to PACU *as Seen from the* PACU Nurses' *View point.* Authors: Kathleen Curtis BSN, RN; Susan P. Joslyn BSN, RN

S. T. Verghese (✉) · K. Curtis · S. P. Joslyn
Children's National Medical Center,
Washington, DC, USA
e-mail: sverghes@cnmc.org; KVyskoci@childrensnational.org; vSJoslyn@childrensnational.org

S. T. Verghese (ed.), *Anesthesia STAT! Acute Pediatric Emergencies in PACU*,
https://doi.org/10.1007/978-3-031-24396-7_1

1 A Safe and Complete PACU Handoff: Why?

1.1 Introduction

The operating room (OR) environment is one of the constant bustling areas with patients' arrival at the pre-op holding area and departure to the assigned OR for anesthesia and surgery. The preoperative nurse welcomes patients after they are registered, directing them and their families to assigned holding bays and evaluating, recording, and transferring information about the patient to surgeon, anesthesiologist, and the OR nurse.

The anesthesiologist is ultimately responsible for assessing each patient for appropriateness for surgery after the pre-op nurse's initial assessment and for administering premedication whenever indicated. The anesthesiologist relies on the preoperative evaluation of each patient, derived from patient's electronic medical records, preoperative interview, and physical examination of the patient, to plan and execute the optimal anesthetic technique for each case. Preoperative planning for induction, monitoring, and pain management with narcotics and/or regional blocks are all discussed with parents, before proceeding with anesthetic induction. When the anesthesiologist, surgeon, OR nurse, technician, and the pre-op nurse are all satisfied with necessary paperwork regarding consent, updated history, and physical and specific tests for the patient, then the induction of anesthesia is signaled to proceed. Anesthetic management, type of airway used, intraoperative use of drugs and intravenous fluids administered, blood loss, and urine output are recorded in the electronic chart during anesthesia in the OR and available for the PACU nurse even before patient reaches the PACU bay.

Patient's vital signs (continuously monitored) and hemodynamic responses during induction, surgery, emergence, and extubation are data that are also recorded in the electronic chart. Even if the information about the anesthesiologist's preoperative assessment, need for premedication, and anesthetic management of each patient is in the electronic record, this is again verbally repeated during handoff to the PACU nurse.

A very busy OR schedule may not allow sufficient time for the anesthesia provider to transfer all the vital information regarding the patient to the receiving PACU nurse. Incomplete and erroneous handoffs are well known to affect patient care and safety adversely. Information without a structured approach can result in the omission of vital patient medical information if the handoff time is brief and rushed. A well-structured method of handoff can assist each member in the perioperative team to focus on vital information related to each patient necessary for continuing care and safety.

1.2 Importance of Checklists: Historical Evidence

Checklists were first developed in aviation industry—a high-risk field that is often compared to the specialty of anesthesia as modalities to help structure complex processes involved in flying. Use of a checklist allows transfer of patient information to be complete, efficient, and safe for continuation of optimal patient care in PACU. Its use during PACU handoff process has become very useful since its benefits became evident following many studies in children and adults.

In a multicenter study by World Health Organization's Safe Surgery Saves Lives program involving 3733 enrolled diverse patients, 16 years and above in 8 hospitals in 8 different cities undergoing noncardiac surgery, implementation of the checklist was shown to reduce the morbidity and mortality [1].

In another study, the researchers' review of literature on transfer of patient care from OR to PACU showed that out of more than 500 papers, there were 31 papers directly assessing postoperative handoffs, and 24 of them had recommendations for a structured processing of information during handoffs, by using protocols and checklists.

Several other broad recommendations included the following:

1. The need to have all relevant team members to be present for handoffs
2. The transfer of information to happen only after completing urgent clinical tasks for the patient safety
3. To focus only on the patient-specific discussion, avoiding spurious discussions not pertaining to patient
4. Emphasis on the need to provide training in improving team skills and communication

An association between poor-quality handovers and adverse events was also demonstrated in this review. [2]

An easy to remember technique named **SBAR** (**S**ituation, **B**ackground, **A**ssessment, **R**ecommendation) was suggested to frame important details about the patient in a concise form by focusing on a stepwise fashion: the situation, followed by a brief background of the present situation and the assessment you were able to make about this problem and your recommendation.

SBAR continues to provide an ease of communication between healthcare team members to focus on precise essential factors to improve patient safety [3].

Ineffective handoffs can occur when multiple handoffs occur in a speedy fashion in PACU increasing the chance to omit transfer of vital information, for example, about patient's allergy or bleeding tendency. Anesthesiologists in Cincinnati Children's Hospital used quality improvement structured processes to facilitate handoff in OR and PACU. Initiating a standardized PACU checklist improved the reliability of their handoffs from 59 to 90% [4].

A pilot study examined the relationship between quality of handoff and PACU length of stay. The authors of this study recommended that more efforts are needed to train anesthesia providers to improve the quality of PACU handoffs [5]. Another study recorded videos of handoffs between anesthesiologist and PACU nurse before and after initiating checklists and recommended that the use of a checklist for post-anesthesia handoff might improve its quality by increasing the quantity of information handed over [6].

In conclusion, there is a need for continuation of increased vigilance in the care of every patient after surgery.

1.2.1 Anesthesia Stat (AS) Calls

Despite the presence of advanced communication capabilities that currently exist, emergency calls or *Anesthesia Stat (AS) calls* are still common in many medical centers.

An interesting study from a tertiary university medical center showed the reason for stat calls in children in the OR and in the PACU after emergence. The researchers of this study collected data prospectively for more than 3 years on the incidence of Anesthesia Stat (AS) calls from pediatric operating rooms and in PACU. Of the 82 Anesthesia Stat calls in children whose ages ranged from 11 days old to 17 years, 60% AS occurred during emergence in OR, and 71% occurred in PACU.

Respiratory events were the cause of 97% of PACU calls and 86% of these calls required the intervention of an anesthesia staff member. Eighty-nine percent *occurred within 30 min of patient arrival.*

The researchers *recommended the presence of an anesthesiologist or a member of the anesthesia staff team with advanced airway management skills to be present and available in PACU.*

In our PACU at Children's National Medical Center, the credit goes to our current chairman, Dr. Eugenie Heitmiller who insisted on a daily assignment for a PACU staff for exactly this reason for improved safety of PACU patients.

Another interesting finding was that 21% of the patients in the PACU AS call *had URI symptoms* and 43% of patients in the PACU AS call group were patients who were slowly emerging because of *deep LMA removal* in OR [7].

The above study reveals what most experienced pediatric anesthesiologists have always known. *PACU emergency or AS calls occur commonly from respiratory events in children and in those who are emerging from a deeper plane of anesthesia.*

Positioning of these patients in the recovery position or the lateral side when possible is a simple efficient way to prevent airway obstruction and aspiration. The presence of preoperative URI symptoms and a history of reactive airway disease in the child can further worsen perioperative respiratory events.

A recent pediatric study evaluated the prevalence and risk factors associated with perioperative respiratory adverse events (PRAE) in 210 pediatric postsurgical patients in university hospitals in Ethiopia. Definition of PRAE included episodes of coughing, breath holding, hypoxemia, laryngospasm, and bronchospasm. Incidence of PRAE was reported as 26.2%, and 89% occurred in the postoperative period with desaturation being the commonest, in age <1 year, presence of recent URI, increased upper airway secretions, ASA status ≥3, and airway-related surgery [8].

The role of the *PACU anesthesiologist is a very important role in evaluating children after surgery for airway safety and pain control and in assessing their readiness for discharge. In addition, there is active involvement in helping the PACU nurses to provide optimal care, administer intravenous medications to decrease emergence agitation in certain children, and discuss any concerns parents may have regarding their children's need for pain and comfort prior to discharge.*

Focus on complete and thorough patient information during handoffs cannot be overemphasized because the lack of it can have deleterious effect on patient care and safety. The relay of patient information starts from the preoperative team to the

OR team and OR team to the PACU team and finally PACU team to the floor inpatient team or the caretakers at home.

Ready, Set, Go! Let the Relay Begin…

1.2.2 What Are the Steps Involved in Passing the Baton Safely?

OR to PACU: Anesthesiologist's View

First Phone Call: First Part of the Relay – *Patient Information Transfer*

The actual handoff begins when the circulating nurse in the operating room calls the PACU charge nurse to give an introductory clinical information about the patient, focusing on the identity of the patient, age, weight, and physical status, expected arrival time, and intra-op events of interest such as reaction to antibiotics and any deviation from planned or scheduled surgery.

If the PACU nurse is assigned, and the location of the PACU bay known ahead, this information is given to the OR nurse to facilitate transfer from OR to the PACU.

If the anesthesiologist would like to make any specific request to have racemic epinephrine mixed and ready in a nebulizer for treatment of croup, then that information will be given to the PACU nurse, assigned to receive the patient. If a young anxious child would benefit from the parents' presence on arrival, then that information is also requested at this time.

1.2.3 Walk; Don't Run: Vigilant Patient Monitoring During Transport Is Vital!

The physical transfer of the patient is normally done with patient lying in the recovery position (lateral position) on the stretcher breathing spontaneously with oxygen supplementation via nasal cannula or face mask with or without an oral airway in place. The transport time is a time of potential danger if vigilance is low. After the stimulation of extubation and movement to the stretcher, the patient can have airway obstruction if ventilation is not monitored and the patient position suboptimal.

1.3 Why Use Recovery or Lateral Position During Patient Transport?

Anesthesia obstructs patient airway mostly by causing a decrease in the anteroposterior dimension. Application of continuous positive airway pressure (CPAP), chin lift, and jaw thrust are some of the main methods utilized to overcome the airway obstruction in children. Jaw thrust maneuver improves airway patency in anesthetized children with enlarged tonsils and adenoid, compared to chin lift and CPAP.

Lateral position results in a dramatic improvement of all the airway maneuvers.

Lateral position also known as the recovery position or tonsillectomy position ***alone*** *improves airway dimensions* [9].

An interesting study by Dr. Ron Litman showed *an increase in the upper airway cross-sectional area and total upper airway volume in the lateral positioning compared to the supine position.* This study was in pediatric patients aged 2–12 years undergoing MRI scan under propofol sedation breathing spontaneously. All non-cartilaginous areas of the airway increased in area in the lateral compared to the supine position. The conclusion of this study was that the upper airway of a sedated, spontaneously breathing child *widens in the lateral position with the area between the tip of the epiglottis and the vocal cords demonstrating the greatest relative percent increase in size* [10].

In children who are emerging from a deeper plane of anesthesia during transport as in patients whose LMA or endotracheal tubes were removed deep and breathing spontaneously, partial or complete airway obstruction can occur resulting in hypoxemia. Opening the patient's airway can be accomplished by jaw thrust and chin lift. Maintaining the sniffing position in the supine position and CPAP application are other well-known maneuvers to open an occluded airway. *Positioning the patient in the lateral position is an efficient effective method to maintain upper airway patency* [11].

In children with enlarged tonsils and adenoids, lateral positioning is a simple maneuver to overcome the obstruction of airway from airway collapsibility of the pharynx under general anesthesia. It is helpful in children and adults with obstructive sleep apnea (OSA). A study looking at airway patency (stridor score by baseline recording) in children 1–10 years of age undergoing adenotonsillectomy under sevoflurane anesthesia showed that common airway maneuvers like chin lift and jaw thrust in the supine position increased airway patency. Lateral position enhanced the effects of these airway maneuvers in a dramatic fashion. *Jaw thrust combined with lateral positioning improved airway patency and eased the airway management for the anesthesiologist* [12].

In some situation the children must lie in a supine position postoperatively and not be able to assume a lateral position. In such situation a small neck roll may be helpful to improve airway patency in sedated children. A neck collar supporting the mandible and keeping the head in a mild extension may be effective in maintaining airway patency in sedated patients.

1.4 Are There Studies to Prove This?

A study evaluating the airway patency in children undergoing propofol sedation for MRI of brain showed the results of placing a small neck roll. The researchers evaluated the upper airway size with and without the placement of a neck collar. Sixty patients 2–4 years of age under propofol sedation for MRI brain were the subjects of this study. Under sedation, T1 3D fast-field echo axial sequence from the nasopharyngeal roof to subglottic region was obtained with and without the placement of a neck collar. Airway dimensions were measured and analyzed at different levels: at the base of the tongue, soft palate, and epiglottis. *At the base of the tongue and soft palate, the cross-sectional area (CSA) and the anteroposterior diameter of the airway were statistically significantly higher with the neck collar in place. However, the CSA at the epiglottis was significantly less with the neck collar placement.* The researchers concluded that application of a soft neck collar in children aged 2–4 years may enhance the retropalatal and retroglossal airway dimensions during pediatric sedation in the supine position [13]. Another study of 125 children 0–16 years of age undergoing sedation under propofol for MRI evaluated the airway size with or without neck roll and confirmed the above results [14].

Experienced pediatric anesthesiologists have always maintained that it is safer to transport the extubated patient in the lateral position to have the maximum airway patency and for oral and nasal secretions to drain by gravity to the side and not to the back of the mouth into the larynx.

During transport, it is not unusual for the patient to continue breathing spontaneously with nasal cannula, attached to the oxygen tank turned on to deliver 2–3 liters of oxygen after total intravenous anesthetic as in endoscopic or brief noninvasive procedures. It is imperative however to have a backup source of ventilation (Jackson Rees circuit) to administer positive pressure ventilation via an appropriately sized mask to be available near the patient during transport.

Regarding **monitoring during transport**, a small portable oxygen saturation measurement device placed on the patient's finger by the anesthesiologist is useful especially if the patient is breathing oxygen via a nasal cannula and not through a mask with a circuit attached.

The Jackson Rees circuit carries oxygen to the patient via a mask which is attached to a rebreathing bag and a pop of valve, enabling easy visualization of the patient's respiratory effort unlike the nasal cannula delivering oxygen from the oxygen tank.

If the oxygen saturation monitor placed on the finger (Fig. 1) is unable to show the oxygen saturation values because of displacement or if the extremity digit is

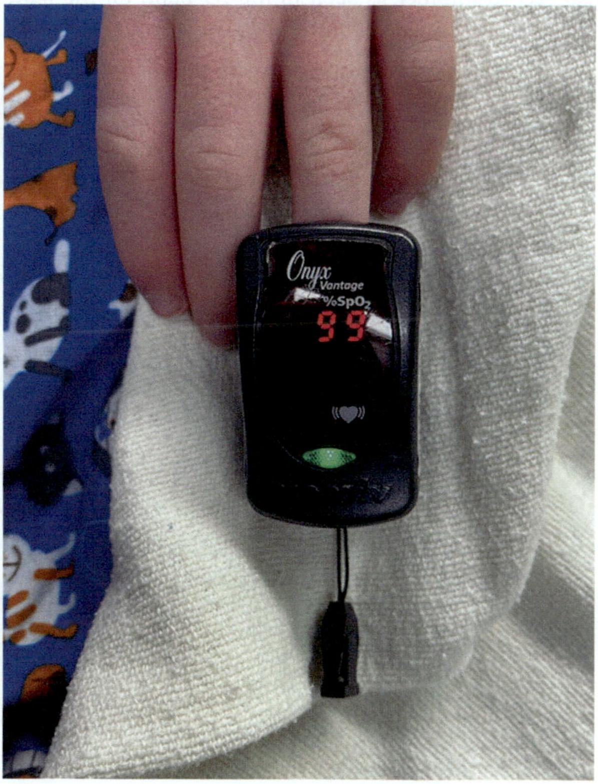

Fig. 1 Portable oxygen monitor for transport

cold, then approximating the face mask tight across the face will give an indication of the depth and rate of the breathing during transport.

Emergency airway medications such as succinyl choline, atropine, and residual narcotics and sedatives like propofol and dexmedetomidine and an oral airway that is appropriate for the patient are additional items taken along by the anesthesia provider for use in PACU if a potential need arises.

During transfer of the patient, the anesthesiologist is always positioned at the head of the stretcher close to the patient's airway to enable assessment of continuous breathing pattern and to hold the mask close to the face if needed and to visualize the heart rate and oxygen saturation shown on the portable oxygen monitor device as the surgical team member leads the stretcher forward.

If the bay number was not assigned before leaving the OR, then it is usually available to the transporting team upon entering the PACU entrance in a large TV screen with patient name, procedure, OR of origin, and the PACU bay destination (Fig. 2).

Once the assigned bay is reached, the patient is reconnected to the PACU bay monitor for continuous recording of EKG, respiratory rate, oxygen saturation by pulse oximetry, and blood pressure by an appropriately sized cuff, after which patient identification is done.

The patient on the stretcher or bed is identified by the receiving nurse with the help of one of the perioperative team members who reads aloud the patient's medical record number as seen in the ID band on the patient's wrist or ankle (as in an

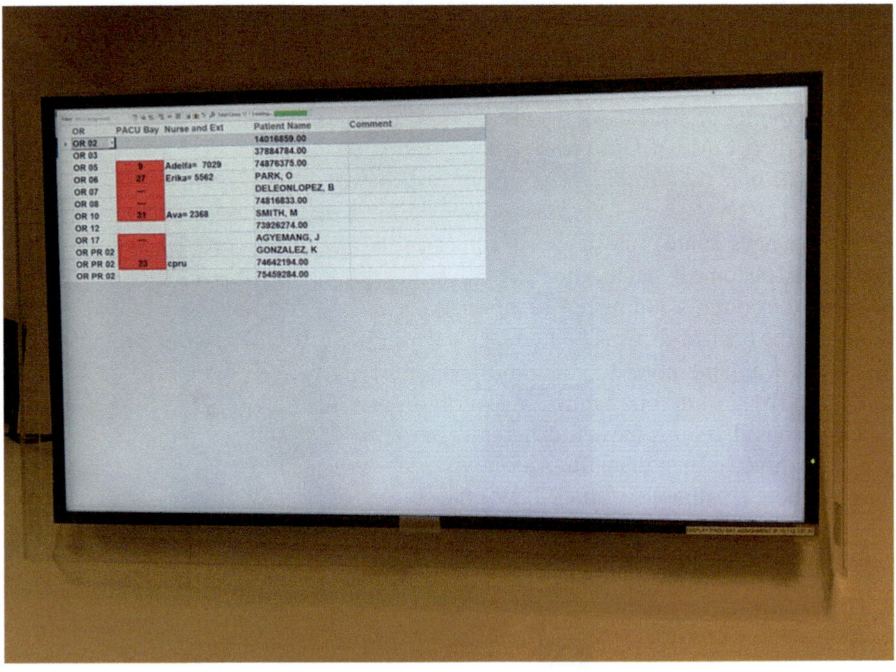

Fig. 2 Patient bay assignment at the PACU entrance

infant) and matches it with the same number available on the patient's chart. The oxygen source attached to the tank on the stretcher is now switched to the source on the wall at the bedside of the patient.

After this identification process, the entire team remains quiet while the PACU nurse is given time to auscultate the patient's chest with her stethoscope to assess the quality and rate of patient's breath sounds as well as the hemodynamic stability of the patient by assessing the vital signs. After the nurse is satisfied with her evaluation of the patient's clinical status, then the surgical team member will begin the surgical handoff by repeating patient's name and the specific disease condition that required the surgical intervention and the anticipated problems pertaining to the surgery.

The surgical team member handoff should be comprehensive, detailing what was done for the patient, patient's allergies, intra-op blood loss if any, and anticipated pain and possible blood loss if drains are present. Intra-op use of antibiotic and need for another dose in the PACU should be clear and same as written orders. It is usual for the surgery team member to expose the patient's operative area to reveal the surgical site covered with a dressing, to show the nurse the current appearance of the dressing, presence of drains beside it, and what to anticipate regarding the volume of blood loss from these drains while in PACU. Any local anesthetic blocks given by the surgeon to alleviate incisional pain and the plan for treating pain anticipated in the postoperative period also should be addressed as agreeing with the anesthesiologist's pain treatment orders at this time. Patient's restrictions for oral intake will be specifically mentioned if the patient is supposed to remain NPO as in a patient who had abdominal surgery or in someone with a nasogastric tube in situ to prevent gastric distension from ileus or intestinal motility problems. Surgical team handoff will conclude with the plan for discharge from PACU to the floor or home, the take-home medications, local antibiotic drops, and specific instructions for the patient's parents regarding activity, bath, wound care, and continuation of antibiotics.

After the surgical handoff is complete, the surgical team member will leave specific phone or pager numbers with the PACU nurse in case of urgent or emergent need to contact the surgical team member.

Anesthesiologist handoff will start with the introduction of the patient and the disease and what was done by the surgeon to correct or repair it. During the introduction of the patient, it is important to emphasize the age of the patient, weight, existing medical problems, and the specific reason for a higher ASA physical status due to deviation from normal health.

For example, in an obese patient with a BMI of 45, complicated with early-onset diabetes mellitus, long-standing hypertension, and somnolence from OSA, it is expected to detail these comorbid conditions to enable the nurse to understand the assignment of the higher ASA status of 3.

The patient's developmental and psychological profile during the preoperative interview and the need for premedication use, parental presence during induction, and type of induction used are detailed to allow the PACU nurse a glimpse of how the patient was on induction. Report continues with description of patient's intraoperative anesthetic course, emphasizing the type of anesthetic chosen: total intravenous anesthesia (TIVA) vs general anesthesia with use of LMA or endotracheal tube, or mask anesthesia with oral airway. The intravenous fluid administered and type of anesthetic emergence specifying if the patient underwent a deep or awake extubation are all significant details that should be transferred to the PACU nurse for her to anticipate potential problems. Any regional blocks performed and the effectiveness intraoperatively should be another area to be detailed at this time.

Other significant details to mention include the type, amount of antibiotic, the patient's response to it, and if there is a need for repeating another dose before discharge from PACU. Even if the surgeon may have mentioned about blood loss, it is important to repeat your assessment about the estimated blood loss during surgery. It is vital to specify if red blood cells were transfused and if a hematocrit value was done post-transfusion in the patient. The total amount of analgesics used, type of antiemetic used, performance of regional blocks (awake or under anesthesia), and the plan for pain management in the PACU are all additional information that should be transferred. It is equally important to emphasize why an antiemetic was omitted and why it should not be used if the patient had prolongation of QT interval and had developed arrhythmias in the past when given Zofran for antiemetic prophylaxis.

Another point to emphasize to the PACU nurse is regarding the patient's sensitivity to pain medication. If the patient demonstrated extraordinary sensitivity to small doses of narcotics in the OR, as in a patient with OSA, a need to titrate small doses of narcotics or for avoiding it completely if other modalities of pain relief are available should be emphasized.

If there is a particular loose tooth in a child that the parent was concerned about before start of anesthesia, it is important to show its presence to the PACU nurse to confirm with the parent later. Taking a quick picture of it may further enable you to show the parent presence of the loose tooth still intact in the mouth after the handoff was completed.

The intended surgery as written in the schedule if different from the performed surgery will also need to be reiterated to allow full understanding of the patient's perioperative course. Detailed information will enable the PACU nurse to anticipate potential pain problems, anticipate emergence delirium, and understand the choice of drugs written for control of pain and/or for delirium as well as the degree of obstructive sleep apnea in an obese patient which was evident intraoperatively.

2 Receiving Team: PACU Nursing Team

2.1 PACU Setup/Highlights

Kathy Curtis and Susan P. Joslyn

2.1.1 Introduction

Who We Are

Children's National Medical Center (CNMC) is a level 1 trauma center, located in the heart of Washington, DC. The PACU (postanesthesia care unit) is a 35-bed unit that provides postanesthesia recovery to all ages from newborns to adults. Being a level 1 trauma center, we provide surgical care covering all pediatric specialties that do not require intensive care monitoring. Our typical OR schedule consists of 80 to 90 surgical cases a day. Our caseload is cared for by nurses with critical care experience combined with the expertise of NPs, PAs, AAs, and anesthesiologists. Bedside nurses that work in the PACU hold a BSN and have current PALS/BLS certification in addition to national certification from various pediatric associations (CPN, CCRN, APON, etc.). PACU RNs work in both surgical prep and postanesthesia care and provide on-call emergency recovery for unscheduled surgeries.

Orientation consists of precepted time in both pre-op and PACU, didactic instruction by the educators, and an airway management skills day with an anesthesiologist providing direct care to pediatric patients undergoing anesthesia. PACU RNs provide hands-on airway skills and manipulation techniques under the direction of an anesthesiologist. Ongoing education is annually necessary consisting of but not limited to 8 h of burn education and 8 h of trauma in a 2-year period.

2.1.2 PACU: Physical Setup

The PACU at CNMC is equipped with telemetry monitoring. Every bay has a monitor for continuously monitoring the heart rate, oxygen saturation, blood pressure, as well as the respiratory rate (Fig. 3).

The pulse oximetry QRS volume is muted, but the alarm limits are set for oxygen saturation, heart rate, and blood pressure for each patient based on the normal values based on the age. All the emergency equipment necessary to rescue airways and

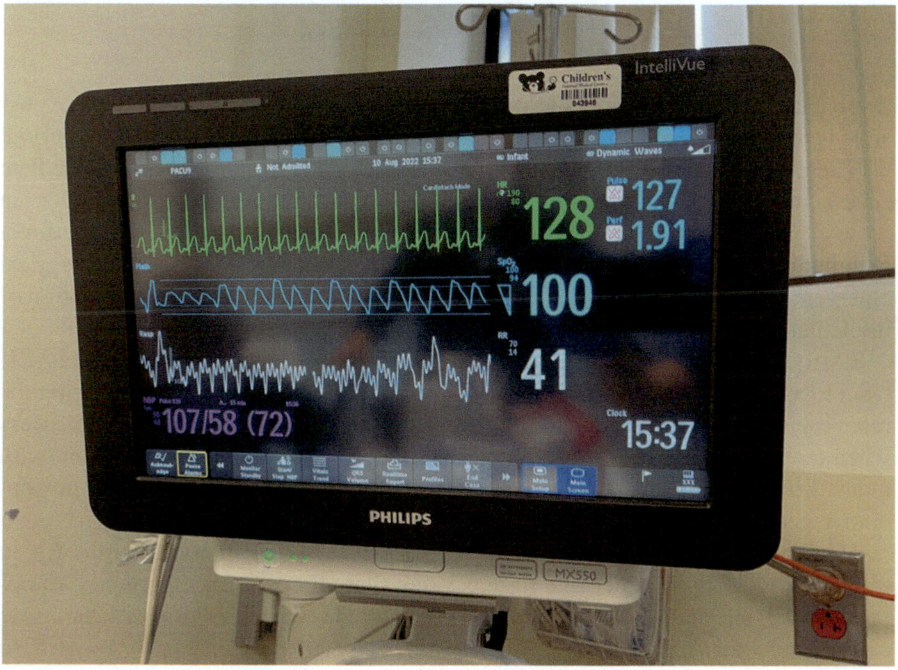

Fig. 3 EKG, O_2 saturation, BP, and ventilation monitor in PACU

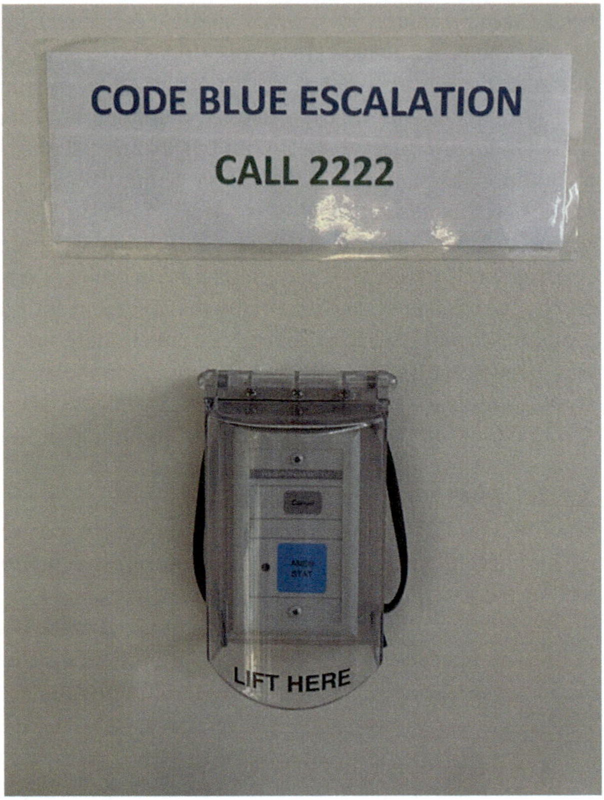

Fig. 4 Code blue button on the wall

respond to cardiopulmonary emergencies and all surgical emergencies that are possible is readily available in the PACU for use in the immediate postoperative period.

There are airway carts and code carts strategically positioned for immediate access in all zones of the PACU. Each bay has an emergency button for an "Anesthesia Stat" in airway emergencies. There is also an intercom device for direct communication with the OR for immediate help from the OR in case of surgical emergencies. A separate "code blue" device is used for hospital-wide notification of immediate assistance in the unit (Fig. 4).

Lastly, but most importantly, an anesthesiologist is assigned as part of the PACU team to assist the bedside RN with urgent/emergent situations that occur during the recovery period. This same anesthesiologist is also part of the discharge process when outpatients are cleared to go home. PACU at CNMC is a very busy unit with many different skill sets necessary to provide safe and efficient care of the postoperative pediatric patient.

Having your PACU bay ready for your patient is the constant role of the RN in the recovery room. It is her role to make sure that all necessary emergency equipment is available and working properly. These include bedside suction with Yankauer and various other (red rubber, sterile suction) catheters, flowmeters for oxygen, to the shift audit of emergency airway and code carts (Fig. 5).

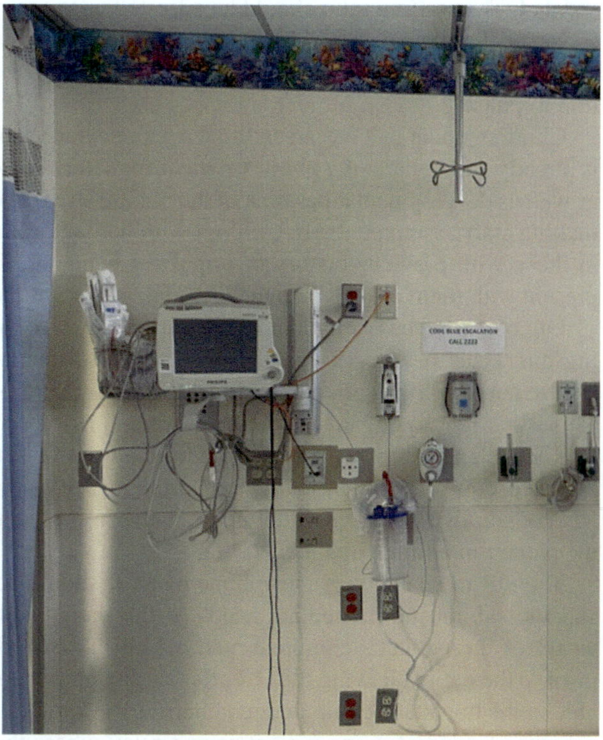

Fig. 5 PACU bay ready for post-op patient

All the staff carry zebra phones that can call, text, and initiate a code. The charge nurse in the PACU oversees the flow of the unit and assigns bays to the PACU nurse and times for lunch breaks, takes reports from the OR nurse, and distributes the patients to individual nurses on a rotation basis. In addition, the charge nurse handles any problems on the unit as they arise and is a resource to assist in the urgent need of a patient in the assigned nurse's care.

In the PACU, patients are either discharged home (SDS (same-day surgery), sent to an inpatient unit, or allowed to stay in the PACU for 3 h or 23 h. There are protocols related to age and condition that determine if a patient is to be SDS or 23-h observation. Our PACU is set up in a manner where phase 1 and phase 2 patients are cared for in the same bay by the same RN.

Phase 1 patients sometimes have oral airways, are sedated, and require close monitoring of vital signs similar to critical care units. This phase lasts until the patient returns to baseline cardiovascular, respiratory, and neurological status and preanesthetic wakefulness.

Phase 2 patients are those that that are in a transitional period of monitoring, instructions are given for postoperative care, and patient is transitioning toward transfer to the inpatient ward or home. Oral hydration is introduced, and oral intake tolerance is monitored. Caregivers are instructed in this phase as well.

Recommended staffing ratios alter according to the level of care the patient needs. Ratios should be 1:1 when the patient has an oral airway and is deeply sedated. The staffing ratio should be adjusted to accommodate the level of care and safety of the patient. Consideration should be given to the age of patient, specific procedure, and amount of pain medication needed to facilitate recovery and transition to phase 2.

Children under age 6 years without a parent should not be assigned to a nurse who is already taking care of a phase 1 patient for safety reasons. The developmental age as well as developmental baseline of the patient should be known beforehand prior to making staff assignments. In children with autism or autism spectrum disorder and in those with previous history of impulsive behavior, the need to have a caregiver present with them on arrival to the PACU is important for patient safety and comfort.

Of note, as a phase 1 patient is being transported to their assigned bay, the receiving nurse has been provided the necessary information about the patient by the charge nurse who has already received the pertinent information from the OR nurse. This is a critically important step that occurs prior to the patient being transported. The bedside RN may need to have additional suction setup for a chest tube or nasogastric decompression, IV fluid pumps, and invasive pressure monitoring. The PCT/RN cooperative role is essential in the gathering of necessary equipment to receive the patient in a timely manner.

The OR to charge nurse telephone handoff should be precise and informative in specifics about the immediate needs of the patient. The receiving RN should be aware of the patient's complete medical history and physical examination results prior to the patient leaving the OR after surgical procedure. All documents are available in the hospital's computerized charting system. There are many handoffs in the process of caring for one patient as in a relay where the baton is passed efficiently from one team member to the other.

Pre-op nurse to OR nurse is the first part of the relay before the start of surgery, and from OR nurse to PACU charge nurse and the anesthesiologist passing patient information to the assigned PACU nurse is the second part of the relay. The passing of this vital information regarding the patient referred to as the "baton" in a relay cannot be allowed to slip and fall on the ground for the safety of our patient. The information needs to be concise and precise, and it is constantly being reevaluated and improved upon by our perioperative management team.

2.1.3 When a Patient Arrives at the PACU Bay After Surgery

Into the bay rolls the stretcher led by the anesthesia-surgical team. The receiving nurse assists with proper alignment of the patient's stretcher with the monitor to ensure easy access to the patient from both sides. After the brakes are applied, we monitor the cardiac/respiratory status, transfer the oxygen source to the wall, and assess the patient's breath sounds. Working suction is available if needed to clear secretions. Temporal temperature monitoring is available in all the bays and is monitored in all our patients. Temperature goal is >36 °C for optimal perfusion and hemodynamic stability in the pediatric patient. Double verification of the patient's ID band with the accompanied chart is done after the patient is situated in the recovery bay, vital signs are stable, and it is safe to proceed. There is always continuous airway monitoring during handoff in the PACU. Assessment of breath sounds and supportive positioning of the airway are crucial for a safe recovery. Many times, especially following any ENT/oral surgery, we will position the patient on the lateral side to prevent laryngospasm especially if there is an oral airway in place. Once the patient is in a satisfactory recovery position (as agreed by the entire team), the process of the surgical handoff is begun. The anesthesiologist remains at the head of the bed during the surgical handoff.

An ideal handoff is depicted in the picture below (Fig. 6) a visual tool available to remind the perioperative team and if the surgical and anesthesia team members

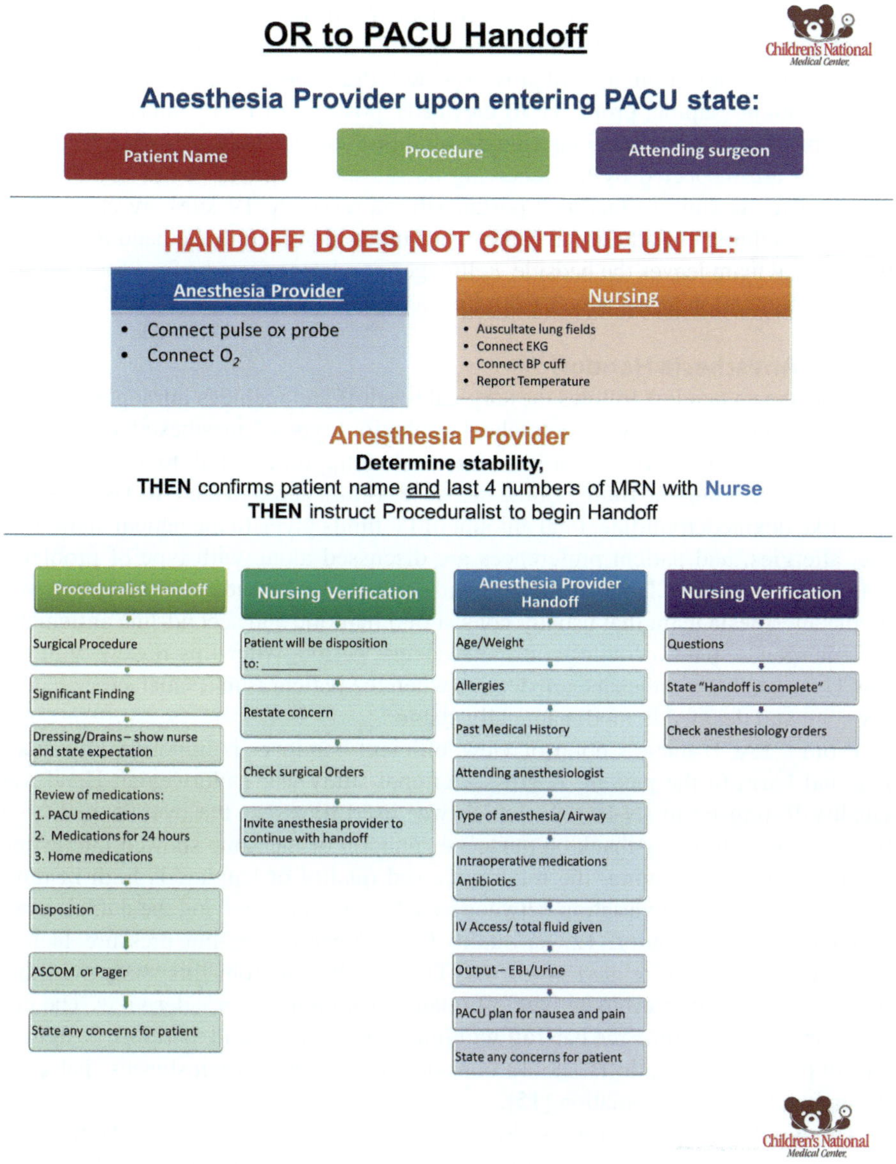

Fig. 6 Visual tool for an ideal handoff developed by Dr. Songyos Valairucha

need to refresh themselves about the process of structured step-by-step handoff. This visual tool was made possible by the effort of one of our anesthesiologists, Dr. Songyos Valairucha who worked on a structured handoff to help the OR to PACU handover to occur in an optimal manner after arrival of the patient to PACU.

2.1.4 Surgical Handoff

Surgical handoff consists of specifying the surgical procedure, findings, tubes/drainage devices, and a multitude of details that are unique to every specialty. It usually involves what type of surgery was done for the patient's diagnosis, what was found, what was placed, and what is to be anticipated in the post-op period. Specifics include but are not limited to what is expected: drainage from a surgical site, position of patient (supine, prone, HOB elevated), position of EVD, hourly rate of IV fluids, post-op diet, medications, and destination (home versus inpatient). The incision sites are inspected by the receiving nurse, and additional warm blankets are provided for warmth to facilitate postanesthesia recovery. IV sites are checked as well as attachment of additional catheters or tubes identified in the handoff. Before the surgical team leaves the bedside, cell/pager numbers are exchanged for immediate communication as necessary from the recovery room.

2.1.5 Anesthesia Handoff

The anesthesia handoff follows the surgical handoff and includes intraoperative airway management LMA vs endotracheal intubation; type of anesthesia; use of muscle relaxants, medications, antiemetics, and antipyretics; and total amount of narcotics, including the timing of the last dose administered in the OR. Use of sedatives like dexmedetomidine, total amount of IV fluids given to the patient, antibiotic use, allergies, and patient preferences are discussed along with type of problems anticipated in the PACU stay. IV access and postanesthesia medications are reviewed by the anesthesia team that usually consist of a narcotic and second-line antiemetic for emergence, pain, or emesis in the recovery period. After this review with the PACU nurse, the anesthesia team departs when the patient is in a satisfactory recovery state and deemed hemodynamically stable.

From a PACU nurse's point of view, efficient handover is important to reduce risk and harm to the patient. A cross-sectional study using Norwegian Handover Quality Rating Form (N-HQRF) which was used to assess the overall quality of handoff and getting feedback on nurse's evaluation of the same showed interesting results. Despite the rating, the total perceived quality of handoff is high in most cases, there was great variation between transferring and receiving the nurse's evaluation of the same handoff. Lower-quality handoff was due to time pressure, lack of certainty, and patient-related problems. The conclusion from this study was that there exists a need to evaluate handoff quality from a much broader view. The circumstances surrounding the handoff will impact the quality, and therefore designing and implementing handoffs should consider the various circumstances that exist during the relay of information [15].

The PACU-assigned anesthesiologist is asked to be present if the case has specific airway concerns during the recovery period (i.e., difficult airway, obstructive sleep apnea, need for bronchodilator during extubation, significant airway secretions, or even waiting for assigned intensive care unit bed).

Some of our patients have an airway surgical "stay" in the PACU for an assigned period as the ENT surgeon desires immediate access to the OR in event of a need to return urgently for a postoperative bleed after T&A. We often receive otherwise healthy children with spinal scoliosis after spinal fusion (anterior or posterior) which is long in duration with significant blood loss who may have already received blood transfusion in the OR. These are 23-h cases in PACU and may have PCA orders for pain control. These are scenarios where it would be ideal for the PACU anesthesiologist to be present for the direct handoff given by the OR team to the PACU team.

2.1.6 PACU Patient and Pain Treatment

The PACU nurse should have a thorough understanding of the patient's pain threshold and response to intraoperative pain management including blocks performed and the assessment of its effectiveness. We have a pain management team in-house that is part of our anesthesia department. Longer and more painful procedures usually involve a postoperative PCA or quite possibly epidural anesthesia. These cases are communicated directly to our pain management team from our anesthesia team in the recovery room. The patient is evaluated while in the PACU before being dispositioned to the inpatient unit.

2.1.7 Kids Are Not Small Adults

Respiratory Obstruction in PACU

Approximately one in ten children presents with respiratory complications in the PACU [16]. The initial postoperative recovery period requires keen assessment skills by an experienced pediatric RN. Many of the early signs of respiratory complications in pediatric recovery can be ominous and elusive. Anticipation, vigilance in monitoring, and early intervention in recognizing obstruction of airway from a large tongue or from laryngospasm developing from secretions when patients are not awake and lying in a supine position are crucial. Oftentimes positioning, oral suctioning, and the use of an oral airway may help to prevent airway obstruction.

An important assessment skill is knowing and being familiar with upper versus lower airway breath sounds. Breath sounds are assessed often to make sure there is no upper airway obstruction as in croup or lower airway obstruction as in asthma with wheezing. One of the most common reasons for an Anesthesia Stat that can be detoured is the positioning of the patient on their side so the secretions drain out of the mouth. This is especially true following oral or ENT surgery, in patients that are at risk for obstruction with large tongue and excess oral secretions and in those patients extubated deep after general (endotracheal or LMA) anesthesia.

Croup

Young children who may have been intubated at birth and dependent on a ventilator for weeks in the NICU may have a history of croup and may develop significant stridor after extubation. The handoff report may include this croup history and the reason for racemic epinephrine by nebulizer in the PACU orders despite the administration of Decadron in the OR. Often allowing parents to participate in this treatment maneuver is helpful to the patient and nursing team. Suctioning the oropharynx and monitoring a patient's respiratory status, the frequency and depth of respirations, use of accessory muscles, and watching for appearance of retractions and/or nasal flaring along with decrease in oxygen saturations are important assessments frequently done by the PACU nurse. Knowing and being familiar with the early warning signs are key to avoiding a potential airway emergency.

Emergence Delirium

Similarly with emergence delirium/agitation, it is important to have information about the patient's anxiety, pre-op reaction to anesthetic induction, and previous history of delirium—which are helpful clues to predict a stormy postoperative period. Identifying and treating a confused agitated child just emerging from anesthesia before they become wild and delirious will prevent a safety event, assault/injury for patient and staff which can affect the existing available manpower. It is vital for the PACU nurse to anticipate and recognize its occurrence early, to call for help to treat this escalating problem with an intravenous drug. Early intervention is important before the IV gets pulled out or nonfunctional in the ensuing struggle with an uncontrollable patient who is thrashing around. We have a PACU anesthesiologist available in the PACU area who usually has these drugs available and can administer dexmedetomidine or propofol to treat emergence delirium rapidly. Anticipation, vigilance, and early recognition and intervention are vital for prevention of delirium in susceptible children.

Development of Shock

A patient with an active infection (appendiceal abscess) may present to the emergency room with subtle signs of sepsis and undergo surgery in OR and may proceed to signs of septic shock in PACU in the immediate post-operative period. This is probably the most ominous sign in the pediatric population because their hemodynamic status can deteriorate very rapidly. Presence of cool clammy extremities is indicative of poor perfusion, along with tachycardia and hypotension with deteriorating oxygen saturation in a patient who is drowsy and lethargic. A patient with potential to develop impending shock needs immediate intervention to prevent morbidity and mortality. Calling for help from the anesthesiologist to help with airway support and oxygenation should be followed by checking a bedside evaluation of acid-base status, serum electrolytes, and sugar and administration of inotropes for improving cardiac output. An anesthesiologist with a team of healthcare providers at the bedside is essential to manage patient's hemodynamic status, if septic shock is suspected. Additional placement of intravenous lines to increase delivery of fluids and inotropes and an arterial line for monitoring blood gases and to monitor the patient's response to ongoing treatment is crucial to first stabilize and then plan for transfer of patient to ICU for continuous observation. If an intravenous line is difficult to access, an intraosseous line placement should be undertaken for immediate volume resuscitation.

Similarly simple hypovolemic shock in a patient who had an uneventful liver biopsy in OR and is now bleeding internally in PACU can be a very subtle presentation. A high degree of suspicion, early intervention, and informing the anesthesia and surgical team members to obtain an ultrasound imaging of the liver at the patient's bedside to confirm a diagnosis while administering fluids and blood are all necessary ways to decrease the possibility of hypovolemic shock from occurring.

2.1.8 Drug Administration in PACU

Additional attention and dual verification of all pediatric dosages of narcotic or other classified medications are mandatory prior to their administration in the PACU. These medications are considered high alert for several reasons, especially in the younger or premature infant. Postoperative apnea after anesthesia is common in the young, particularly premature infants, and can be potentiated with use of opioids/benzodiazepines. Barbiturates and opioids also have a longer duration of action due to an infant's slower metabolism and immature hepatic system.

Temperature regulation is a challenge post-anesthesia in the younger child and infant due to the large surface area to weight ratio and minimal subcutaneous fat. This can lead to bradycardia and hemodynamic instability. Infants and small children also have poorly developed sweating and shivering mechanisms. Heat loss can be exaggerated in this age group and active measures should be taken to prevent hypothermia. In the PACU we often use warm blankets but also have access to IV fluid warmers as well as forced warm air devices.

Hypoglycemia

Low blood sugar is common in the premature babies, stressed infants, newborns of diabetic mothers, as well as those pediatric patients with mitochondrial or metabolic disorders. For this reason, we monitor the glucose regularly in all patients that are at high risk for alterations in glucose metabolism and use specific infusions to prevent it. These include children who have been fasting for a prolonged period or have a history of failure to grow as well as those who are vomiting.

2.1.9 Autism and Autism Spectrum Disorders

Special consideration is given to our autistic and autistic spectrum disorder patients in both the pre-op arena and in the PACU. Referred to as the *Keep Me Calm* initiative, these patients are identified by our child life specialists with a screening tool that is done prior to surgery. Some children on waking up from anesthesia often complain of noises around them being loud. Loud noises can produce autonomic changes as in a stress reaction and can aggravate their discomfort. In children with autism, the preoperative experience itself begins in a quiet room with the goal of decreasing sensory stimulation. All team members are briefed by the child life specialist leading the transition to the OR, sometimes allowing parents to accompany the patient until induction of anesthesia. The PACU is aware of the patient's status and all efforts are made to recover these children in a quieter, less stimulating manner.

The nurses at CNMC PACU work in a very collegial cohesive manner with the anesthesia and surgical team to improve the care of each patient after surgery.

Anecdotally, it was the PACU nurses at CNMC who brought a significant clinical finding to children's anesthesia team about caudal block effectiveness in the children postoperatively. *They said almost with certainty that they could predict which of their patients had a good caudal block by one single repeatedly observed phenomenon. Every patient who had a very lax anal sphincter tone when the nurse inserted a Tylenol suppository invariably did not mind the insertion and woke up comfortable without needing any pain medicine in PACU.* This finding by these clinically astute PACU nurses prompted the anesthesia team to prospectively study this phenomenon occurring in children undergoing caudal blocks, and the results were affirmatory and therefore published in a paper in *Anesthesia & Analgesia* [17].

The days of rectal suppositories in PACU are gone and forgotten, but this clinical observation by the PACU team and follow-up with anesthesia team are an example of harmonious supportive perioperative teamwork at CNMC which is invaluable for optimal patient care!

Finally, the perioperative team at CNMC who care for our pediatric patients include many people in the hospital. It takes a multitude of hospital employees and health workers to undertake the care and safety of each patient scheduled for surgery. There are numerous perioperative services to plan, organize, and implement the safe arrival and departure of our young patients who need to undergo their surgical procedures under general anesthesia in a timely, efficient, and safe manner. Open communication among perioperative team members, constant vigilance in monitoring our patients during their surgical and PACU stay, and working as a strong dedicated team are the essential factors needed to provide premier care to all our patients at CNMC.

3 Conclusion

Handoff must be complete and efficient describing the patient's pre-op medical condition, ASA status, drug allergies, intra-op course, drugs administered and anticipated airway problems, pain thresholds, and specific written orders for PACU. Certain critical patient information can be repeated for emphasis during OR to PACU transfer. PACU staff members often write down these in a piece of paper during the verbal handoff. In critical clinical situations, it may be necessary to ask the nurse receiving this information or specific instructions to repeat it back to assure that the message was clearly understood as in a closed-loop communication. Finally, for our patients' continuing care, each of us in the perioperative team must identify our role in running this relay race with the baton of information to the finish line by focusing on that single prize: our patients' comfort and safety.

References

1. Haynes AB, Weiser TG, Berry WR, Lipsitz SR, Breizat AH, Dellinger EP, Herbosa T, Joseph S, Kibatala PL, Lapitan MC, Merry AF, Moorthy K, Reznick RK, Taylor B, Gawande AA, Safe Surgery Saves Lives Study Group. A surgical safety checklist to reduce morbidity and mortality in a global population. N Engl J Med. 2009;360(5):491–9. https://doi.org/10.1056/NEJMsa0810119. Epub 2009 Jan 14. PMID: 19144931.
2. Segall N, Bonifacio AS, Schroeder RA, Barbeito A, Rogers D, Thomlow DK, Emery J, Kellum S, Wright MC, Mark J, On behalf of the Durham VA patient safety Centre of Inquiry. Can we make postoperative patient handovers safer? A systematic review of the literature. Anesth Analg. 2012;115:102–15.
3. Institute for Healthcare Improvement. SBAR technique for communication. www.ihi.org/IHI/Topics/PatientSafety/SafetyGeneral/Tools. Accessed 16 Jan 2012.
4. Boat AC, Spaeth JP. Handoff checklists improve the reliability of patient handoffs in the operating room and postanesthesia care unit. Paediatr Anaesth. 2013;23(7):647–54. https://doi.org/10.1111/pan.12199. Epub 2013 May 18. PMID: 23683085.
5. Bittner EA, George E, Eikermann M, Schmidt U. Evaluation of the association between quality of handover and length of stay in the post anaesthesia care unit: a pilot study. Anaesthesia. 2012;67:548–489.
6. Salzwedel C, Bartz HJ, Kühnelt I, Appel D, Haupt O, Maisch S, Schmidt GN. The effect of a checklist on the quality of post-anaesthesia patient handover: a randomized controlled trial. Int J Qual Health Care. 2013;25:176–81.
7. Vishneski SR, Nagatsuka M, Smith LD, Templeton TW, Downard MG, Goenaga-Diaz EJ, Templeton LB. It's not over till it's over: a prospective cohort study and analysis of "Anesthesia stat!" emergency calls in the Pediatric Post-Anesthesia Care Unit (PACU). Cureus. 2021;13(8):e17571. https://doi.org/10.7759/cureus.17571. PMID: 34646626; PMCID: PMC8480442.
8. Wudineh DM, Berhe YW, Chekol WB, Adane H, Workie MM. Perioperative respiratory adverse events among pediatric surgical patients in university hospitals in Northwest Ethiopia; a prospective observational study. Front Pediatr. 2022;10:827663. https://doi.org/10.3389/fped.2022.827663. PMID: 35223702; PMCID: PMC8873930.
9. Chapter 14. The pediatric airway. In: Fiadjoe EJ, Litman SR, Serber FJ, Stricker AP, Cote JC, editors. Cote and Lerman's a practice of anesthesia for infants and children, 6th ed. Elsevier. pp. 297–339.
10. Litman RS, Wake N, Chan LM, McDonough JM, Sin S, Mahboubi S, Arens R. Effect of lateral positioning on upper airway size and morphology in sedated children. Anesthesiology. 2005;103(3):484–8. https://doi.org/10.1097/00000542-200509000-00009. PMID: 16129971.
11. von Ungern-Sternberg BS, Erb TO, Frei FJ. Management der oberen Atemwege beim spontan atmenden Kind. Eine Herausforderung für den Anästhesisten [Management of the upper airway in spontaneously breathing children. A challenge for the anaesthetist]. Anaesthesist. 2006;55(2):164–70. German. https://doi.org/10.1007/s00101-005-0946-7. PMID: 16252114.
12. Arai YP, Fukunaga K, Hirota S, Fujimoto S. The effects of chin lift and jaw thrust while in the lateral position on stridor score in anesthetized children with adenotonsillar hypertrophy. Anesth Analg. 2004;99(6):1638–41. https://doi.org/10.1213/01.ANE.0000135637.95853.1C. PMID: 15562046.
13. Moustafa MA, Emara DM, Nouh MR. Effect of a neck collar on upper airway size in children sedated with propofol-midazolam combination during magnetic resonance imaging. Paediatr Anaesth. 2015;25(4):421–7. https://doi.org/10.1111/pan.12593. Epub 2015 Jan 12. PMID: 25581094.

14. Yilmaz G, Varol K, Esen O, Kayhan A, Salihoglu Z. Airway patency in children undergoing magnetic resonance imaging using neck collars: a single center, randomized, double-blind, prospective study. Braz J Anesthesiol. 2021;71(1):11–6. https://doi.org/10.1016/j.bjane.2020.12.002. Epub 2020 Dec 26. PMID: 33712246; PMCID: PMC9373510.
15. Reine E, Ræder J, Manser T, Småstuen MC, Rustøen T. Quality in postoperative patient handover: different perceptions of quality between transferring and receiving nurses. J Nurs Care Qual. 2019;34(1):E1–7. https://doi.org/10.1097/NCQ.0000000000000031.
16. von Ungern-Sternberg BS. Respiratory complications in the pediatric postanesthesia care unit. Anesthesiol Clin. 2014;32(1):45–61. https://doi.org/10.1016/j.anclin.2013.10.004. Epub 2013 Dec 8. PMID: 24491649.
17. Verghese ST, Mostello LA, Patel RI, Kaplan RF, Patel KM. Testing anal sphincter tone predicts the effectiveness of caudal analgesia in children. Anesth Analg. 2002;94:1161–4.

Anaphylaxis After Antibiotics in PACU

Giuliana Geng-Ramos

Objectives
- Define anaphylaxis and its clinical manifestations.
- Describe the pathophysiology of anaphylaxis.
- Recognize the symptoms and triggers of anaphylaxis.
- Describe the management of anaphylaxis.
- Describe how to prevent anaphylaxis in a patient with history of anaphylaxis.

1 Case Presentation

A 5-year-old female with past medical history of asthma presents for hand exploration following a dog bite injury. After an uneventful surgery, she is transported to the postanesthesia care unit (PACU). Given the extensity of her wound, the surgeon orders antibiotics to be administered postoperatively. Intravenous amoxicillin/clavulanate was administered slowly. Ten minutes later, the patient is noted to have swelling of her face and tongue, and urticaria. Her oxygen saturation decreases, and wheezing is audible upon auscultation.

What is your differential diagnosis for this patient?
What is your immediate next step?

You provide supplemental oxygen using a non-rebreather face mask at 10 liters per minute. Oxygen saturation via pulse oximetry remains in the 80s. The patient becomes hypotensive with blood pressure 42/20; tachycardia ensues. You place her

G. Geng-Ramos (✉)
Children's National Hospital, The George Washington University School of Medicine, Washington, DC, USA
e-mail: ggengramos@childrensnational.org

S. T. Verghese (ed.), *Anesthesia STAT! Acute Pediatric Emergencies in PACU*,
https://doi.org/10.1007/978-3-031-24396-7_2

in recumbent position with lower extremities elevated to maximize perfusion of vital organs. The patient becomes weak and loses consciousness.

What is your next intervention?
How will you manage the low oxygen saturation? Will you intubate?
What is at the top of your differential diagnosis? How do you proceed?

Anaphylaxis is suspected. You call for help and intubate the patient. The waveform on capnography reveals a sawtooth slope and carbon dioxide value of 74.

What is anaphylaxis and how common is it?
Why is the incidence of anaphylaxis less common in children compared to adults?
What is the pathophysiology of anaphylaxis?
What are the clinical manifestations of anaphylaxis?
Does the patient's asthma history place her at risk for anaphylaxis?
What are the associated risk factors?
Identify the most common causes of anaphylaxis in the perioperative period.
How do you diagnose anaphylaxis?
How do you treat anaphylaxis?
What interventions are applied if the patient remains hypotensive?
How will you monitor this patient in PACU?

The child is stable and transferred to the intensive care unit (ICU). You update her parents about her condition and prognosis. The parents are shocked to hear that this unexpected reaction has occurred, since their child has had antibiotics in the past without any problems. They want to know why she needed to be intubated and how long she will have to stay in the hospital.

How do you manage the airway during anaphylaxis?
How long should the patient be observed?
What is the mortality rate of anaphylaxis?

Her parents are grateful after they see she remains stable in the ICU after this unusual event. They request guidance on what they can do to prevent this from happening again.

What can be done to prevent anaphylaxis?

2 Discussion

2.1 What Is Anaphylaxis and How Common Is It?

Anaphylaxis is an unanticipated severe, life-threatening generalized or systemic hypersensitivity reaction after exposure to an allergen which manifests as respiratory and cardiovascular compromise [1, 2]. Perioperative anaphylaxis is relatively uncommon with an incidence of 1 in 37,000 pediatric anesthetics, which is less than the estimated incidence of 1 in 10,000 to 20,000 anesthetics in adults [3, 4]. However, the exact prevalence is unclear as the incidence of perioperative anaphylaxis in children is not comprehensively reported worldwide [2].

2.2 Why Is the Incidence of Anaphylaxis Less Common in Children Compared to Adults?

The rate of perioperative anaphylaxis in children is about one quarter of that in adults. The lower incidence rate may be influenced by the type of procedures children undergo as well as the differing anesthetic techniques used in children compared to adults. Hospital-wide efforts to increase awareness and reduce exposure to known triggers, such as latex, have reduced the rate of perioperative anaphylaxis. Children may also be less sensitized to allergens and less exposed to allergens in the perioperative period as compared to adults. Neuromuscular blocking agents and antibiotics are not used as frequently during a general anesthetic in children compared to adults. Furthermore, a study found 14% of children received only sevoflurane as their anesthetic induction and maintenance, which is a low anaphylaxis-risk anesthetic [4].

2.3 What Is the Pathophysiology of Anaphylaxis?

After exposure to an allergen, there is sudden release of substances and mediators from mast cells and basophils into circulation. Allergens can trigger anaphylaxis via IgE-dependent mechanisms, known as allergic anaphylaxis, or direct mast cell activation known as nonallergic anaphylaxis or anaphylactoid reaction [1]. IgE-dependent mechanism involves an initial sensitizing exposure after which IgE antibodies are produced and bind to receptors on mast cells and basophils. Upon subsequent exposure to the same or chemically similar antigen, the IgE antibodies bind the allergen forming an antigen-antibody complex that induces basophil and mast cell degranulation. Nonallergic anaphylaxis does not necessitate prior sensitization. Regardless of the triggering mechanism, both result in release of mediators including histamine, tryptase, and inflammatory leukotrienes and prostaglandins leading to immediate anaphylaxis symptoms [2]. Mast cells then release additional chemokines that recruit and activate additional inflammatory cells [5].

2.4 What Are the Clinical Manifestations of Anaphylaxis?

Symptoms typically occur shortly after exposure to an allergen and progress rapidly. The release of vasoactive mediators results in increased capillary permeability and peripheral vasodilation and extravasation of intravascular fluid into the extracellular fluid space, leading to hypovolemic shock. Organs involved include the skin, mucous membranes, cardiovascular system, respiratory system, and gastrointestinal tract [6]. In the pediatric population, severe anaphylaxis most often presents with bronchospasm or high airway pressure [4].

2.5 Clinical Manifestations of Anaphylaxis by Organ System [6]

Affected organ system	Clinical manifestation
Skin	Pruritis, flushing, urticaria, angioedema
Eyes	Conjunctivitis
Respiratory	Upper: rhinitis, laryngeal edema
	Lower: bronchoconstriction, wheezing, dyspnea, cyanosis
Intestinal tract	Abdominal pain, nausea, vomiting, diarrhea
Cardiovascular	Tachycardia, hypotension, arrhythmias, shock
Renal	Decreased urine output
Hematologic	Disseminated intravascular coagulation (DIC)

Children on beta-blocker therapy can have an atypical presentation of anaphylaxis characterized by hypotension and bradycardia [7]. The clinical severity of anaphylaxis is graded using clinical manifestations and can be used to guide clinical care.

2.6 Anaphylaxis Grading Adapted from Ring and Messmer Grading Scale [5, 8]

	Clinical manifestations based on organ system			
Grade	Cutaneous-mucous	Gastrointestinal tract	Respiratory system	Cardiovascular system
1	Pruritis, erythema, *±angioedema*			
2	Pruritis, erythema, ±angioedema	Nausea, abdominal cramps	Dyspnea, cough, rhinorrhea	Hypotension tachycardia or bradycardia, ±cardiac dysrhythmia
3	Pruritis, erythema, ±angioedema	Emesis, diarrhea	Wheezing, cyanosis, laryngeal edema	Cardiovascular collapse/ shock
4	Pruritis, erythema, ±angioedema	Emesis, diarrhea	Respiratory arrest	Cardiac arrest

2.7 Does the Patient's Asthma History Place Her at Risk for Anaphylaxis? What Are the Associated Risk Factors?

There are several risk factors found in children who develop perioperative anaphylaxis. A history of asthma, atopy, food allergies, undergoing multiple operations, and family history of atopy are risk factors for anaphylaxis in children. While there is no sex difference found in children, anaphylaxis is more common in adult females compared to male counterparts [2].

2.8 Identify the Most Common Causes of Anaphylaxis in the Perioperative Period

Antibiotics account for the highest incidence of perioperative anaphylaxis, of which cephalosporins, followed by penicillins, have been recognized as the most frequently reported culprits [2, 3]. Cephalosporins are commonly used in surgical prophylaxis creating a challenge for the anesthesiologist caring for a child with reported penicillin or cephalosporin allergy. Penicillins and cephalosporins share a beta-lactam ring that when attached to similar R1 side chains can result in potential cross-reactivity. Certain cephalosporins, such as cephazolin, contain a unique side chain structure that does not react with penicillins, while ampicillin, cefaclor, and cephalexin share an R1 group side chain. Data in perioperative settings are limited but suggest very low incidence of anaphylaxis to cephazolin in patients with penicillin allergy; there is no clear evidence of an increased risk of anaphylaxis in a cefazolin-naïve, penicillin-allergic patients [9].

Neuromuscular blocking agents (NMBA) were previously identified as the most common cause of anaphylaxis in the perioperative period and are now second to antibiotics [3]. Succinylcholine has the highest rate of anaphylaxis, followed by rocuronium and atracurium [10]. It's important to note that because of the low number of cases reported in children, it is not possible to make definitive conclusions concerning risk rates with different drugs, and this varies among countries. However, there appears to be a proportionate number of cases of atracurium and succinylcholine exposures [4].

Many common over-the-counter medications and daily-use cosmetics and products contain the same allergenic epitopes found in NMBA that could lead to sensitization; therefore a prior exposure to an NMBA is not required to develop anaphylaxis [2, 6].

Sugammadex, widely used worldwide, is a cyclodextrin compound used for the reversal of neuromuscular blocking agents such as rocuronium and vecuronium. Sugammadex is generally thought to be a safe and well-tolerated drug; however, confirmed cases of anaphylaxis to sugammadex have been recently reported. Little is known about the mechanism of sugammadex-induced anaphylaxis as there is a lack of IgE-specific antibodies, and skin prick testing is still in development. In reported cases, none of the patients had prior exposure to sugammadex, suggesting cross-reactivity between sugammadex and another substance. Cyclodextrins are present in various foods, which may partly explain sensitization and cross-reaction with sugammadex. [2, 11]

Chlorhexidine is an emerging cause of anaphylaxis when applied to mucous membranes or the skin. It can also occur when the skin or mucus membrane comes in contact with it from a chlorhexidine-impregnated device. When applied to mucous membranes or the skin, chlorhexidine may produce a delayed reaction; conversely, when inserted as part of a chlorhexidine-impregnated device, it can lead to rapid and severe anaphylaxis [2].

Latex has historically been cited as a prominent trigger for anaphylaxis in the perioperative period. Exposure to latex has reduced significantly over recent years, drastically decreasing sensitization and, in turn, reducing the incidence of latex-induced anaphylaxis [4]. Children with spina bifida are at highest risk for anaphylaxis from latex exposure with a reported prevalence as high as 70% [12]. Children with known allergies to tropical fruits, such as papaya, banana, kiwi, and avocado, are at risk for allergic reaction to latex due to cross-reactivity [5].

2.9 What Is the Differential Diagnosis?

The diagnosis of anaphylaxis may be challenging when only a few or nonspecific symptoms are present. The differential diagnosis includes hypovolemia, sepsis, embolism, vasovagal reaction, asthma, tension pneumothorax, aspiration, or foreign body in the airway [2].

2.10 How Do You Diagnose Anaphylaxis?

The initial diagnosis is clinical, based on the history and physical examination. Serologic and skin testing can provide confirmation of the diagnosis. Tryptase is a neutral protease stored in mast cells that is released during anaphylactic reactions. An increased plasma tryptase level within 1–2 h of suspected reaction confirms mast cell activation and mediator release occurrence, signaling an immune-mediated mechanism. It does not differentiate between anaphylaxis and anaphylactoid reactions [6]. Skin testing performed by prick and intradermal techniques 4–6 weeks after an anaphylaxis episode can help identify the offending antigen. [6]

2.11 How Do You Treat Anaphylaxis?

Anaphylaxis must be recognized and treated immediately. Management consists of immediate withdrawal of suspected triggers, interrupting the effects of the released vasoactive and inflammatory mediators, and averting further mediator release. Resuscitation involves reversing airway obstruction and increasing intravascular volume and tone, for which epinephrine is the drug of choice since its alpha-1 effect induces vasoconstriction and beta-2 effect causes relaxation of bronchial smooth muscle. Early administration of epinephrine is critical. If the child is in cardiac arrest, the arrest dose of 10 mcg/kg IV should be given. For hypotension or impending cardiac arrest, give epinephrine 1–10 mcg/kg IV, and this can be repeated every 1–2 min as needed if unresponsive. An epinephrine infusion of 0.02–0.2 μg/kg/min may be necessary for refractory hypotension. Intravascular depletion is treated with multiple boluses of 20 mL/kg of intravenous crystalloid, such as normal saline, given rapidly. The child should be placed on 100% oxygen to increase oxygen delivery. In case of severe airway obstruction, early intubation by a skilled practitioner should be performed. Inhaled bronchodilators can be given for treatment of bronchospasm. To decrease the histamine-mediated effects, antihistamines such as diphenhydramine 1 mg/kg and ranitidine 1 mg/kg are given. Corticosteroids should be administered to help decrease mediator release, decrease airway swelling, and prevent recurrence of symptoms [2, 6].

2.12 Management of Anaphylaxis

Organ system	Treatment	Effect
Airway	100% oxygen Early intubation if severe airway obstruction	Increase oxygen delivery
Respiratory	Albuterol and ipratropium bromide nebulization	Reverse bronchoconstriction
Circulation	Epinephrine 1–10 mcg/kg bolus PRN Epinephrine infusion 0.02–0.2 mcg/kg/min	Increase intravascular tone Bronchial smooth muscle relaxation Decrease mediator release
	IV crystalloid 20 mL/kg boluses	Restore intravascular volume
Cellular cutaneous	Diphenhydramine 1 mg/kg IV Ranitidine 1 mg/kg IV	Decrease effects of histamine
	Corticosteroids	Decrease mediator release Decrease airway swelling Prevent recurrence

2.13 What Interventions Are Applied if the Patient Remains Hypotensive?

For resistant hypotension, consider administering norepinephrine or vasopressin infusions. The cause for resistant hypotension may be due to desensitization of adrenergic receptors for which vasopressin may be useful since it has vasoactive effects mediated by non-adrenergic vascular V^1 receptors. It's important to note that vasopressin administered alone in the early course of anaphylaxis may be detrimental and should be reserved for patients experiencing anaphylaxis refractory to epinephrine or norepinephrine [5]. Patients who are taking beta-blocker therapy, alone or in combination with angiotensin-converting enzyme inhibitors, may be resistant to standard treatment and have severe anaphylaxis. If a patient taking beta-blockers is refractory to epinephrine, isoprenaline and glucagon should be considered [2]. Glucagon has inotropic and chronotropic effects that are not mediated through beta-receptors [13].

2.14 How Will You Monitor This Patient in PACU?

Continuous noninvasive monitoring of blood pressure, heart rate, and oxygenation via pulse oximetry should be performed. An intra-arterial catheter should be placed for arterial pressure monitoring in children receiving vasoactive infusions. A urinary catheter should be placed to monitor urine output. Central venous pressure monitor should be placed in children with fluid and catecholamine-resistant shock [14].

2.15 How Do You Manage the Airway During Anaphylaxis?

The initial management of anaphylaxis involves assessment of the patient's airway. If the airway is not edematous, supplemental oxygen can be administered via non-rebreather oxygen. Severe anaphylaxis can lead to angioedema and bronchospasm, which is the most common presenting symptom in children [4]. Anaphylaxis can result in significant edema of the tongue and oropharyngeal tissues, leading to rapid airway compromise and difficult intubation. Intubation should be performed urgently if stridor or respiratory distress is present.

If bronchospasm is present, albuterol and ipratropium bromide nebulizers should be administered to allow bronchial smooth muscle relaxation. Administration of corticosteroids should be considered to reduce airway edema and prevent late and delayed symptoms. Hydrocortisone is the preferred steroid because of its fast onset. Because airway swelling and inflammation may continue for 24 h, extubation should be delayed [6].

2.16 How Long Should the Patient Be Observed?

Following stabilization, the patient should be observed in the intensive care unit because airway swelling and inflammation may persist or the patient may exhibit a biphasic response [2, 6]. Biphasic responses involve an initial reaction meeting criteria for anaphylaxis, followed by a period of 1 h or more without symptoms, and subsequent return of symptoms meeting criteria for anaphylaxis without further exposure to the antigen. The time period between the resolution of the first reaction and initiation of biphasic response ranges from 1 h to up to 48 h [15]. The incidence of biphasic reactions in pediatric patients is 6% and is associated with delayed administration of epinephrine. Given that biphasic reactions occur with significant frequency, a 24-h period of observation is recommended [16].

2.17 What Is the Mortality Rate of Anaphylaxis?

Mortality is relatively rare but has occurred [3]. The observed mortality rate is 3.8% and is associated with increased age, increased ASA physical status, morbid obesity, coronary artery disease, and concomitant use of beta-blocker and angiotensin-converting enzyme inhibitor [4].

A case report described the occurrence of atypical stress-induced cardiomyopathy associated with cephalosporin-induced anaphylaxis in a young adult. Stress-induced cardiomyopathy may be triggered by anaphylaxis via two mechanisms. Simultaneous multivessel coronary artery spasms by anaphylactic mediators may initiate stress-induced cardiomyopathy. Secondly, excessive rise of systemic catecholamines activates cardiac catecholamine receptors, precipitating stress-induced cardiomyopathy. Anaphylaxis leads to compensatory release of catecholamines. This, combined with administration of catecholamines for hemodynamic support in anaphylactic shock, may provoke stress-induced cardiomyopathy. Although life-threatening, the prognosis of stress-induced cardiomyopathy is generally favorable [17].

2.18 What Can Be Done to Prevent Anaphylaxis?

The most effective measure to prevent anaphylaxis is to identify and avoid the known triggering agent. Children with suspected allergic reaction should be referred to an allergy testing center, 4–6 weeks after symptom resolution for a diagnostic workup. Any drug with a high clinical suspicion of causing anaphylaxis but negative testing should be avoided [2]. Premedication with antihistamines or corticosteroids has little benefit and may blunt the early signs of anaphylaxis leading to delay in recognition and management [6]. Children with documented anaphylaxis to a medication should be referred for a medical alert bracelet to alert medical professionals should the child be found unconscious or unaccompanied by a guardian [2].

3 Summary

Although perioperative anaphylaxis is relatively rare in children, most drugs used in the perioperative setting can lead to anaphylaxis. Perioperative anaphylaxis is most commonly caused by antibiotics and neuromuscular blocking agents, and prior exposure to the drug is not often necessary. The most common presenting symptom of anaphylaxis in children is bronchospasm. Management involves early recognition, removal of the triggering agent, administration of epinephrine, and aggressive fluid resuscitation. The airway can become edematous quickly; therefore early intubation should be considered if angioedema is observed. Patients should be monitored for refractory anaphylaxis for at least 24 h. Children with suspected anaphylaxis should be referred to a specialized allergy testing center for follow-up to identify the causative agent and prevent recurrence in the future. Medical alert bracelets are imperative to identify life-threatening agents that should be avoided during medical emergencies.

References

1. Johansson SG, Bieber T, Dahl R, et al. Revised nomenclature for allergy for global use: report of the Nomenclature Review Committee of the World Allergy Organization, October 2003. J Allergy Clin Immunol. 2004;113(5):832–6. https://doi.org/10.1016/j.jaci.2003.12.591.
2. Stepanovic B, Sommerfield D, Lucas M, von Ungern-Sternberg BS. An update on allergy and anaphylaxis in pediatric anesthesia. Paediatr Anaesth. 2019;29(9):892–900. https://doi.org/10.1111/pan.13703.
3. Wakimoto M, Miller R, Kim SS, et al. Perioperative anaphylaxis in children: a report from the wake-up safe collaborative. Paediatr Anaesth. 2021;31(2):205–12. https://doi.org/10.1111/pan.14063.
4. Harper NJN, Cook TM, Garcez T, et al. Anaesthesia, surgery, and life-threatening allergic reactions: management and outcomes in the 6th National Audit Project (NAP6). Br J Anaesth. 2018;121(1):172–88. https://doi.org/10.1016/j.bja.2018.04.015.
5. Dewachter P, et al. Anaphylaxis and anesthesia: controversies and new insights. Anesthesiology. 2009;111(5):1141–50.
6. Hepner DL, Castells MC. Anaphylaxis during the perioperative period. Anesth Analg. 2003;97(5):1381–95. https://doi.org/10.1213/01.ANE.0000082993.84883.7D.
7. Momeni M, Brui B, Baele P, Matta A. Anaphylactic shock in a beta-blocked child: usefulness of isoproterenol. Paediatr Anaesth. 2007;17(9):897–9. https://doi.org/10.1111/j.1460-9592.2007.02276.x.
8. Ring J, Messmer K. Incidence and severity of anaphylactoid reactions to colloid volume substitutes. Lancet. 1977;1(8009):466–9.
9. Vorobeichik L, et al. Misconceptions surrounding penicillin allergy: implications for anesthesiologists. Anesth Analg. 2018;127(3):642–9.
10. Tacquard C, Collange O, Gomis P, et al. Anaesthetic hypersensitivity reactions in France between 2011 and 2012: the 10th GERAP epidemiologic survey. Acta Anaesthesiol Scand. 2017;61(3):290–9. https://doi.org/10.1111/aas.12855.
11. Takazawa T, et al. Three suspected cases of sugammadex-induced anaphylactic shock. BMC Anesthesiol. 2014;14:92.
12. Bernardini R, et al. Prevalence of and risk factors for latex sensitization in patients with spina bifida. J Urol. 1998;160:1775–8.
13. Thomas M, Crawford I. Best evidence topic report. Glucagon infusion in refractory anaphylactic shock in patients on beta-blockers. Emerg Med J. 2005;22(4):272–3.
14. Waltzman M. Initial management of shock in children. UpToDate. 2020. https://www.uptodate.com/contents/initial-management-of-shock-in-children?search=anaphylaxis%20urine%20output&source=search_result&selectedTitle=4~150&usage_type=default&display_rank=4#H23.
15. Lieberman P. Biphasic anaphylactic reactions. Ann Allergy Asthma Immunol. 2005;95(3):217–26; quiz 226, 258.
16. Lee JM, Greenes DS. Biphasic anaphylactic reactions in pediatrics. Pediatrics. 2000;106(4):762–6.
17. Suk EH, et al. Stress-induced cardiomyopathy following cephalosporin-induced anaphylactic shock during general anesthesia. Can J Anaesth. 2009;56(6):432–6.

Somnolence After V-P Shunt Revision in an Infant

Nina Deutsch

1 Stem Case

A 13-month-old infant weighing 8 kg with a history of hydrocephalus is admitted to the postanesthesia care unit (PACU) after a revision of a ventriculoperitoneal (VP) shunt. She was admitted to the hospital the previous day secondary to altered mental status at home. Her mother reports that she vomited several times over the prior 24 h as well. Workup demonstrated that her shunt was no longer functioning properly.

Her past medical history is significant for birth at 27 weeks' gestation via spontaneous vaginal delivery and very low birth weight. She had a grade III intraventricular hemorrhage (IVH) with subsequent hydrocephalus. She was diagnosed with a patent ductus arteriosus that required surgical closure at 1 month of age. She had bronchopulmonary dysplasia (BPD) for which she was intubated for approximately 4 weeks following birth. She was discharged home on oxygen, NG feeds, and apnea monitor. She also required sildenafil for elevated pulmonary pressures for the first 9 months of life. However, the apnea monitor has been discontinued, and she has had no oxygen requirements for the last 4 months. Her baseline CBC laboratory values demonstrated a hemoglobin of 10 g/dL and hematocrit of 31%.

She underwent initial VP shunt placement for her hydrocephalus at 3 months of age. She has been on NG feeds for 9 months and growing slowly. Her only medication currently is GE reflux medications and albuterol as needed.

Key Questions

- What is an IVH and how is it graded?
- What causes hydrocephalus following an IVH?
- What is the treatment of hydrocephalus?

N. Deutsch (✉)
Children's National Hospital, Washington, DC, USA
e-mail: ndeutsch@childrensnational.org

S. T. Verghese (ed.), *Anesthesia STAT! Acute Pediatric Emergencies in PACU*,
https://doi.org/10.1007/978-3-031-24396-7_3

- What are the anesthetic concerns of an infant with a history of prematurity?
- What is the anesthetic management of an infant undergoing VP shunt revision?

Case continued: Her vital signs on arrival to the PACU are as follows: BP 74/38, HR 120/mt, sat 98%, and temp 36.3 °C.

Physical examination demonstrates a somnolent infant. She has a dressing in place on her head, and the fontanelle appears normal. She has poor muscle tone.

- What are the signs and symptoms of VP shunt malfunction? How likely is it with her current presentation?
- Apart from issues with the VP shunt, what are other potential causes of her somnolence?

Case continued: In reviewing the anesthetic, you note that the patient had a general anesthetic with an endotracheal tube. Sevoflurane, fentanyl (5 mcg), rocuronium, and acetaminophen have been administered. The rocuronium was reversed with glycopyrrolate and neostigmine and the patient was extubated awake per the anesthesiologist that did the case. She received a total of 80 cc of normal saline during the case and her blood loss was minimal. How does general anesthesia affect formerly premature infants in the recovery period?

- What would be the most common presentation in the PACU if an excessive amount of opioid was administered to the infant? How would you treat this?
- How would her presentation differ if inadequate reversal of the neuromuscular blocking agent was suspected? How would this scenario be treated?

Case continued: Further evaluation of the patient reveals that residual anesthetic agents are not the likely cause of the patient's current presentation.

- What are the other important diagnoses for somnolence to rule out immediately?
- What tests or studies can help in the differential diagnosis?

Case continued: On physical exam, the patient responds to pain when stimulated; however, she is still difficult to arouse. She looks more lethargic with poor muscular tone. Her temperature has drifted down to 35.1 despite being swaddled up in blankets. An electrolyte panel and arterial blood gas are sent to the lab. Vital signs remain stable.

- What findings on an arterial blood gas could result in the patient's somnolence?
- What electrolyte abnormalities could be the cause of her current condition?
- If the patient's electrolyte panel demonstrated hyponatremia, what would be the treatment? How should the treatment be carried out?
- What are the concerns with treatment of hyponatremia?

Case continued: The laboratory study findings are as follows:

Test	Result
pH	7.34
pCO_2	53
pO_2	154
BE	−2
Sodium	142
Potassium	3.8
Glucose	40
Hemoglobin	9.9
Hematocrit	30

- What are the implications of her hemoglobin and hematocrit values?
- Which finding on the above labs is *most* likely the cause of the somnolence?
- What is the treatment of this?
- What treatment during the case could have helped to avoid this?

Case continued: The patient is administered 10% dextrose 2 mL/kg (16 mL) and has improvement in her mental status. She is now awake and crying. Vital signs remain normal. In review of the patient's preoperative fluids and the anesthetic record, the patient received normal saline without dextrose from the time of her admission.

- What maintenance fluids should she be given now?
- If the laboratory values were all within normal limits (i.e., no electrolyte abnormalities), what would be the appropriate next step in the diagnosis and treatment of her somnolence?
- At what point should neurosurgery be notified of the patient's condition?

2 Discussion

2.1 What Is an IVH and How Is It Graded?

IVH is the leakage of blood into the cerebral ventricular space secondary to vascular fragility of the germinal matrix and changes in cerebral blood flow. Approximately 20% of preterm and very low birth weight (VLBW) newborns will develop an IVH, with more extensive bleeds more likely the smaller and more premature the infant. More than 50% of IVH will occur in the first 24 h after birth, while 90% will occur within the first week of life [1].

Diagnosis is made with the use of cranial ultrasound. The extent of the bleeding will determine the grade of IVH, as summarized in Table 1.

Table 1 Intraventricular grade based on ultrasound findings

Grade of IVH	Findings
I	Confined to the subependymal germinal matrix
II	Hemorrhage within the lateral ventricle without dilation and/or occupying less than 50% of the ventricle
III	Hemorrhage with distention resulting in ventricular dilation and/or hemorrhage occupying more than 50% of the ventricle
IV	Intraventricular hemorrhage that extends into the surrounding parenchyma

Clinical presentation of IVH can vary depending on the speed of onset of the bleeding. Acute neurologic deterioration will be seen with significant large, rapidly expanding IVH and is associated with poor outcomes. A slower IVH that evolves over hours to days will present as decreased alertness and activity, hypotonia, abnormal eye movements, and alterations in respiratory effort [1].

2.2 What Causes Hydrocephalus Following an IVH?

While the mechanism of posthemorrhagic hydrocephalus is not certain, it is thought that blood clots obstruct the flow of cerebrospinal fluid at the cerebral aqueduct or fourth ventricle outlets, resulting in obstructive hydrocephalus [2]. This is followed by a delayed communicating hydrocephalus secondary to abnormal cerebrospinal fluid absorption [1]. Ultimately, ventricular dilation can result in hypoxia, ischemia, decreased cerebral perfusion, increased development of free radicals, and destruction of the white matter [2].

2.3 What Is the Treatment of Hydrocephalus?

To prevent long-term sequelae of hydrocephalus, the definitive treatment is placement of a ventriculoperitoneal (VP) shunt. While this is the definitive treatment, it is typically not performed immediately secondary to the high risk of complications in very low birth weight infants, including skin ulceration, shunt malfunction, and the need for revisions. Often, temporizing measures such as lumbar punctures or external ventricular drains will allow for drainage of fluid and prevent significant dilation until the infant is older [1].

2.4 What Are the Anesthetic Concerns of an Infant with a History of Prematurity?

Babies born prior to 37 weeks' gestation have an increased risk of developing several complications, the severity of which increases with lower gestational age at birth. These include but are not limited to the conditions listed in Table 2.

Table 2 Complications of prematurity

Complications of prematurity
Bronchopulmonary dysplasia (BPD)
Anemia of prematurity
Intraventricular hemorrhage
Patent ductus arteriosus (PDA)
Retinopathy of prematurity (ROP)
Neurologic abnormalities (cerebral palsy)

Multiple studies have demonstrated an increased risk for adverse events related to anesthesia or sedation for preterm children, children under 3 years of age, and those with significant comorbidities [3]. Furthermore, infants less than 60 weeks post-gestational age are at higher risk of developing postanesthesia apnea [4].

2.5 What Is the Anesthetic Management of an Infant Undergoing VP Shunt Revision?

Infants requiring VP shunt revision typically require a general anesthetic due to the need to potentially access the cranial and abdominal portions of the catheter. Most practitioners will elect to intubate the infant with an endotracheal tube to allow for control of ventilation and protection of the airway while the intra-abdominal portion of the procedure is done.

Revisions of the shunt can occur in the portion in the head, in the tubing between the head and the abdomen, or in the abdomen. If the entire shunt needs to be replaced, the tunneling of the new catheter is extremely stimulating and may require an opioid. If the patient otherwise meets extubation criteria at the end of the procedure, the infant is extubated to allow for a neurologic exam in the postoperative period.

2.6 What Are the Signs and Symptoms of VP Shunt Malfunction? How Likely Is It with Her Current Presentation?

VP shunt malfunction can present with an array of signs and symptoms. Bulging fontanelle, fluid collection along the shunt, depressed level of consciousness, irritability, abdominal pain, nausea and vomiting, and headache were found to be strongly associated with shunt failure [5]. Other signs of increased intracranial pressure, such as seizures, sunsetting eyes, and papilledema, can also be present. Fever is strongly associated with a shunt infection [5].

While this patient does have a common sign of shunt malfunction (depressed level of consciousness), she does not have a bulging fontanelle or vomiting in this postoperative period. While an issue with the shunt cannot be ruled out, other causes of her current presentation should be investigated as well.

Table 3 The differential diagnosis of delayed awakening following anesthesia

Patient factors	**Surgical and anesthetic factors**
Extremes of age (former premature infant)	Long surgery and anesthetic
Gender	Muscle relaxant used
Genetic variation	Hypotension
Comorbidities (i.e., apnea of prematurity)	Hypoxia
Body habitus (i.e., obesity)	Embolism
Cognitive dysfunction	Cardiac/neurosurgery
Seizures	Regional techniques with sedation
Stroke	Painful stimulation
Drug factors	**Metabolic factors**
Dosage	Hypo-/hyperglycemia
Time of administration	Hypo-/hypernatremia
Blood-gas solubility	Hypothermia
Metabolism	Hypothyroidism
Excretion	Hepatic and/or renal failure
Drug interactions	Central anticholinergic syndrome
Fluid overload	Acidosis
Local anesthetic toxicity	Coagulation defects

2.7 Apart from Issues with the VP Shunt, What Are Other Potential Causes of Her Somnolence?

The differential diagnosis of delayed awakening following anesthesia can be divided into four main categories as outlined in Table 3 [6].

It is imperative to confirm that the most life-threatening conditions, such as hypotension and hypoxia, are not present. Maintenance of the airway, breathing, and circulation are important for initial management. Once these are ruled out, a systematic review of the most common or likely issues should occur to begin appropriate therapy. In this scenario, the patient is maintaining her airway with normal vital signs. Therefore, other factors need to be evaluated promptly.

2.8 What Would Be the Most Common Presentation in the PACU if an Excessive Amount of Opioid Was Administered to the Infant? How Would You Treat This?

With the administration of opioids, it is imperative to monitor the patient for potentially harmful side effects. Excessive sedation has been shown to predict opioid-related respiratory depression and should be always monitored for while a pediatric patient is receiving opioid therapy [7]. Opioids also cause constriction of the pupils and can help in the differential diagnosis. Formerly premature infants such as this patient are at particular risk of apnea in the perioperative period [4]. Other known side effects of opioids include emesis, pruritis, ileus, and chest wall rigidity.

If excessive opioids are suspected, naloxone (0.1 mg/kg/dose) should be administered with titration to effect (i.e., reversal of sedation or respiratory depression).

Support of the airway and ventilation should also be done to prevent excessive accumulation of carbon dioxide from the resulting hypoventilation that opioids induce. In this case she received 5 mcg of fentanyl at the time of surgical incision but no further opioids after the surgical procedure. Clinically significant dose variation can occur when drug volumes ≤0.5 mL are injected. Pediatric anesthesiologists must be aware of this possible unintended medication error when drawing small volumes of drugs to be administered to smaller patients [8].

Although the dose administered could have been more than intended unless drawn up in a small syringe and precise amount given, she was awakened and extubated fully awake at the end of the surgical procedure and then slowly became somnolent in PACU.

2.9 How Would Her Presentation Differ if Inadequate Reversal of the Neuromuscular Blocking Agent Was Suspected? How Would This Scenario Be Treated?

Inadequate reversal of a neuromuscular blocking agent will present with poor respiratory effort (shallow breathing or weak, rocking breaths), difficulty opening the eyes, and weakness of the extremities. The patient will also be difficult to arouse and not fully responsive to stimulation. Residual paralysis has been shown to increase the risk of passive regurgitation of gastric contents, worsen atelectasis, and interfere with hypoxic ventilatory control [9].

Train-of-four monitoring (TOF) is the standard to determine the presence of residual neuromuscular blockade. Importantly, a ratio of 0.9 is necessary to ensure the patient can protect their airway following extubation [9]. Despite this, in a recent survey of pediatric anesthesiologists, a minority of survey respondents always assess TOF, and the use of it was less in those who used sugammadex as their primary reversal agent [10].

If prolonged neuromuscular blockade is suspected, a reversal agent should be administered. The cholinesterase inhibitor neostigmine (0.07 mg/kg/dose) can be given with the anticholinesterase glycopyrrolate (0.01 mg/kg). However, it is inappropriate to administer these agents with the expectation of full reversal before at least T2 has been detected on the TOF. Alternatively, sugammadex, an agent that forms a 1:1 inclusion complex around steroidal neuromuscular blocking agent and thereby terminates its action (4–16 mg/kg), can be given despite the presence of a profound block [9].

2.10 What Are Other Important Diagnoses for Somnolence to Rule Out Immediately?

At this point, hemodynamic instability (hypotension, hypoxia, dysrhythmia) and side effects from the anesthetic and residual medications have been ruled out as potential causes of the patient's somnolence. The patient's temperature should also be taken to confirm that she does not have hypothermia, which can cause abnormal slowing of her metabolism and drug clearance. Since the patient's temperature was normal on arrival to PACU, metabolic factors and underlying neurologic causes must now be taken into consideration.

Infants are at risk for developing hypothermia during transport and in recovery if warming measures are not taken to prevent it. Complications of perioperative hypothermia include coagulopathy and increased transfusion requirement, surgical site infection, delayed drug metabolism, prolonged recovery, and, in older patients, shivering and thermal discomfort [11].

2.11 What Tests or Studies Can Help in the Differential Diagnosis?

Electrolyte abnormalities can be determined with the use of point-of-care testing for sodium, potassium, and glucose levels. The presence of acidosis (either respiratory or metabolic) should also be investigated with analysis of an arterial blood gas (ABG). If these values are within normal limits, more rare but potential conditions such as renal and hepatic failure and hypothyroidism should then be considered.

2.12 What Findings on an Arterial Blood Gas Could Result in the Patient's Somnolence?

Significant respiratory depression can result in hypercarbia. In preterm infants, the ventilatory response to carbon dioxide is significantly reduced. However, this improves with advancing age [12]. Elevations in carbon dioxide can result in somnolence if they are extremely high. Similarly, extreme hypoxia can decrease consciousness and should be evaluated as well.

2.13 What Electrolyte Abnormalities Could Be the Cause of Her Current Condition?

Abnormal levels of plasma sodium and glucose can cause significant somnolence. This can be determined with point-of-care testing or the analysis of a basic metabolic panel. A heel stick measurement of blood glucose is a rapid and readily available bedside test that can be performed as well.

2.14 If the Patient's Electrolyte Panel Demonstrated Hyponatremia, What Would Be the Treatment? How Should the Treatment Be Carried Out?

Severe hyponatremia (less than 120 mEq/L) can result in cerebral edema, altered mental status, or coma [13]. This can be secondary to severe vomiting, medications such as diuretics, kidney or liver disease, syndrome of inappropriate antidiuretic hormone (SIADH), or iatrogenic causes, such as excessive administration of hypotonic intravenous fluids [14]. Once this has been determined, treatment should be undertaken.

In patients with severe symptoms such as vomiting, deep somnolence, seizures, coma, or cardiac arrest, 3% saline is administered to correct 4–6 mEq/L within 1–2 h, followed by a slower correction over the subsequent days to normal. Less severe clinical pictures should be corrected by 8 mEq/L/day or slower [13].

2.15 What Are the Concerns with Treatment of Hyponatremia?

Importantly, if correction of hyponatremia is too rapid, patients are at risk of central osmotic demyelination in which protein aggregation, DNA fragmentation, and programmed cell death lead to destruction of myelin. Evidence has shown that in patients with hyponatremia for less than 24 h, a more rapid correction is generally well tolerated compared to more chronic (greater than 48 h) hyponatremia [13].

2.16 What Are the Implications of Her Hemoglobin and Hematocrit Values?

The patient has a baseline hemoglobin and hematocrit that are indicative of anemia and could be a result of her poor feeding habits. The values that are obtained in the postoperative labs do not indicate that there has been significant perioperative bleeding. However, the presence of anemia in premature infants has been shown to be associated with an increased incidence of postoperative apnea compared to premature infants with a normal hematocrit [15]. This is less likely in this patient considering her age at the time of the procedure.

2.17 Which Finding on the Above Labs Is MOST Likely the Cause of the Somnolence?

Based on the reported laboratory values, the patient appears to have hypoglycemia. Age-based definitions of hypoglycemia in young children are presented in Table 4 [16].

Signs and symptoms of hypoglycemia include lethargy, change in level of consciousness, hypothermia, seizures, poor feeding, and hypotonia.

Table 4 Age-based definitions of hypoglycemia in young children

Age	Plasma glucose level
Neonate <48 h old	<47 mg/dL
Neonates >48 h old, infants, and children unable to communicate	<50–70 mg/dL

2.18 What Is the Treatment of This?

The patient should receive 200 mg of glucose per kg and 2 mL/kg dextrose 10% in water [$D_{10}W$], intravenously.

2.19 What Treatment During the Case Could Have Helped to Avoid This?

Hyperglycemia can be seen in the perioperative period, prompting many anesthesiologists to infuse non-glucose-containing fluids such as normal saline or lactated Ringer's solution intraoperatively. However, in this child, there are many risk factors for hypoglycemia. Riegger and colleagues studied the risk factors for intraoperative hypoglycemia in children and determined that these included young age, weight for age less than fifth percentile, ASA status greater than III, having a gastric or jejunal tube, poor feeding, and abdominal surgery [17].

This patient is an infant with a history of poor feeding and poor weight gain requiring gastric tube feeds. She also had recent vomiting associated with her shunt malfunction. These factors all put her at risk for having low glycogen stores and subsequent hypoglycemia. Therefore, monitoring of blood glucose is recommended either preoperatively with a heel stick glucose level, intraoperatively, or in the recovery room. Infusion of a glucose containing solution for maintenance fluids is indicated when hypoglycemia is likely.

2.20 What Maintenance Fluids Should She Be Given Now?

Postoperatively, a continuous infusion of glucose ($D_{10}W$ at 80–100 mL/kg per day) should be given with routine measurement of plasma glucose levels until the patient is taking fluids by mouth.

2.21 If the Laboratory Values Were All Within Normal Limits (i.e., No Electrolyte Abnormalities), What Would Be the Appropriate Next Step in the Diagnosis and Treatment of Her Somnolence?

If there were no electrolyte abnormalities found and the ABG was within normal limits, there should be an extremely low threshold to obtain a head CT scan. Considering her recent neurosurgical procedure, she is at increased risk of intracranial hemorrhage, stroke, or air embolus that warrants further evaluation. The possibility of subclinical seizures, potentially seen on an EEG, should also be considered.

2.22 At What Point Should Neurosurgery Be Notified of the Patient's Condition?

Considering that this has occurred in the immediate postoperative period, the neurosurgeons should be notified earlier rather than later to discuss concerns related to the surgical procedure. Consultation with a neurologist to help guide further workup and management of the patient's continued somnolence is important as well.

2.23 Where Should This Patient Be Monitored? And for How Long a Period?

The patient should be monitored overnight at the very minimum. She should be placed on a monitor that has pulse oximetry and EKG capabilities. Depending on the hospital's monitoring capabilities on the inpatient floor, this can be done either there or in the intensive care unit if necessary.

2.24 What Would You Discuss with the Parents and the New Surgeons Who Are Going to Be Managing Her Overnight Stay and Discharge?

Postoperatively, a continuous infusion of glucose ($D_{10}W$ at 80–100 mL/kg per day) should be given with routine measurement of plasma glucose levels until the patient is taking fluids by mouth. Regular neurologic checks will be important as well to look for any clinical changes that would point to an issue with the new shunt.

3 Summary

Ex premature patients with GE reflux who are poor eaters, often seen to have low weight gain, have a high chance of developing hypoglycemia in the perioperative period. The history of vomiting in an infant with failure to thrive clinical scenario should alert the anesthesiologist of the possibility of perioperative hypoglycemia. If a blood glucose level is not done preoperatively, one should be checked intraoperatively, and appropriate therapy should be initiated.

References

1. Sandoval PV, Hernández Rosales P, Quiñones Hernández DG, et al. Intraventricular hemorrhage and posthemorrhagic hydrocephalus in preterm infants: diagnosis, classification, and treatment options. Childs Nerv Syst. 2019;35(6):917–27.
2. Strahle J, Garton HJL, Maher CO, Muraszko KM, Keep RF, Xi G. Mechanisms of hydrocephalus after neonatal and adult intraventricular hemorrhage. Transl Stroke Res. 2012;3:25–38.

3. Havidich JE, Beach M, Dierdorf SF, et al. Preterm versus term children: analysis of sedation/anesthesia adverse events and longitudinal risk. Pediatrics. 2016;137(3):e20150463.
4. Coté CJ, Zaslavsky A, Downes JJ, et al. Postoperative apnea in former preterm infants after inguinal herniorrhaphy. A combined analysis. Anesthesiology. 1995;82(4):809–22.
5. Piatt JH, Garton HJL. Clinical diagnosis of ventriculoperitoneal shunt failure among children with hydrocephalus. Pediatr Emerg Care. 2008;24:201–10.
6. Misal US, Joshi SA, Shaikh MM. Delayed recovery from anesthesia: a postgraduate educational review. Anesth Essays Res. 2016;10:164–72.
7. Cravero JP, Agarwal R, Berde C, et al. The Society for Pediatric Anesthesia recommendations for the use of opioids in children in the perioperative period. Paediatr Anaesth. 2019;29:547–71.
8. Muffly MK, Chen MI, Claure RE, Drover DR, Efron B, Fitch WL, Hammer GB. Small-volume injections: evaluation of volume administration deviation from intended injection volumes. Anesth Analg. 2017;125(4):1192–9. https://doi.org/10.1213/ANE.0000000000001976. PMID: 28338490.
9. Srivastava A, Hunter JM. Reversal of neuromuscular block. Br J Anaesth. 2009;103:115–29.
10. Faulk DJ, Austin TM, Thomas JJ, et al. A survey of the Society for Pediatric Anesthesia on the use, monitoring, and antagonism of neuromuscular blockade. Anesth Analg. 2021;132:1518–26.
11. Sessler DI. Perioperative thermoregulation and heat balance. Lancet. 2016;387:2655–64.
12. Matthew OP. Apnea of prematurity: pathogenesis and management strategies. J Perinatol. 2011;31:302–10.
13. Sterns RH. Treatment of severe hyponatremia. Clin J Am Soc Nephrol. 2018;13(4):641–9.
14. Mercier JC, Titomanlio L, Basmaci R, Gaschignard J. Risks of severe hyponatremia in children receiving hypotonic fluids. Arch Pediatr. 2020;27(8):474–9.
15. Welborn LG, Hannallah RS, Luban NL, Fink R, Ruttimann UE. Anemia and postoperative apnea in former preterm infants. Anesthesiology. 1991;74:1003–6.
16. Casertano A, Rossi A, Fecarotta S, et al. An overview of hypoglycemia in children including a comprehensive practical diagnostic flowchart for clinical use. Front Endocrinol (Lausanne). 2021;12:684011. https://doi.org/10.3389/fendo.2021.684011.
17. Riegger LQ, Leis AM, Golmirzaie KH, Malviya S. Risk factors for intraoperative hypoglycemia in children: a multicenter retrospective cohort study. Anesth Analg. 2021;132:1075–83.

Emergence Delirium in a Toddler

Chaitanya Challa

A full-term healthy 3-year-old male 18 kg patient presented for an elective circumcision. At the age of 9 months, he had bilateral myringotomy and tube placements under anesthesia without any issues. There are no history of allergies and no significant family history of issues under anesthesia. Patient had premedication with midazolam (0.5 mg/kg) in the preoperative setting, as his parents stated he would become anxious prior to induction. He had a mask induction, and his airway was managed by an LMA which was placed after an intravenous line was secured. This was followed by an uneventful injection of 10 cc of ropivacaine 0.2% via the caudal space after sterile preparation of the caudal area while the patient was in the lateral position. Caudal anesthesia is very useful for providing pain relief during and after the surgery as well as decreasing the use of narcotics intraoperatively. The duration of surgery was 30 min and the patient's LMA was removed deep while he was still anesthetized, and then he was taken to PACU. About 15 min later, the patient woke up combative, attempting to rip off the intravenous line, screaming, and unable to be calmed down. The parents who were at the bedside and the PACU nurse are now unable to calm him and attempt to hold him from hurting himself. You are called back to de-escalate this erratic behavior of the 3-year-old young boy!

Could he be in pain? Was the caudal block effective? "Are you sure?", the mother asks. "He may be in pain," she says.

C. Challa (✉)
Children's National Medical Center, Washington, DC, USA
e-mail: CChalla@childrensnational.org

S. T. Verghese (ed.), *Anesthesia STAT! Acute Pediatric Emergencies in PACU*,
https://doi.org/10.1007/978-3-031-24396-7_4

1 What Is the Differential Diagnosis for This Behavior?

First it is important to rule out that he is not in pain from the surgical incision and bladder distention and fear of waking up alone in a new place without his parents. Since he had an excellent effect from the caudal anesthesia during surgery and he had peed after the surgery, we can safely rule out the first two possibilities. Since his parents are both near him and are attempting to hold him, the third possibility is also ruled out. Lastly, consider emergence delirium or agitation as a diagnosis of exclusion [1].

The first thing to do in this scenario is to ask for an alcohol wipe and inject 1–2 mg per kilogram of propofol and explain to the parents that what you are doing is to help the patient go back to sleep. Once he is asleep lying on his side, with stable vital signs and oxygen blow-by near his face via a face mask, you can direct your attention to the distressed parents and explain the problem of emergence delirium. You explain that this is a common problem in young children and that he should be waking up much better after the effect of the propofol has worn out. It is only after administering the intravenous propofol treatment that you can explain to the parents the phenomenon of emergence delirium in children which they witnessed in their son. They might ask you if he will wake up again and exhibit the same distress as he showed on first emergence. If the heart rate is high, then additional drugs like dexmedetomidine in small doses may be titrated to prolong the sleep and allow slow wake up with parents by his bedside.

The father then asks the question as to why his son was not given this same drug at the end of the case if this phenomenon is known to occur in PACU. Your thoughtful and insightful response at this time includes that not all patients display this behavior and that you would have proactively given the drug if there was a history of emergence delirium in the past after placement of bilateral ear tubes. You also emphasize that you are very glad that he raised this question because since this was his second anesthetic and he woke up with delirium, it is important to mention this phenomenon to the future anesthesiologist. The anesthesiologist then can give these drugs prophylactically to slow his wake up in PACU and avoid emergence delirium after the surgical procedure. It is also important to mention that additional drugs can indeed delay emergence and discharge, and that is why it is not given to all children at a certain age to treat anticipated delirium. In about 35 min, the patient wakes up and looks happy to see his parents and begins to play with his toy. He is smiling and drinking apple juice when you see him again, and the parents are very grateful for his smooth wake up a second time. You reiterate to the parents that they mention this incident to the next anesthesiologist and request the need for premedication if he is anxious before surgery again and the need for additional dose of propofol or dexmedetomidine prior to emergence. You can give them a piece of paper to describe his emergence delirium incident after circumcision and recommend that he may benefit from premedication as well as preventive measures against delirium prior to emergence.

2 What Is Emergence Delirium and What Are Its Risk Factors?

Emergence delirium (ED) is a state of restlessness, agitation, hyperactivity, and confusion in patients after an anesthetic procedure [1]. It was first described in the 1960s when Dr. Eckenhoff's team at the University of Pennsylvania reviewed the records of 14,436 patients over 4 years [2]. They noted, at that time, that a higher risk of emergence delirium exists with younger children, with the specific type of procedure and the temperament of the patient playing a contributing role. The patient may be combative, pulling out intravenous lines and patient monitor accessories, removing dressings, and attempting to cause harm to themselves or their caretakers with sudden movements using their torso, head, and limbs.

3 Are There Specific Factors That Can Predict ED in Children?

3.1 Risk Factors for Emergence Delirium

The earliest reports of emergence delirium indicate a relation to head and neck surgeries, as patient's wake up with a feeling of strangulation.

The primary risk factors include: [3]

- Patient age between 2 and 6 years
- Head, neck, and throat surgery
- Inhalational anesthesia
- Male gender
- Preoperative anxiety
- Parental anxiety
- Child's temperament (nervous, anxious)
- Rapid awakening from anesthesia [3]

Emergence delirium usually starts about 5–10 min after emergence and can last up to 45 min. It is important to remember that usually emergence delirium does not recur once it has resolved [4].

4 What Clinical Measurement Tools Are Used to Assess Emergence Delirium?

The *Pediatric Anesthesia Emergence Delirium (PAED) scale* is the most commonly used diagnostic tool in children between the ages of 18 months and 6 years of age. [5]

The child is evaluated against the five questions in Table 1 and the point values associated with each answer are aggregated. The higher the score, the more likely

Table 1 The pediatric anesthesia emergence delirium scale

Point	Description	Not at all	Just a little	Quite a bit	Very much	Extremely
1	The child makes eye contact with the caregiver	4	3	2	1	0
2	The child's actions are purposeful	4	3	2	1	0
3	The child is aware of his/her surroundings	4	3	2	1	0
4	The child is restless	0	1	2	3	4
5	The child is inconsolable	0	1	2	3	4

the child has emergence delirium [4]. The scale has a maximum score of 20 and a score greater than 12 is indicative of emergence delirium. Postoperatively, the FLACC scale (Face, Leg, Activity, Cry, Consolability scale) and the PAED scale can be used to help differentiate pain from emergence delirium [5].

5 Which Types of Anesthesia Increase the Risk of Emergence Delirium?

Inhalational anesthesia, specifically sevoflurane, has been known to have the highest incidence of emergence delirium.

5.1 Volatile Anesthetics

Inhalational anesthetics have been used for more than 150 years in pediatrics. Sevoflurane, one of the most popular inhalation anesthetics used today, was developed in Japan in 1992 and became available worldwide in 1995. Several studies have demonstrated that the rapid wake up with the use of sevoflurane in the pediatric population has increased the incidence of emergence delirium. [6] In a study comparing sevoflurane with halothane published by T. Foesel, it was evident that sevoflurane had significantly more post behavioral changes despite the type of induction, pain therapy, or surgery [7]. Although all inhalational agents can cause emergence delirium, sevoflurane has the highest propensity. Interestingly, Driscoll et al. compared children undergoing ENT procedures using desflurane and sevoflurane and did not see a significant difference in the rate of ED. [8] Cohen et al. reported that children undergoing general anesthesia with desflurane exhibited shorter recovery time but had similar emergence delirium as the patients with sevoflurane [9].

5.2 General Anesthesia Vs. Total Intravenous Anesthesia (TIVA)

In a study comparing the use of sevoflurane and TIVA on dental patients between the ages of 3 and 7 years, Kocaturk and Keles found that there was a lower incidence of emergence delirium in the TIVA group as well as higher patient and parent satisfaction [10].

Chandler et al. studied the rate of emergence delirium in 112 children undergoing strabismus surgery with inhalational versus intravenous anesthesia and noted a reduction in emergence delirium in the TIVA group (propofol and remifentanil) compared to sevoflurane, as well as a reduction in pain score. [11]

6 What Treatments and Preventative Measures Are Available for Emergence Delirium?

Emergence delirium will typically self-resolve; however there are pharmacological and non-pharmacological techniques that can be utilized for treatment and prevention.

At low doses, propofol has been demonstrated to reduce the risk of emergence delirium [12]. The drug has several mechanisms of action, including binding to GABA(A) receptors, thereby inhibiting the release of acetylcholine, causing sedative effects [13]. Its fast onset of action and short half-life make it very appealing to use in the pediatric ambulatory setting. Clearance for propofol is mostly through the liver, but due to the extreme speed of metabolism, there is evidence to suggest that it is also metabolized outside of the hepatic system. In addition to reducing the risk of emergence delirium, several studies have reported that propofol at low doses (such as 1 mg/kg at the conclusion of the case) can also cut down the rate of postoperative nausea and vomiting (PONV) without increasing PACU recovery time [14].

Dexmedetomidine has been used as an agent to help aid in reducing the rates of emergence delirium under general anesthesia with sevoflurane. Dexmedetomidine is a selective adrenoceptor alpha 2 agonist that is used for its anxiolytic, sedative, and analgesic properties [15]. It works by binding to alpha 2 receptors in the locus coeruleus of the pons causing sedation and in the dorsal horns of the spinal cord to improve analgesia [16]. Side effects of dexmedetomidine include bradycardia and hypotension. Mengzhu Shi et al. conducted a double-blind study comparing children undergoing tonsillectomy with or without the use of dexmedetomidine (0.5 mcg/kg) after induction. Significant reduction in emergence delirium was noted in the group receiving dexmedetomidine; however a longer time to extubation and discharge from PACU was observed [17].

Dexmedetomidine can be used as a premedication and for reducing emergence delirium. Yao et al. studied the effects of intranasal dexmedetomidine vs. oral midazolam, noting a decrease in emergence delirium, improvement in patient satisfaction, and reduction in PONV in the group with dexmedetomidine [18].

Tan et al. conducted a meta-analysis which demonstrated that sevoflurane in combination with dexmedetomidine, ketamine, fentanyl, propofol, sufentanil, remifentanil, and clonidine were synergistic in reducing the incidence of emergence delirium for pediatric ophthalmic surgery. Dexmedetomidine was proven to be superior to all others in reducing the risk of emergence delirium with the least side effects [19]. In a study by Song et al., it was shown that dexmedetomidine reduced emergence delirium without increasing the oculo-cardiac reflex although the mechanism is still unclear. The additional benefit noted in this meta-analysis result was that dexmedetomidine infusion could reduce the risk of post-op nausea and vomiting and opioid consumption [20].

6.1 Fentanyl/Ketamine and Regional Anesthesia

Emergence delirium can occur despite pain after inhalational and intravenous anesthesia. A risk factor for emergence delirium can be postoperative pain control, but the use of fentanyl, opioids, or regional anesthesia techniques can be used to reduce the risk of agitation after anesthesia.

Kim et al. performed a meta-analysis on the effects of fentanyl on emergence delirium which demonstrated that it could reduce the risk of agitation if given 10–20 min before the conclusion of anesthesia. If given at the end of the case, it can increase PACU recovery time, respiratory depression, and postoperative nausea and vomiting [21]. Intravenous and intranasal (IN) fentanyl have been proven to reduce the rate of emergence delirium in ophthalmologic and ENT procedures, but it has been associated with respiratory depression.

Children receiving a caudal block after anesthesia had reduced rates of emergence delirium and pain in the PACU. [22] Aouad, in his double-blind prospective study on children undergoing inguinal hernia with caudal anesthesia vs. IV fentanyl, noted a significant reduction in agitation in the group receiving caudal anesthesia only. Similarly, peripheral nerve blocks can be helpful to reduce pain as well as emergence delirium. Kim et al. studied the effects of fascia iliaca nerve blocks on emergence agitation in children undergoing orthopedic surgery. Agitation scores using the PAED scale were far higher in the group that did not receive the fascia iliaca nerve block [23].

7 What Are Some of the Non-pharmacological Techniques to Reduce ED?

7.1 Non-pharmacological Techniques

Anxiety has a strong correlation to postoperative complications such as emergence delirium and negative behavior up to 1 week after surgery. Kim et al. demonstrated in a study of 100 preschoolers ages 2–7 years undergoing elective surgery that those who were diagnosed with emergence delirium had higher incidences of preoperative anxiety and postoperative behavioral changes up to 1 week after surgery [24]. Behavioral changes can include sleep disturbances, enuresis, poor appetite, and tantrums. As they did not complete a long-term follow-up, it is unclear how long these behavioral changes can persist after surgery. It is important for healthcare providers to inform families of the risk associated with negative behavior after anesthesia.

Involving child life specialists to engage children in lessening their anxiety may help them to participate in the induction of anesthesia if parents are not able to accompany them. Virtual reality (VR) provides a unique opportunity to gradually expose children to all aspects of the operating theater. Virtual reality exposure (VRE) is available now and may become a remarkable tool to help relax anxious children who are uncomfortable with new surroundings by preparing them psychologically for surgery. Ryu et al. studied whether virtual reality tours in children would reduce anxiety and/or post-op behavioral changes. In the final analysis, it was clearly illustrated that preoperative VR tours were helpful to alleviate preoperative anxiety for patients undergoing surgery; however they did not result in a reduction in emergence delirium [25].

Monochromatic blue light (MBL) is yet another non-pharmacologic method that was found to reduce the incidence of emergence delirium and PAED scores in children [26]. Monochromatic light is associated with wakefulness and alertness, reduced reaction times, and enhanced cognition. In Adler's study it was evident that patients waking up after adenotonsillectomy with monochromatic light had reduced emergence delirium post-sevoflurane general anesthesia [26].

Martin et al. studied EEG patterns in children undergoing surgery and compared it to those with emergence delirium. Results demonstrated an increase in frontal lobe network connectivity preceding emergence delirium after sevoflurane use [27]. This correlates with an hyperexcitable cortical activity to internal and external stimuli.

7.2 Hypoactive Delirium

Children can present with hyperactive, hypoactive, or mixed delirium. Patients with hypoactive delirium appear similarly to hyperactive patients in having confusion and disorientation and not making eye contact. However, they make minimal movements and do not respond to any social interactions [28]. Similar to how the PAED scale is used to assess hyperactive delirium after anesthesia, the Cornell Assessment of Pediatric Delirium, shown in Table 2, can be helpful to assess hypoactive delirium [20, 29]. Hypoactive delirium is exceedingly rare after anesthesia; however it's important to evaluate if this phenomenon is present after a postoperative encounter in a child who seems unable to respond to social interactions.

Table 2 Cornell assessment of pediatric delirium revised

	Never 4	Rarely 3	Sometimes 2	Often 1	Always 0	Score
1. Does the child make eye contact with the caregiver?						
2. Are the child's actions purposeful?						
3. Is the child aware of his/her surroundings?						
4. Does the child communicate needs and wants?						
	Never 0	Rarely 1	Sometimes 2	Often 3	Always 4	Score
5. Is the child restless?						
6. Is the child inconsolable?						
7. Is the child underactive—very little movement while awake?						
8. Does it take the child a long time to respond to interactions?						
Total						

RASS Richmond Agitation and Sedation Scale

8 Summary

Clinical signs of emergence delirium include disorientation sometimes accompanied by aggressive behavior, usually occurring within 5–15 min after anesthesia has ended. Emergence delirium (ED) is a diagnosis of exclusion, and it's important to first rule out bladder distension, gastric distension due to air trapping (occurring during mask anesthesia), and incisional pain. ED is now more common with the increased use of inhalational agents with low blood-gas solubility coefficient such as sevoflurane and desflurane, which lead to a rapid emergence in children. Some key risk factors associated with emergence delirium are preschool age, head and neck surgeries, and history of anxiety. Treatment of ED typically consists of opioids, propofol, midazolam, and dexmedetomidine. Actions that can be taken to reduce the likelihood of ED can include use of child life specialists, premedication, and preoperative preparation such as virtual reality tours.

References

1. Mason L. Pitfalls of pediatric anesthesia. 2004. https://www2.pedsanesthesia.org/meetings/2004winter/pdfs/mason_Pitfalls.pdf. Accessed December 2021.
2. Eckenhoff JE, Kneale DH, Dripps RD. The incidence and etiology of postanesthetic excitement. A clinical survey. Anesthesiology. 1961;22:667–73. https://doi.org/10.1097/00000542-196109000-00002. PMID: 13889092.
3. Lee SJ, Sung TY. Emergence agitation: current knowledge and unresolved questions. Korean J Anesthesiol. 2020;73(6):471–85. https://doi.org/10.4097/kja.20097. Epub 2020 Mar 25. PMID: 32209961; PMCID: PMC7714637.

4. Jooma Z, et al. Emergence delirium in children undergoing dental surgery under general anesthesia. Pediatr Anesthesia. 2020;30(9):1020–6.
5. Sikich N, Lerman J. Development and psychometric evaluation of the pediatric anesthesia emergence delirium scale. Anesthesiology. 2004;100:1138–45. https://doi.org/10.1097/00000542-200405000-00015.
6. Voepel-Lewis T, Malviya S, Tait AR. A prospective cohort study of emergence agitation in the pediatric postanesthesia care unit. Anesth Analg. 2003;96(6):1625–30. https://doi.org/10.1213/01.ANE.0000062522.21048.61.
7. Foesel T, Reisch HJ. Postoperative behavioural changes in children: comparison between halothane and sevoflurane. Paediatr Anaesth. 2001;11(6):719–23. https://doi.org/10.1046/j.1460-9592.2001.00720.x. PMID: 11696150.
8. Driscoll JN, Bender BM, Archilla CA, Klim CM, Hossain MJ, Nd GM, Wei JL. Comparing incidence of emergence delirium between sevoflurane and desflurane in children following routine otolaryngology procedures. Minerva Anestesiol. 2017;83(4):383–91. https://doi.org/10.23736/S0375-9393.16.11362-8. Epub 2016 Nov 30. PMID: 27901329; PMCID: PMC5685164.
9. Cohen IT, Finkel JC, Hannallah RS, Hummer KA, Patel KM. Rapid emergence does not explain agitation following sevoflurane anaesthesia in infants and children: a comparison with propofol. Paediatr Anaesth. 2003;13(1):63–7. https://doi.org/10.1046/j.1460-9592.2003.00948.x. PMID: 12535042.
10. Kocaturk O, Keles S. Recovery characteristics of total intravenous anesthesia with propofol versus sevoflurane anesthesia: a prospective randomized clinical trial. J Pain Res. 2018;11:1289–95. https://doi.org/10.2147/JPR.S164106. PMID: 30013385; PMCID: PMC6038881.
11. Chandler JR, Myers D, Mehta D, Whyte E, Groberman MK, Montgomery CJ, Ansermino JM. Emergence delirium in children: a randomized trial to compare total intravenous anesthesia with propofol and remifentanil to inhalational sevoflurane anesthesia. Paediatr Anaesth. 2013;23(4):309–15. https://doi.org/10.1111/pan.12090. PMID: 23464658.
12. Dahmani S, Stany I, Brasher C, et al. Pharmacological prevention of sevoflurane- and desflurane-related emergence agitation in children: a meta-analysis of published studies. Br J Anaesth. 2010;104(2):216–23.
13. Khan KS, Hayes I, Buggy DJ. Pharmacology of anaesthetic agents I: intravenous anaesthetic agents. Contin Educ Anaesthesia Crit Care Pain. 2014;14(3):100–5. https://doi.org/10.1093/bjaceaccp/mkt039.
14. Abu-Shahwan I. Effect of propofol on emergence behavior in children after sevoflurane general anesthesia. Paediatr Anaesth. 2008;18:55–9.
15. Weerink MAS, Struys MMRF, Hannivoort LN, et al. Clinical pharmacokinetics and pharmacodynamics of dexmedetomidine. Clin Pharmacokinet. 2017;56:893–913. https://doi.org/10.1007/s40262-017-0507-7.
16. Coursin DB, Coursin DB, Maccioli GA. Dexmedetomidine. Curr Opin Crit Care. 2001;7(4):221–6.
17. Shi M, Miao S, Gu T, Wang D, Zhang H, Liu J. Dexmedetomidine for the prevention of emergence delirium and postoperative behavioral changes in pediatric patients with sevoflurane anesthesia: a double-blind, randomized trial. Drug Des Devel Ther. 2019;13:897–905. Published 2019 Mar 15. https://doi.org/10.2147/DDDT.S196075.
18. Yao Y, Sun Y, Lin J, Chen W, Lin Y, Zheng X. Intranasal dexmedetomidine versus oral midazolam premedication to prevent emergence delirium in children undergoing strabismus surgery: a randomised controlled trial. Eur J Anaesthesiol. 2020;37(12):1143–9. https://doi.org/10.1097/EJA.0000000000001270. PMID: 32976205.
19. Tan D, Xia H, Sun S, Wang F. Effect of ancillary drugs on sevoflurane related emergence agitation in children undergoing ophthalmic surgery: a Bayesian network meta-analysis. BMC Anesthesiol. 2019;19(1):138. https://doi.org/10.1186/s12871-019-0810-y. PMID: 31370793; PMCID: PMC6670177.

20. Song J, Liu S, Fan B, Li G, Sun Q. Perioperative dexmedetomidine reduces emergence agitation without increasing the oculocardiac reflex in children: a systematic review and meta-analysis. Medicine (Baltimore). 2021;100(18):e25717. https://doi.org/10.1097/MD.0000000000025717. PMID: 33950954; PMCID: PMC8104235.
21. Kim N, Park JH, Lee JS, Choi T, Kim MS. Effects of intravenous fentanyl around the end of surgery on emergence agitation in children: systematic review and meta-analysis. Paediatr Anaesth. 2017;27(9):885–92. https://doi.org/10.1111/pan.13181. Epub 2017 Jul 4. PMID: 28675609.
22. Aouad MT, Kanazi GE, Siddik-Sayyid SM, Gerges FJ, Rizk LB, Baraka AS. Preoperative caudal block prevents emergence agitation in children following sevoflurane anesthesia. Acta Anaesthesiol Scand. 2005;49(3):300–4. https://doi.org/10.1111/j.1399-6576.2005.00642.x. PMID: 15752392.
23. Kim HS, Kim CS, Kim SD, Lee JR. Fascia iliaca compartment block reduces emergence agitation by providing effective analgesic properties in children. J Clin Anesth. 2011;23(2):119–23. https://doi.org/10.1016/j.jclinane.2010.08.007. PMID: 21377075.
24. Kim J, Byun SH, Kim JW, Kim JY, Kim YJ, Choi N, Lee BS, Yu S, Kim E. Behavioral changes after hospital discharge in preschool children experiencing emergence delirium after general anesthesia: a prospective observational study. Paediatr Anaesth. 2021;31(10):1056–64. https://doi.org/10.1111/pan.14259. Epub 2021 Aug 6. PMID: 34309126.
25. Ryu JH, Oh AY, Yoo HJ, Kim JH, Park JW, Han SH. The effect of an immersive virtual reality tour of the operating theater on emergence delirium in children undergoing general anesthesia: a randomized controlled trial. Paediatr Anaesth. 2019;29(1):98–105. https://doi.org/10.1111/pan.13535. Epub 2018 Nov 25. PMID: 30365231.
26. Adler AC, Nathanson BH, Chandrakantan A. Monochromic light reduces emergence delirium in children undergoing adenotonsillectomy; a double-blind randomized observational study. BMC Anesthesiol. 2021;21(1):217. https://doi.org/10.1186/s12871-021-01435-1. PMID: 34496743; PMCID: PMC8424999.
27. Martin JC, Liley DT, Harvey AS, Kuhlmann L, Sleigh JW, Davidson AJ. Alterations in the functional connectivity of frontal lobe networks preceding emergence delirium in children. Anesthesiology. 2014;121:740–52.
28. Lee-Archer PF, von Ungern-Sternberg BS, Reade MC, Law KC, Long D. An observational study of hypoactive delirium in the post-anesthesia recovery unit of a pediatric hospital. Paediatr Anaesth. 2021;31(4):429–35. https://doi.org/10.1111/pan.14122. Epub 2021 Feb 7. PMID: 33405250.
29. Traube C, Silver G, Kearney J, et al. Cornell assessment of pediatric delirium: a valid, rapid, observational tool for screening delirium in the PICU*. Crit Care Med. 2014;42(3):656–63. https://doi.org/10.1097/CCM.0b013e3182a66b76.

Cardiac Arrest After Central Line Placement in a Child

Chinwe Unegbu

1 Case

A 5-year-old boy with Trisomy 21 (Down syndrome) arrives to the postanesthesia care unit (PACU) after placement of a Broviac central venous catheter (CVC). He was admitted to the hospital 2 days prior with several weeks of fever, lethargy, and poor po intake. His complete blood count was concerning for leukemia, and he subsequently underwent a lumbar puncture and bone marrow aspiration with confirmation of diagnosis of acute lymphoblastic leukemia (ALL). He requires central venous access for initiation of chemotherapy. He has been NPO since midnight. He has a history of snoring and has developed some sniffles with the onset of fever and lethargy and does not have an appetite.

On pre-op examination he is cooperative and able to come to the surgical procedure room for his Broviac placement without any need for premedication. He has some facial petechiae. Parents say that he has not had any epistaxis or bleeding from gums with brushing his teeth.

His weight is 18 kg.

His labs show Hb/Hct of 8.5/28 and platelets 40 K.

Past Medical History: Full term, spontaneous vaginal delivery, prenatal diagnosis of Trisomy 21.

Past Surgical History: Tonsillectomy and Adenoidectomy at age 3 for obstructive sleep apnea.

Medications: Acetaminophen and Ondansetron.

Vital Signs on Arrival to PACU: BP 80/40, HR 130, sat 89%, temp 36.3 °C.

Physical Examination: Agitated, inconsolable, and limited cardiopulmonary examination.

C. Unegbu (✉)
Division of Cardiac Anesthesiology, Children's National Hospital, Washington, DC, USA
e-mail: cunegbu@childrensnational.org

S. T. Verghese (ed.), *Anesthesia STAT! Acute Pediatric Emergencies in PACU*,
https://doi.org/10.1007/978-3-031-24396-7_5

Key Questions

- What is a Broviac CVC?
- What are the broad indications for a CVC?
- How does a Broviac catheter differ from the other types of CVCs?
- In this patient who is s/p tunneled line insertion, what is your differential diagnosis for hypoxia?
- Why is aspiration on your differential diagnosis for hypoxia in this patient?
- Why are airway obstruction and pulmonary edema on your differential diagnosis?
- Any procedure-specific concerns that may be contributing to the clinical picture?
- Why are you concerned about a congenital heart defect?

Case continued: The patient's oxygen saturations are intermittently decreasing to 70%. BP is 60/40 and HR 160 bpm. CXR is obtained and echo ordered. Attempts to place oxygen mask on the face are difficult and oxygen saturations are still in the range of 70–75%.

- If you suspected a venous air embolism, what would you do?
- How could you prevent a venous air embolism?
- How could an inadvertent arterial puncture lead to this clinical presentation?
- If an arterial puncture was suspected intraoperatively, what should have been done?
- Which CVC insertion site is more prone to hematoma formation with accidental arterial puncture? Which site is more prone to cause airway compromise?
- Any late complications that you are concerned about with accidental arterial puncture?
- Could a dysrhythmia account for this clinical picture? Any preventative steps?
- Would you order any diagnostic studies in this patient?
- What are the expected chest x-ray findings for aspiration, pulmonary edema, and pneumothorax?
- What are the expected echocardiographic findings for tamponade?

Case continued: Patient becomes unresponsive. Pulse oximeter is intermittently reading; BP by NIBP reading shows a mean of 30. HR is 170 bpm.

- What is a tension pneumothorax?
- How do you diagnose a tension pneumothorax?
- What are the chest x-ray findings of tension pneumothorax?

Case continued: No pulse is detected on palpation. Attempts at auscultation reveal no heart sounds. There is no detectable blood pressure, and the patient is minimally responsive. EKG demonstrates normal sinus rhythm with a heart rate in the 70s.

- Which PALS algorithm will you use?
- If the child is in PEA arrest, what is your next step?
- What is considered good-quality CPR?
- What are the reversible causes of PEA arrest that you consider?
- What are the interventions for these reversible causes of PEA arrest?
- If you are suspecting a tension pneumothorax, how would you perform a needle decompression?
- How does the needle decompression in a pediatric patient differ from an adult patient?
- Should the patient be intubated prior to needle decompression?

Case continued: Needle decompression is performed. BP is 80/40 and HR 100 bpm.

- Should a chest tube be inserted following needle decompression?
- Any concerns with rapid lung re-expansion?
- What are the possible procedural factors which may have contributed to the development of a pneumothorax?
- How would you differentiate a pneumothorax from a cardiac tamponade?
- Any preventative measures to reduce the likelihood of causing a pneumothorax?
- What are the pros and cons of the various CVC access sites?

2 Discussion

2.1 What Is a Broviac CVC?

A Broviac CVC is a tunneled small-bore soft silicone catheter. It has a cuff that provides anchorage into the subcutaneous tract and allows subcutaneous tissues to grow into it. The design of the Broviac catheter and Hickman catheter is similar, and both are tunneled CVCs with the major difference being inner luminal diameter. The Broviac catheter has an inner luminal diameter of 1 mm when compared to Hickman catheter's inner luminal diameter of 1.6 mm.

2.2 What Are the Broad Indications for a CVC?

A CVC may be needed to deliver multiple medications including chemotherapeutics, vesicant drugs, and antibiotics. Additional indications include administration of parenteral nutrition and need for repeated blood transfusions.

2.3 How Does a Broviac Catheter Differ from the Other Types of CVCs?

A Broviac catheter is a tunneled CVC. Tunneled catheters are preferred when intravenous access is needed for a longer duration of time. They have the benefit of having a lower infection rate when compared to non-tunneled catheters [1]. Catheters that are non-tunneled are used most frequently in emergency and acute situations primarily because of their simplicity and the ease of insertion. Non-tunneled catheters are intended for a short duration of use, so these should be removed as soon as possible in order to prevent complications like infections or thrombosis. When compared to tunneled and non-tunneled catheters, implanted ports are preferred as they have better cosmetic results and less infection risk; however, they take more time and skill to implant.

2.4 In This Patient Who Is S/P Tunneled Line Insertion, What Is Your Differential Diagnosis for Hypoxia?

Airway/respiratory
Airway obstruction
Pulmonary edema
Pneumothorax
Aspiration
Cardiac
Myocardial perforation/tamponade
Arrhythmia
Venous air embolism
Pulmonary embolism
Congenital heart defect
Others
Arterial puncture
Hemothorax

2.5 Why Is Aspiration on Your Differential Diagnosis for Hypoxia in This Patient?

Although perioperative aspiration is a rare event that occurs more commonly in children undergoing emergency surgery, it should always be a consideration in any patient presenting postoperatively with hypoxia. Aspiration events typically occur peri-induction of anesthesia, but in this case no emesis was noted intraoperatively. Patients with suspected aspiration and respiratory symptoms within 2 h of the event are more likely to develop respiratory sequelae and require further respiratory support [2]. Symptoms of aspiration include cough, wheezing, low oxygen saturation, and a chest x-ray infiltrate.

2.6 Why Are Airway Obstruction and Pulmonary Edema on Your Differential Diagnosis?

This patient has Trisomy 21, and patients with Down syndrome are prone to airway obstruction because of micrognathia, a short neck, hypotonia, and macroglossia. Patients with Down syndrome can also have small nares and a narrower trachea, and there is an increased incidence of subglottic stenosis in this population [3]. Sleep-disordered breathing, including upper airway obstruction and obstructive sleep apnea, is seen in 30–60% of children with Down syndrome. A component of this obstructive sleep apnea is adenotonsillar hypertrophy, but the patient in question is status post tonsillectomy and adenoidectomy.

Post-obstructive pulmonary edema (also known as negative pressure pulmonary edema) is a well described but infrequent complication of upper airway obstruction [4]. It often develops following extubation when subatmospheric pressure is generated in the alveolus and most often occurs in young, muscular, adult male patients who experience acute airway obstruction. It is less common in neonates and infants because their musculature is not yet fully developed and their chest wall is very compliant, thereby limiting their ability to generate extremely negative intra-alveolar pressure in the presence of airway obstruction [5]. Clinical signs of post-obstructive pulmonary edema include agitation, tachypnea, tachycardia, pink frothy pulmonary secretions, and progressive oxygen desaturation.

2.7 Any Procedure Specific Concerns That May Be Contributing to the Clinical Picture?

Pneumothorax is a potentially serious complication of central line insertion which results from inadvertent puncture of the lung apex. Central venous catheterization, specifically the internal jugular and subclavian sites, is the most common cause of iatrogenic pneumothorax [6, 7]. The incidence of central access-related pneumothorax varies not only with access site but also with the presence of underlying risk factors such as lung disease, operator experience, and the setting (elective versus emergency) [6, 7].

Pericardial tamponade is another possibility given the presenting symptoms especially with tunneled hemodialysis catheter insertion. Although a rare complication, tamponade results from atrial perforation, which can lead to severe bleeding into the pericardium. Clinical signs and symptoms associated with tamponade include tachycardia, tachypnea, respiratory distress, hypoxemia, narrow pulse pressure, hypotension, and pulsus paradoxus.

Arterial injury due to inadvertent needle puncture of the associated artery instead of the targeted vein (e.g., the femoral artery, carotid artery, or subclavian artery) is another possibility. Hematomas that may form after an inadvertent arterial puncture can compress associated structures and lead to life-threatening airway obstruction [8]. Unrecognized arterial puncture with subsequent dilation and catheter placement can lead to life-threatening bleeding into the chest, retroperitoneum, or thigh, depending on the access site. Ultrasound use reduces but does not eliminate this risk. Immediate recognition and management of arterial puncture usually prevent subsequent complications. Late recognition of arterial catheterization increases the risk of hemorrhagic or thrombotic complications, which may require surgical intervention. Accidental catheterization of the carotid or subclavian artery by a large-bore catheter (>7 Fr) can cause arterial thrombosis, hemorrhage, stroke, pseudoaneurysm, or death [9].

Periprocedural arrhythmias are also a consideration and are universally the result of guidewire or catheter placement into the right heart [10, 11]. Premature atrial and ventricular contractions as well as ventricular dysrhythmias and bundle branch block are possible complications during central venous access procedures. Their initial presentation would include abnormal rhythm on the electrocardiogram with associated hypotension. Respiratory insufficiency likely would not be the initial presentation.

Venous air embolism is a rare yet potentially lethal complication associated with central venous access. It is often poorly recognized but more common with large-lumen catheters. Venous air embolisms typically occur at the time of CVC insertion but can also occur during catheter use or at the time of catheter removal [12]. With a venous air embolism, air is entrained into the venous system when either a needle or catheter is left open to the atmosphere or by inadvertent injection of air into the vessel. Risk factors for developing a venous air embolism during catheter insertion include upright positioning, hypovolemia, and spontaneous inhalation during instrumentation. Placement of a patient in Trendelenburg position, if possible, may reduce the risk of air embolization. The effect of venous air embolization depends upon the rate and volume of air introduced into the venous circulation, but the lethal dose for humans has been theorized to be 3–5 mL/kg [13]. Affected patients can suffer both cardiovascular and pulmonary symptoms including tachyarrhythmias, chest pain, coughing, dyspnea, hypoxemia, respiratory distress, and cardiovascular collapse. This patient became progressively less stable in the recovery room, and the CVC had not been utilized prior to the decompensation making inadvertent air entrainment into the venous circulation unlikely.

Lastly, recurrent laryngeal nerve injuries can occur with CVC insertion and have had an incidence of 1.6%. It is due to accidental trauma or perineural hematoma formation [14]. This would result in hoarseness and possibly some respiratory distress, but it would not account for the hemodynamic perturbations seen in this patient.

2.8 Why Are You Concerned About a Congenital Heart Defect?

Congenital heart defects occur in approximately 40–50% of children with Trisomy 21. Atrioventricular septal defects (AVSD) have a particular association with this population and children with Down syndrome account for 70% of AVSD cases. Pulmonary vascular disease may also occur in children with trisomy 21 due to an unrepaired cardiac lesion such as an AVSD. Pulmonary vascular disease can lead to reversal of a left to right shunting through an AVSD resulting in cyanosis. Pulmonary vascular disease may also occur in the absence of cardiac lesions because of chronic hypoxemia and hypoventilation due to muscle hypotonia and obstructive sleep apnea and is associated with a high perioperative mortality. It should be a consideration in any child with Trisomy 21.

2.9 If You Suspected a Venous Air Embolism, What Would You Do?

The suspicion for venous air embolism is very low since the patient decompensated post-procedure and the CVC was not being used in the PACU. However, if a venous air embolism was suspected, positioning the patient in left lateral decubitus with Trendelenburg would in theory help trap the air in the right ventricular apex. Supportive measures such as administration of 100% inspired oxygen concentration could help increase the speed of air resorption. Fluid resuscitation and administration of adrenergic agonists can also aid in hemodynamic support and air resorption [15].

2.10 How Could You Prevent a Venous Air Embolism?

Venous air embolism can occur at any time such as during CVC insertion or while the catheter is in place and during catheter removal [16, 17]. During catheter insertion, Trendelenburg positioning, Valsalva maneuver, prompt needle/catheter occlusion, and tight intravenous connections can help to avoid this complication [18]. CVC removal should be performed during exhalation when intrathoracic pressure is greater than atmospheric pressure. Firm pressure should be applied for at least 1 min following removal.

2.11 How Could an Inadvertent Arterial Puncture Lead to This Clinical Presentation?

Serious blood loss associated with CVC placement is uncommon; however, hematomas can develop after inadvertent arterial puncture which can compress associated structures. In the case of inadvertent carotid puncture, this can obstruct the airway and be life-threatening [19]. Unrecognized arterial puncture with subsequent dilation of the arteriotomy and catheter placement, particularly of large-bore catheters (i.e., greater than 7 Fr), can lead to life-threatening bleeding into the chest, retroperitoneum, or thigh, depending on the access site.

2.12 If an Arterial Puncture Was Suspected Intraoperatively, What Should Have Been Done?

Once an arterial stick is suspected, the needle should be immediately withdrawn and direct, but nonocclusive, pressure applied to the site continuously for 15 min to prevent hematoma formation. Bleeding usually resolves within 10–15 min with direct compression, which is more easily performed at the femoral and jugular sites as compared with the subclavian site. Because tunneled hemodialysis and pheresis catheters can be quite large (often greater than 12 Fr), inadvertent arterial placement of either of these catheters mandates emergency consultation with a vascular surgeon. Removal of these catheters should not be attempted without surgical oversight since removal of such large-bore devices risks serious hemorrhage and almost always requires vascular repair [9, 20].

2.13 Which CVC Insertion Site Is More Prone to Hematoma Formation with Accidental Arterial Puncture? Which Site Is More Prone to Cause Airway Compromise?

Mechanical complications are more common after attempted insertion of a CVC into the subclavian vein compared with the other sites. The subclavian site is least amenable to direct compression and therefore more prone to hematoma formation.

The carotid artery is near critical airway structures and more prone to cause airway compromise when inadvertently punctured such as during attempted internal or external jugular venous cannulation. The rate of mechanical complications is significantly decreased with the use of dynamic ultrasound-guided venous access [21].

2.14 Any Late Complications That You Are Concerned About with Accidental Arterial Puncture?

Late recognition of arterial catheterization increases the risk of hemorrhagic or thrombotic complications, and in this patient with ALL, preoperative attention to platelet count and coagulation profile would be indicated. Inadvertent catheterization of the carotid or subclavian artery with a large-bore catheter (>7 Fr) can cause arterial thrombosis, hemorrhage, stroke, pseudoaneurysm, or death.

2.15 Could a Dysrhythmia Account for This Clinical Picture? Any Preventative Steps?

Non-tunneled CVCs positioned deep into the right atrium are more likely to cause dysrhythmias. Catheter movement of up to 3 cm is common with patient movement and this repositioning may cause delayed symptoms. During insertion, direct visualization of the wire/catheter under fluoroscopy and limiting the depth of guidewire insertion help avoid this complication.

2.16 Would You Order Any Diagnostic Studies in This Patient?

A chest radiograph and echocardiogram were ordered given the patients clinical decompensation. One could also consider ordering an ultrasound of the chest.

2.17 What Are the Expected Chest X-ray Findings for Aspiration, Pulmonary Edema, and Pneumothorax?

The radiographic findings of aspiration depend on the positioning of the patient at the time of the event. The right lower lung lobe is the most common site of an infiltrate due to the larger caliber and more vertical orientation of the right mainstem bronchus; however, patients lying in the left lateral decubitus position during an aspiration event are more likely to have left-sided infiltrates. Other suggestive chest x-ray findings for aspiration pneumonia include lobar pneumonia, areas of opacity, and/or unilateral consolidation. With pulmonary edema, a chest x-ray often demonstrates increased fluid within the alveolar walls as well as increased vascular filling, Kerley B lines, and peribronchial cuffing. In a patient with a suspected pneumothorax, the chest x-ray will demonstrate ipsilateral lung collapse and possible mediastinum shift away from pneumothorax.

2.18 What Are the Expected Echocardiographic Findings for Tamponade?

The echocardiographic findings of tamponade include presence of a pericardial effusion, diastolic right ventricular collapse (high specificity), systolic right atrial collapse (earliest sign), a plethoric inferior vena cava with minimal respiratory variation (high sensitivity), and exaggerated respiratory cycle changes in mitral and tricuspid valve inflow velocities as a surrogate for pulsus paradoxus [22, 23].

2.19 What Is a Tension Pneumothorax?

A pneumothorax is lung collapse that is secondary to air accumulation between the parietal and visceral pleura of the lung. A tension pneumothorax is a more severe condition whereby the pleural space is under pressure leading to displacement of mediastinal structures which compromises cardiopulmonary function. In a tension pneumothorax, air enters into the pleural space but cannot fully exit (similar to a one-way valve mechanism) [24].

2.20 How Would You Diagnose a Tension Pneumothorax?

Clinical signs of a tension pneumothorax include absence of unilateral breath sounds, asymmetric lung expansion, hypoxia, respiratory failure, and evidence of hemodynamic compromise including hypotension, tachycardia, and/or cardiac arrest [24]. Chest x-ray, chest CT, or ultrasonography can be used, but if clinically unstable and the clinical suspicion is high, then intervention should not be withheld to await imaging [25].

2.21 What Are the Chest X-ray Findings of a Tension Pneumothorax?

Chest X-ray findings include ipsilateral lung collapse, mediastinum shift away from pneumothorax, subcutaneous emphysema, tracheal deviation to the contralateral side of the pneumothorax, and flattening of hemidiaphragm on the ipsilateral side.

2.22 Which PALS Algorithm Will You Use?

The patient meets criteria for a pulseless electrical activity (PEA) arrest. Pulseless electrical activity (PEA) is a life-threatening and unshockable rhythm. PEA may include any pulseless EKG waveform except ventricular fibrillation, ventricular tachycardia, or asystole.

2.23 If the Child Is in PEA Arrest, What Is Your Next Step?

You should begin CPR immediately. Push hard and fast at 100–120 beats per minute. Ventilate with a bag-mask and attach to supplemental oxygen (assuming that there is no significant cardiac disease that would preclude use of 100% oxygen). Two-person CPR for a child without a definitive airway should begin at a ratio of 15 compressions to 2 breaths. Attach a monitor/defibrillator as soon as possible and check for a shockable rhythm. If no shockable rhythm is detected (asystole/PEA), give epinephrine 0.01 mg/kg every 3–5 min. Continue CPR and treat the reversible causes. If a shockable rhythm is detected, defibrillate with a shock of 2 J/kg and resume CPR immediately after the shock. Continue CPR and check for a shockable rhythm every 2 min. Increase the joules to 4 J/kg, increasing with every shock up to 10 J/kg or to an adult dose. Consider an advanced airway and place the patient on a capnography monitor. Amiodarone IV/IO 5 mg/kg and bolus of lidocaine 1 mg/kg can be given for ventricular fibrillation or pulseless ventricular tachycardia. Consider and treat the reversible causes.

2.24 What Is Considered Good Quality CPR?

Good-quality CPR includes rotating compressors every 2 min, maintaining a compression-ventilation ratio of 15:2 without an advanced airway, or performing continuous chest compressions and ventilating at 8–10 breaths per minute with an advanced airway in place. In addition, when performing chest compressions, push at least 1/2 of the anterior-posterior diameter of the chest wall and allow for complete recoil of the chest.

2.25 What Are the Reversible Causes You Consider with PEA Arrest?

Reversible causes for PEA arrest include acidosis (hydrogen ion), hypoxia, hypovolemia, hypothermia, hypo-/hyperkalemia, hypoglycemia, toxins, cardiac tamponade, tension pneumothorax, coronary thrombosis, and pulmonary thrombosis.

2.26 What Are the Interventions for These Reversible Causes of PEA Arrest?

Hs	Etiology	Treatment
	Hydrogen ion (acidosis)	• Provide adequate ventilation • Administer sodium bicarbonate
	Hypovolemia	• Intravenous fluid administration
	Hypoxia	• Ensure airway patency • Ensure adequate ventilation • Administer supplemental oxygen
	Hypoglycemia	• Administer dextrose
	Hyperkalemia	• Glucose/insulin • Bicarbonate • Intravenous calcium • Beta-agonist
	Hypokalemia	• Potassium replacement
	Hypothermia	• External rewarming • Warm intravenous fluids • Antibiotic administration • Humidified oxygen administration
Ts	Coronary thrombosis	• Acute coronary syndrome algorithm • Oxygen • Aspirin • Nitroglycerin • Thrombolytics
	Pulmonary thrombosis	• Thrombolytics
	Cardiac tamponade	• Pericardiocentesis
	Tension pneumothorax	• Needle decompression
	Trauma	• IV fluids • Transfusion • Surgery
	Toxicosis	• Reversal of toxin (if possible)

2.27 If You Are Suspecting a Tension Pneumothorax, How Would You Perform a Needle Decompression?

Needle decompression is an important and life-saving maneuver in the management of a tension pneumothorax. Needle decompression involves placing an angiocatheter into the second intercostal space midclavicular line, along the anterior chest wall and just above the third rib. This results in re-expansion of the collapsed lung.

2.28 How Does the Needle Decompression in a Pediatric Patient Differ from an Adult Patient?

In adults and children older than 15 years of age, the fifth intercostal space, anterior axillary line can be used. However, the second intercostal space, midclavicular line remains an option.

2.29 Should the Patient Be Intubated Prior to Needle Decompression?

Endotracheal intubation, if performed prior to needle decompression, can lead to the rapid accumulation of intrathoracic air, thereby converting a simple pneumothorax to tension physiology. As a result, prior to needle decompression, positive pressure ventilation should be avoided as it will contribute to increasing the size of the pneumothorax. However, administration of 100% supplemental oxygen is advisable as this will help reduce the size of the pneumothorax by decreasing the alveolar partial pressure of nitrogen [24, 26].

2.30 Should a Chest Tube Be Inserted Following Needle Decompression?

Needle decompression is the first step and must be followed by the placement of a chest tube to allow for the evacuation of the presumed ongoing air leak. Chest x-ray is done to assess for resolution of the pneumothorax.

2.31 Any Concerns with Rapid Lung Re-expansion?

Rapid lung re-expansion increases the risk of pulmonary edema.

2.32 What Are the Possible Procedural Factors Which May Have Contributed to the Development of a Pneumothorax?

Multiple attempts for supradiaphragmatic lines are associated with an increased rate of complications such as the development of pneumothoraces. The rate of complications is significantly decreased with the use of ultrasound-guided venous access. Dynamic ultrasound-guided puncture of the vein with imaging of the wire in the vein prior to dilation and catheter placement along with fluoroscopic guidance of the wires and catheter have been shown to increase technical success and reduce mechanical complication rates [21].

2.33 How Would You Differentiate Pneumothorax from Cardiac Tamponade?

It can be difficult to differentiate pneumothorax from cardiac tamponade since the clinical findings can be similar. Cardiac tamponade is a rare complication of central line insertion. The classic triad of low systemic blood pressure, jugular venous distension, and muffled/distant heart sounds, which is also known as Beck's triad, may be seen in some children with tamponade. Additional clinical findings of cardiac tamponade include tachycardia, tachypnea, respiratory distress, tachypnea, and hypoxemia. A narrow pulse pressure and pulsus paradoxus can also be seen. Chest x-ray may demonstrate an enlarged cardiac silhouette, and the EKG may show low voltage complexes, electrical alternans, and sinus tachycardia. Echocardiography is the primary diagnostic tool and may demonstrate cardiac chamber collapse and increased atrioventricular valve inflow respiratory variation. The definitive treatment for cardiac tamponade is pericardiocentesis with possible pericardial drain placement [27].

2.34 Any Preventative Measures to Reduce the Likelihood of Causing a Pneumothorax?

Limiting the number of attempts can reduce the likelihood of causing a pneumothorax since line-associated mechanical complications increase with the number of attempts. In a prospective cohort study, the incidence of mechanical complications was sixfold higher when there were more than three insertion attempts, compared with successful insertion on the first attempt [28]. As a result, it is reasonable for an operator to seek assistance if a CVC cannot be successfully inserted after three attempts.

In addition, real-time ultrasound guidance is superior to blind, landmark-guided techniques particularly for CVC insertion into the internal jugular vein. Confirming CVC positioning with a chest radiograph x-ray is also advisable. Failure to confirm the position can be problematic since clinician judgment does not consistently predict catheter malposition or other mechanical complications [29].

2.35 What Are the Pros and Cons of the Various CVC Access Sites?

Pros		Cons
Internal jugular vein	Minimal risk of pneumothorax (Especially with US guidance) Head-of-table access Procedure-related bleeding amenable to direct pressure Lower failure rate with novice operator Excellent target using US guidance	Risk of carotid artery puncture Uncomfortable Thoracic duct injury possible on left Poor landmarks in obese/edematous patients Potential access and maintenance issues with concomitant tracheostomy (non-tunneled) Vein prone to collapse with hypovolemia Difficult access during emergencies when airway control being established
External jugular vein	Superficial vessel that is often visible Coagulopathy not prohibitive Minimal risk of pneumothorax (especially with US guidance) Head-of-table access Rapid venous access	Not ideal for prolonged venous access Poor landmarks in obese patients High rate of malposition Catheter may be difficult to thread
Subclavian vein	Easier to maintain dressings More comfortable for patient (non-tunneled) Better landmarks in obese patients Accessible when airway control is being established Associated with lower incidence of catheter-related infection	Increased risk of pneumothorax Procedure-related bleeding less amenable to direct pressure Decreased success rate with inexperience Longer path from skin to vessel Catheter malposition more common (especially right SCV) Interference with chest compressions Risk for stenosis/occlusion, which impacts future hemodialysis arteriovenous access
Femoral vein	Rapid access with high success rate Does not interfere with CPR Does not interfere with intubation No risk of pneumothorax Trendelenburg position not necessary during insertion	Delayed circulation of drugs during CPR Prevents patient mobilization Difficult to keep site sterile with increased risk of infection Difficult for PA catheter insertion

Case continues:

Our patient had a pneumothorax which was suspected by clinical signs in PACU and confirmed by chest x-ray. Since this was diagnosed rapidly and the air was removed by percutaneous needle decompression followed by chest tube insertion, the patient was resuscitated successfully. He was intubated after the evacuation of pneumothorax and was sent to PICU for ventilation and continuous assessment of hemodynamic status. There was a small amount of blood draining out when the pneumothorax was first evacuated however, this resolved after he was treated with 4 units of platelets. He was extubated a few days after the event and transferred to the oncology floor for chemotherapy. He had a reassuring neurological evaluation before discharge and was advised to return as an outpatient for further therapy of his ALL.

3 Summary

Acute pneumothorax is a life-threatening emergency which needs prompt diagnosis and treatment to avoid further hemodynamic deterioration and death. This young boy with a diagnosis of ALL with low hematocrit and platelet count should not undergo needle entry into any major vessels, solely guided by anatomic landmarks. The ideal method is to select a superficial vessel like internal jugular vein, to enter it by a small surgical cut down or with a small needle inserted under ultrasound guidance or fluoroscopy. After successful atraumatic entry into the vessel, a guidewire can be inserted to help navigate the large-bore double lumen central line into the ideal central location.

In conclusion, this case scenario of postoperative complication of pneumothorax could have been avoided if the central venous entry was guided by real-time ultrasonography or fluoroscopic guidance. In addition, a confirmatory chest x-ray should always be obtained postoperatively before the patient is awakened and transferred to PACU. In the practice of medicine, this following dictum is well known: "Prevention of a complication is better than diagnosing it and treating it immediately." Therefore, the perioperative team members should focus on providing the safest and best care to these fragile patients by entering the vein on the first attempt by *seeing* the vessel with ultrasound or fluoroscopic guidance and thus avoiding inadvertent entry into adjacent structures.

References

1. Bannon MP, Heller SF, Rivera M. Anatomic considerations for central venous cannulation. Risk Manag Healthc Policy. 2011;4:27–39. https://doi.org/10.2147/RMHP.S10383.
2. Warner MA, Warner ME, Warner DO, et al. Perioperative pulmonary aspiration in infants and children. Anesthesiology. 1999;90:66.
3. Kubacki T, Haché M. Down syndrome. In: Houck PJ, Haché M, Sun LS, editors. Handbook of pediatric anesthesia. New York: McGraw Hill; 2015.
4. Oswalt CE, Gates GA, Holmstrom MG. Pulmonary edema as a complication of acute airway obstruction. JAMA. 1977;238:1833–5.
5. Lang SA, Duncan PG, Shephard DA, Ha HC. Pulmonary oedema associated with airway obstruction. Can J Anaesth. 1990;37:210–8.

6. Celik B, Sahin E, Nadir A, Kaptanoglu M. Iatrogenic pneumothorax: etiology, incidence and risk factors. Thorac Cardiovasc Surg. 2009;57:286.
7. Larsson AS, Jørgensen IM. [Acupuncture-induced bilateral pneumothorax in a 16-year-old boy]. Ugeskr Laeger. 2018;180.
8. Nicholson T, Ettles D, Robinson G. Managing inadvertent arterial catheterization during central venous access procedures. Cardiovasc Intervent Radiol. 2004;27:21.
9. Guilbert MC, Elkouri S, Bracco D, et al. Arterial trauma during central venous catheter insertion: case series, review and proposed algorithm. J Vasc Surg. 2008;48:918.
10. Boyd R, Saxe A, Phillips E. Effect of patient position upon success in placing central venous catheters. Am J Surg. 1996;172:380.
11. Tripathi M, Dubey PK, Ambesh SP. Direction of the J-tip of the guidewire, in Seldinger technique, is a significant factor in misplacement of subclavian vein catheter: a randomized, controlled study. Anesth Analg. 2005;100:21.
12. Toung TJ, Rossberg MI, Hutchins GM. Volume of air in a lethal venous air embolism. Anesthesiology. 2001;94:360.
13. Brull SJ, Prielipp RC. Vascular air embolism: a silent hazard to patient safety. J Crit Care. 2017;42:255.
14. Khouzam RN, Soufi MK, Weatherly M. Heparin infusion through a central line misplaced in the carotid artery leading to hemorrhagic stroke. J Emerg Med. 2013;45:87–9. https://doi.org/10.1016/j.jemermed.2012.12.026.
15. McCarthy CJ, Behravesh S, Naidu SG, Oklu R. Air embolism: practical tips for prevention and treatment. J Clin Med. 2016;5:93.
16. Roberts S, Johnson M, Davies S. Near-fatal air embolism: fibrin sheath as the portal of air entry. South Med J. 2003;96:1036.
17. Laskey AL, Dyer C, Tobias JD. Venous air embolism during home infusion therapy. Pediatrics. 2002;109:E15.
18. Ely EW, Hite RD, Baker AM, et al. Venous air embolism from central venous catheterization: a need for increased physician awareness. Crit Care Med. 1999;27:2113.
19. Kander T, Frigyesi A, Kjeldsen-Kragh J, et al. Bleeding complications after central line insertions: relevance of pre-procedure coagulation tests and institutional transfusion policy. Acta Anaesthesiol Scand. 2013;57:573.
20. Shah PM, Babu SC, Goyal A, et al. Arterial misplacement of large-caliber cannulas during jugular vein catheterization: case for surgical management. J Am Coll Surg. 2004;198:939.
21. Stone MB, Nagdev A, Murphy MC, Sisson CA. Ultrasound detection of guidewire position during central venous catheterization. Am J Emerg Med. 2010;28:82.
22. Armstrong WF, et al. Diastolic collapse of the right ventricle with cardiac tamponade: an echocardiographic study. Circulation. 1982;65(7):1491–6.
23. Singh S, et al. Right ventricular and right atrial collapse in patients with cardiac tamponade–a combined echocardiographic and hemodynamic study. Circulation. 1984;70(6):966–71.
24. Jalota R, Sayad E. Tension pneumothorax. Treasure Island: StatPearls; 2021.
25. Williams K, Baumann L, Grabowski J, Lautz TB. Current practice in the management of spontaneous pneumothorax in children. J Laparoendosc Adv Surg Tech A. 2019;29(4):551–6.
26. Vallee P, Sullivan M, Richardson H, Bivins B, Tomlanovich M. Sequential treatment of a simple pneumothorax. Ann Emerg Med. 1988;17(9):936–42.
27. Li SS, Rossfeld Z, Basu SK. Cardiac tamponade in a child with fever of unknown origin. Hosp Pediatr. 2017;7(11):692–6.
28. Britt RC, Novosel TJ, Britt LD, Sullivan M. The impact of central line simulation before the ICU experience. Am J Surg. 2009;197:533.
29. Abood GJ, Davis KA, Esposito TJ, et al. Comparison of routine chest radiograph versus clinician judgment to determine adequate central line placement in critically ill patients. J Trauma. 2007;63:50.

Lost Tooth After EGD in a 6-Year-Old Child

Jonathan Maxwell Teets

1 Case Discussion

A 7-year-old 20 kg boy with a history of moderate persistent asthma and eosinophilic esophagitis presents for a routine surveillance esophagoduodenoscopy (EGD) with biopsies. He has no drug allergies but has seasonal allergies and takes oral budesonide at home and albuterol as needed. He underwent an uneventful anesthetic induction with inhalational anesthetic and had an intravenous line placed for fluids and infusion of propofol for maintenance of anesthesia. The only difficulty was when the oral bite block was placed, the patient had a bout of coughing which was treated with a bolus of propofol. The remainder of the case proceeded without any problems.

The anesthesiologist reports to the PACU nurse during the handoff that he underwent an uneventful mask induction and easy mask ventilation, followed by spontaneous ventilation with nasal cannula oxygen while the anesthetic was maintained with a propofol infusion through a left-hand peripheral intravenous line. The patient had tolerated the procedure well and he was brought to the PACU lying on his side with the nasal cannula and in a clinically stable condition. In PACU his vital signs are stable and he is sedated, still lying on the left lateral side with oxygen flowing via the nasal cannula.

After 15 min in the PACU, the patient is awake spontaneously and the nasal cannula is pulled out by him on awakening. The PACU nurse notices that he has a persistent dry cough. On examination there are bilateral breath sounds with no wheezing and all vital signs are stable on room air. As the patient takes sips of apple juice, his parents notice a missing front tooth. They would like to see this tooth.

The PACU nurse calls you to the bedside and asks for your assessment.

J. M. Teets (✉)
Department of Anesthesiology, Pain and Perioperative Medicine,
Children's National Hospital, Washington, DC, USA
e-mail: jteets@childrensnational.org

S. T. Verghese (ed.), *Anesthesia STAT! Acute Pediatric Emergencies in PACU*,
https://doi.org/10.1007/978-3-031-24396-7_6

2 What Are Some of the Questions You May Have to Answer to Explain This Unexpected Tooth Loss?

1. Was there any trauma with oral airway/oral bite block insertion? Yes/**No**
2. Was the placement of the endoscope difficult? Yes/**No**
3. Was any blood or tooth noticed in the mouth, vallecula, or esophagus when the video of the endoscope entry was visible? Yes/**No**
4. Did the tooth come lose when the scope was removed? Yes/**No**
5. If so, were the front four teeth examined and found to be intact prior to ending anesthesia? **Yes**/No
6. If the tooth was missing, could you have continued to look for it in the stomach to see if it had been pushed into it? **Yes**/No
7. Did the mother specifically tell you that her son's front tooth was quite loose and he was waiting for the tooth fairy to come every day? **Yes**/No
8. Was there a history of a loose tooth before the procedure, available to the pre-op nurse, surgeon, and the interviewing anesthesia provider? **Yes**/No

Assuming the answers to the eight questions are in the bold letters, did you show the intact teeth to the PACU nurse after handoff before leaving the patient lying on his side? **Yes**/No

9. Therefore, are you convinced that the tooth loss occurred after the procedure when the patient woke up? **Yes**/No
10. Did you have a chance to bring the parents to the PACU bay to show that the tooth is still intact in the presence of the PACU nurse as the patient is slowly emerging from the anesthetic? Yes/**No**
11. If your answers to the last two questions were **Yes,** then did you and the PACU nurse both document these in the perioperative and anesthetic chart? Yes/**No**

The clinical scenario above highlights the significance of timely **documentation** in the chart about the presence of *loose but not lost tooth* in the patient on emergence to protect yourself from potential future medicolegal problems that can arise.

It is important to identify the correct missing tooth with the parent. A thorough examination of the mouth should be compared with the preoperative dental exam. Two universal systems are used to identify primary teeth and permanent teeth. The first system designates 20 primary teeth. Primary teeth may be referred to as milk teeth or baby teeth. Primary teeth are identified by a sequence of letters starting with the primary maxillary right second molar designated tooth A and continuing alphabetically to the contralateral teeth of the maxilla ending on the left second molar, tooth J. The mandibular teeth then continue from the primary mandibular left second molar, tooth K, all the way around to the mandibular right second molar, tooth T. The second system to identify teeth is a numeric system designated for 32 permanent teeth. This numeric system begins with the maxillary right third molar and then continues around the mouth in the same fashion as the primary teeth (Fig. 1) [1].

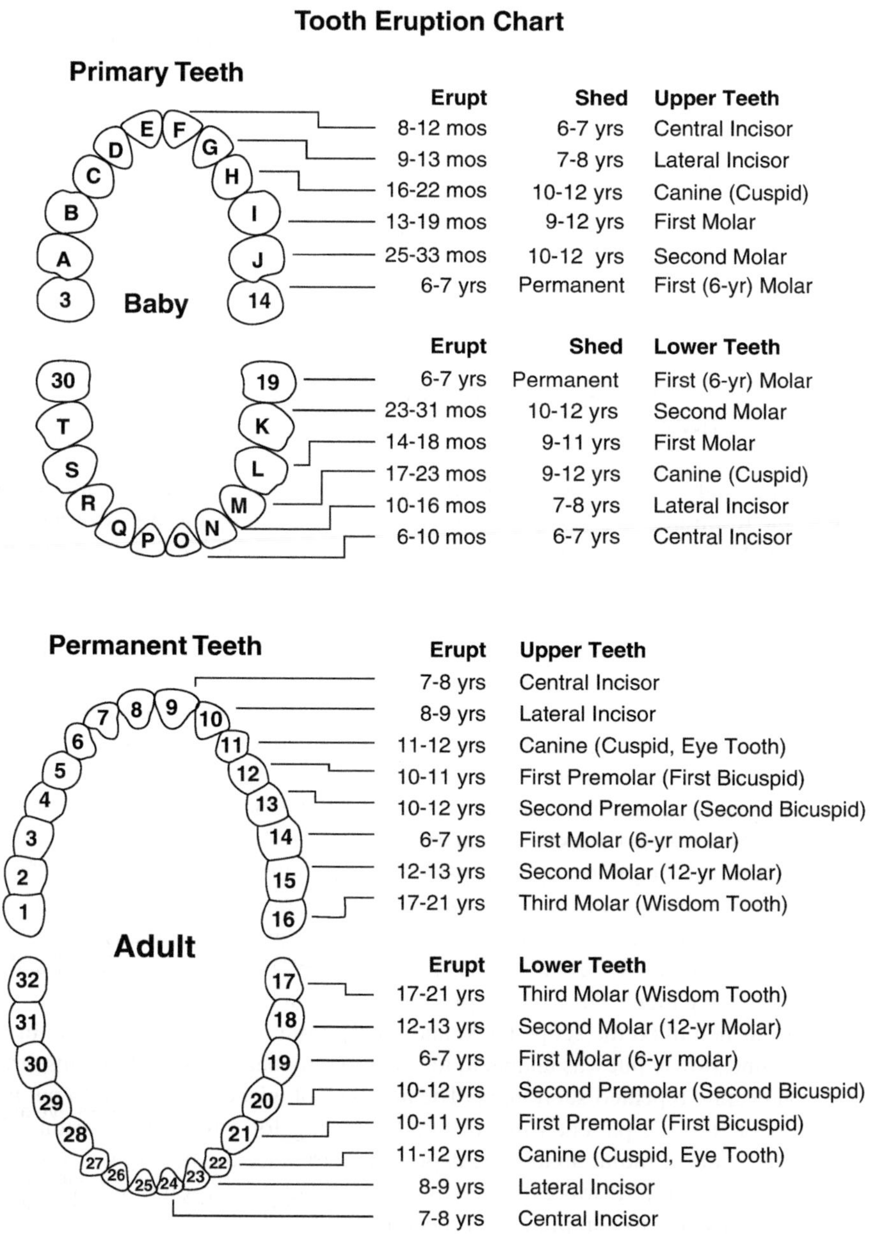

Fig. 1 A universal system for identifying teeth is used for children as well as adults. The chart includes the names of each tooth as well as the approximate age teeth erupt. (*Figure reprinted with permission from* https://templaterepublic.com/medical/dental-chart-forms/)

Primary teeth usually begin to erupt around 6–7 months of age and continue until age 2–2.5 years. Around age 6–7 years, the primary teeth will begin to erupt usually starting with the "6-year molars" which are permanent teeth 3, 14, 19, and 30. Children frequently start to lose primary teeth beginning around age 6 or 7.

The missing tooth has been identified as the primary right lateral incisor (tooth D). The child's parent suggests that since it is "just a baby tooth," they are not very concerned. They were initially disappointed that they could not get the tooth to take home to put under his pillow but are not alarmed about its possible other location. The parents ask if it is safe for him to be discharged home now that the coughing seems to be less.

3 What Is the Appropriate Response You Should Give the Parent?

The missing tooth must first be identified within the oropharynx, the gastrointestinal tract, or the respiratory tract to determine whether it is safe or not to be discharged. If a tooth is lost during induction of anesthesia, then laryngoscopy may assist with visualization and extraction of the foreign body from the oropharynx. Laryngoscopy while the patient is under anesthesia may also be useful if the tooth becomes dislodged during placement of an oral airway or from a rigid bite block during endoscopy cases.

The incident in the past in our institution about a missing tooth during the procedure was quite different. In this case everyone was aware of a loose front tooth and its loss was discovered shortly after introduction of the endoscope. This was prompted by the endoscopist's question "where is all the blood in the mouth coming from?". In answer to this unexpected query about the etiology of bleeding, the anesthesiologist asked the endoscopist to pause so she could check on the loose front tooth. A front tooth was missing, and the bleeding source was from the base of the avulsed tooth. At this juncture it was important for the OR team to focus on retrieving this tooth that was detached and has the risk of entering the respiratory tract in this anesthetized patient. The endoscopist looked first in the stomach and then in the esophagus as he pulled the scope back, and after pulling it back into the mouth, he looked around slowly but was unable to locate it mainly because the blood obscured his vision despite repeated suctioning. The anesthesiologist decided then to put her gloved finger into the patient's mouth blindly feeling for a tooth and fortunately encountered it in the molar area in the dependent part since the patient was lying in the left lateral position. It was extracted manually intact to everyone's relief and the endoscopist was able to complete the procedure.

If a tooth is not retrieved from the oropharynx, then a chest x-ray should be completed. Both PA and lateral view of the chest films must be obtained to avoid any ambiguity as to whether a foreign body is in the respiratory versus gastrointestinal tract. A tooth in the GI tract should naturally pass and will not necessitate endoscopy. However, a tooth in the respiratory tract presents risk of chronic irritation, cough, infection, and obstruction. Patients with tooth aspiration present with a variety of symptoms including nonproductive cough, dyspnea, wheezing, hemoptysis, or cyanosis [2]. As a result, an aspirated tooth must be safely retrieved by a specialist qualified to perform bronchoscopy for foreign body removal.

PA and lateral films have identified the tooth within the right side of the lung. A surgeon is consulted to assist with removal. Imaging from a different patient demonstrates teeth fragments in the right lung (Fig. 2).

The surgeon asks if it is necessary to wait 2 h since the patient just had apple juice in the PACU.

It is important to weigh risks and benefits of NPO guidelines. Although ASA fasting guidelines recommend 2 h for clears, there has been debate over the evidence to liberalize these guidelines to 1 h for pediatric patients [3]. By the time the chest x-ray has been completed and interpreted by the radiologist, 1 h has passed since clears were ingested. Risks and benefits of proceeding at this point should be agreed upon by the surgeon and anesthesiologist and should be made on a case-by-case basis. If the patient at any point developed respiratory distress, then it would be prudent to proceed emergently to the operating room for rigid bronchoscopy regardless of the NPO status. Although unlikely from a primary tooth, foreign bodies may be at risk to cause more complete occlusion as they move proximally within the airway. The case proceeded with IV induction. He received albuterol for bronchodilation as well as dexamethasone to alleviate swelling in the oropharynx due to repeated instrumentation from EGD and rigid bronchoscopy. Intravenous ondansetron was administered prophylactically to prevent post-op nausea. The surgical team retrieves the tooth uneventfully. The patient was extubated awake given the repeated instrumentation to the oropharynx from multiple procedures on a single day.

The parents are thankful that there were no major issues from the aspirated tooth. Two weeks later there are an incident report in your email inbox and a request to attend a root cause analysis meeting to discuss safety concerns regarding perioperative dental injuries.

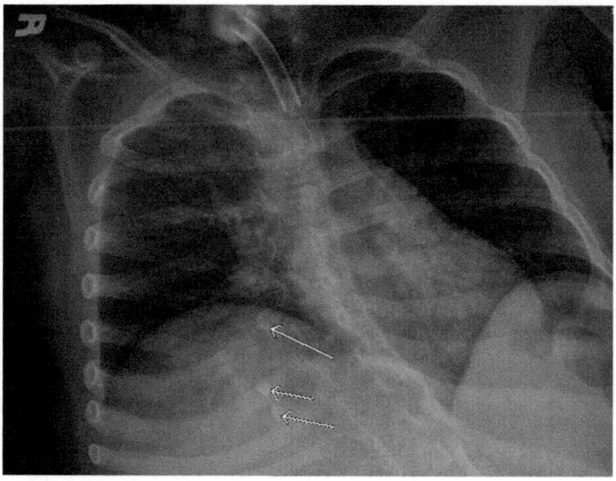

Fig. 2 Teeth or teeth fragments that appear in the right lung of a patient with history of seizures and tracheostomy

4 At the Meeting the Chief Safety Officer Asks: How Common Are Perianesthetic Dental Injuries and Which Patients Are at Highest Risk for Dental Injuries?

Retrospective data estimates the incidence of perioperative dental damage to be 0.02–0.07%. A survey of 133 anesthesiology training programs reported an average incidence of 1:1000 dental injuries during or after over one million tracheal intubations in a year [4].

Congenital craniofacial anomalies associated with cleft palates, Treacher Collins syndrome, Pierre Robin sequence, and Goldenhar syndrome may lead to difficult intubations increasing risk of dental injury. Congenital dental anomalies like amelogenesis imperfecta or dentinogenesis imperfecta also lead to increased risk of dental fracture since even the slightest airway manipulation may injure the tooth [1].

Patients with neurologic impairments or Down syndrome also are at higher risk of aspiration of foreign bodies because of decreased gag reflex or other problems with airway protective mechanisms. They may also have delayed diagnosis if they do not complain of their symptoms, if they present with nonspecific symptoms, or when they are asymptomatic. The case report of a 4-year-old boy with Down syndrome who aspirated his maxillary incisor during a dental extraction procedure should be a caution to everyone not to assume that the missing tooth is in the stomach without radiological confirmation prior to discharge. Since this young child had shown no signs of respiratory distress, he was sent home without a diagnosis of the tooth's location only to be readmitted through the ER because of pneumonia from the aspiration of that tooth into his respiratory tract. After general anesthesia for two bronchoscopies, the foreign body or tooth in the bronchial tree was eventually extracted. The case report signifies the importance of obtaining a radiological confirmation of the tooth location in the stomach after it was seen missing during the procedure prior to discharge [2].

5 What Should Be Done to Prevent Perioperative Dental Injury?

Although many perioperative dental injuries may be minor and easily repaired, these injuries are estimated to make up one third of all medicolegal anesthetic claims. Dental injury is the adverse event responsible for the greatest number of malpractice claims brought against anesthesiologists [4]. In order to prevent harm to patients and avoid an increasingly litigious medicolegal environment, the anesthesia team should conduct a thorough preoperative dental evaluation. Identifying and documenting which teeth may be loose or damaged and documenting this is essential. Especially loose teeth should be evaluated with a glove by the anesthesiologist to test the degree of mobility and formulate a plan of action. Poor dentition may not only put teeth at risk for avulsion or aspiration, but untreated dental abscess can contribute to extended postoperative treatment and potentially compromise surgical outcome. If an area of the mouth is concerning for infection, then the patient should have a dental consult prior to proceeding with an elective case. The need to establish a heightened awareness of dental abnormalities like loose, chipped, and missing conditions cannot be overemphasized. Documentation of the preoperative dental condition and the potential perioperative risk factors regarding these may help reduce medicolegal expenses from claims of dental damage that can arise after an uneventful anesthetic. Anesthesiologists should document the intactness of the teeth after laryngoscopy, intubation, and extubation to protect him-/herself from legal conundrums at a later stage [4].

Dental injuries include enamel fracture, subluxation (loosening of the tooth), luxation (partial displacement of tooth from socket), avulsion (complete displacement of the tooth from the socket), or crown and root fractures. In addition, damages to fillings, crowns, permanent dentures, bridges, and veneers are all possible as a consequence of airway manipulation [5].

A review of over 160,000 cases in a 14-year time period identified that dental injury occurred in 1 per 2073 anesthetics. Perianesthetic dental injury was defined as any significant change to the patient's dentition during the perianesthetic period that may or may not have required dental consultation or treatment. Factors predictive of dental injury associated with anesthesia were patients that had poor dentition or reconstructive work as well as those patients considered to be moderately difficult to intubate. Patients with poor dentition and who are moderately difficult to intubate are at a 20-fold higher risk of dental injury. Maxillary central incisors were the most likely teeth to be injured according to this case-control study [5].

Since it is not practical to obtain a dental consultation for every loose tooth prior to surgery, a discussion of the risk of dental injury should occur preoperatively. Discussing these risks with parents and patients in the presence of another medical professional before surgery and documenting this conversation or modified informed consent will reduce dissatisfaction should inadvertent dental complications occur [1].

Some practitioners suggest a loose tooth may be secured with a silk suture and taped to the ipsilateral cheek so in the event it becomes dislodged during airway manipulation, it will not be lost [6]. If tooth extraction is discussed with parents preoperatively, then many pediatric anesthesiologists will remove "extremely mobile" primary teeth after induction of anesthesia. A gauze barrier should be placed lingually to prevent accidental introduction of the tooth more distally. Then another gauze should be used to help extract the tooth using a twisting and snapping action [1].

A review of foreign body aspiration (FBA) in 157 children over a 10-year period showed that most children with FB aspiration were diagnosed accurately. In 80% of cases despite a history of witnessed choking, only 46% were diagnosed early (within 24 h). The clinical triad of wheezing, coughing, and diminished breath sounds was more prevalent in late diagnoses (47%) (later than 24 h) than in early diagnoses (31%). Right-sided FB were more common (56%) than left-sided FB aspiration (35%) [7]. A witnessed choking event is the most important historical information to make an early diagnosis of FBA [8]. Diagnosis of foreign body location can be made by radiography and CT scan, and a rigid bronchoscopy is necessary to retrieve the foreign body under general anesthesia. Complications from bronchoscopic retrieval include bronchial irritation, tracheitis, atelectasis, and pneumonia if the FB has been lodged for a long time [9]. Rigid bronchoscopy is the gold standard procedure for removal of pediatric airway foreign bodies [10].

Dental injury can occur during direct laryngoscopy (DL). In a recent review of adult patients, DL was found to cause a higher rate of dental injury (4.86%) compared to suspension laryngoscopy (1.7%) by an otolaryngologist. The use of a dental guard and the technique and tools used may explain this difference [11, 12].

6 Summary

Dental injury from anesthetic care causes patient dissatisfaction, added medical expenses, additional procedures, and harm to patients. Understanding dental anatomy and physiology will help the anesthesia team conduct a more thorough preoperative dental examination. Identifying patients with preoperative dental anomalies should alert the team to take additional precautions and care during airway manipulation. During endoscopy procedures, the entire team should be aware of loose teeth to ensure that placement of the bite block and the endoscope is performed with caution. In addition, checking for the presence and intactness of known loose teeth is essential before the completion of the procedure. Dental guards should be considered to avoid dental injury in cases where difficult laryngoscopy and intubation are anticipated.

References

1. Herlich A, Cladis FP, Vecchione L, Martin B. Anesthesia for pediatric dentistry. In: Davis J, Cladis FP, editors. Smith's anesthesia for infants and children. 9th ed. Philadelphia: Elsevier; 2017. p. 1018–34.
2. Canceill T, et al. Misdiagnosed tooth aspiration in a young, handicapped boy: case report and recommendations. Case Rep Dent. 2019;(2019):8495739.
3. Disma N, Frykholm P, Cook-Sather SD, Lerman J. Pro-con debate: 1- vs 2-hour fast for clear liquids before anesthesia in children. Anesth Analg. 2021;133(3):581–91.
4. Yasny JS. Perioperative dental considerations for the anesthesiologist. Anesth Analg. 2009;108(5):1564–73.
5. Newland MC, et al. Dental injury associated with anesthesia: a report of 161,687 anesthetics given over 14 years. J Clin Anesth. 2007;19:339–45.
6. Lee BB, Jiang N. Loose—but not lost—tooth. Anesth Analg. 2005;101(3):920.
7. Wiseman NE. The diagnosis of foreign body aspiration in childhood. J Pediatr Surg. 1984;19(5):531–5. https://doi.org/10.1016/s0022-3468(84)80097-4. PMID: 6502421.
8. Chiu CY, Wong KS, Lai SH, Hsia SH, Wu CT. Factors predicting early diagnosis of foreign body aspiration in children. Pediatr Emerg Care. 2005;21(3):161–4. PMID: 15744193.
9. Zur KB, Litman RS. Pediatric airway foreign body retrieval: surgical and anesthetic perspectives. Paediatr Anaesth. 2009;19(Suppl 1):109–17. https://doi.org/10.1111/j.1460-9592.2009.03006.x. PMID: 19572850.

10. Ozdemir S, Surmelioglu O, Tarkan O, Tuncer U, Kiroglu M, Dagkiran M. The utility of endoscope-assisted rigid bronchoscopy in pediatric airway foreign body removals. J Craniofac Surg. 2020;31(2):e217–9. https://doi.org/10.1097/SCS.0000000000005660. PMID: 31188250.
11. Wilson CP, Romano E, Vasan NR. Comparison of dental injury rates in perioperative intubation and suspension laryngoscopy for otolaryngology procedures. OTO Open. 2021;5(4):2473974X211065021. https://doi.org/10.1177/2473974X211065021. PMID: 34926975; PMCID: PMC8671680.
12. Bowcock EB, Goonan P. A cheap fix for an expensive problem: the use of a thermoplastic mouthguard to reduce the risk of dental trauma during orotracheal intubation. Anaesth Intensive Care. 2016;44(5):643. https://doi.org/10.1177/0310057X1604400515. PMID: 27608354.

Intractable Cardiac Arrhythmias After Bone Marrow Biopsy in a Child with Leukemia

Andrew Matisoff

1 Stem Case

A 4-year-old male with newly diagnosed B-cell acute lymphoblastic leukemia presents to the operating room for bone marrow biopsy under general anesthesia. He undergoes mask induction of anesthesia with sevoflurane and nitrous oxide, and after placement of an intravenous catheter, a propofol infusion is started at 250 μg/kg/min, and the sevoflurane is discontinued. Airway management consists of a nasal cannula at 2 L/min with end-tidal carbon dioxide ($ETCO_2$) monitoring. For antiemetic prophylaxis, he is given ondansetron 0.1 mg/kg and dexamethasone 0.5 mg/kg.

What are the common presenting signs and symptoms of leukemia in a child?

What important information should be obtained from the medical history?

Describe the anesthetic concerns in a child with newly diagnosed leukemia?

What lab studies and radiological studies are needed prior to anesthesia?

Discuss common medications and their appropriate dosages for prevention of nausea and vomiting.

The bone marrow biopsy is performed successfully, and the child is brought to the recovery room on 2 L of oxygen via a nasal cannula in stable condition. Approximately 20 min after arrival, the child is noticed to have increased work of breathing, nasal flaring, and decreased oxygen saturation to 89%.

Discuss the evaluation and management of a hypoxic child in the recovery room.

What are the differential diagnoses of hypoxia in an oncology patient after a simple procedure like BMA/biopsy?

A. Matisoff (✉)
Division of Cardiac Anesthesia, Children's National Hospital, Washington, DC, USA
e-mail: amatisof@childrensnational.org

S. T. Verghese (ed.), *Anesthesia STAT! Acute Pediatric Emergencies in PACU*,
https://doi.org/10.1007/978-3-031-24396-7_7

Upon examination, the child appears lethargic with some agitation. He has nasal flaring and increased work of breathing. Auscultation of the lungs reveals crackles at the bases bilaterally. His vital signs are heart rate of 145 beats/min, respiratory rate 40 breaths/min, blood pressure 80/50, temperature 37.1 °C, and oxygen saturation 89% on 2 L of oxygen. A face mask with 100% oxygen is applied with improvement in the oxygen saturation to 93%.

What Are the Indications for Reintubation of a Child in the Recovery Room?

Despite mild improvement in oxygenation, a decision is made to intubate the child due to respiratory muscle exhaustion and altered mental status.

Which medications would you use for induction of anesthesia and intubation in this child?

What is the risk of attempting an intubation in this child without any medications?

Is succinylcholine contraindicated in this patient?

In securing an airway rapidly in this patient, it is important to intubate without any risk of trauma to the airway because of the thrombocytopenia or thrombasthenia even if the quantity of platelets is normal. Avoidance of intravenous succinylcholine is prudent because of its tendency to produce hyperkalemia.

Upon administration of propofol 3 mg/kg, the patient becomes pulseless, and the following rhythm is seen on the monitor:

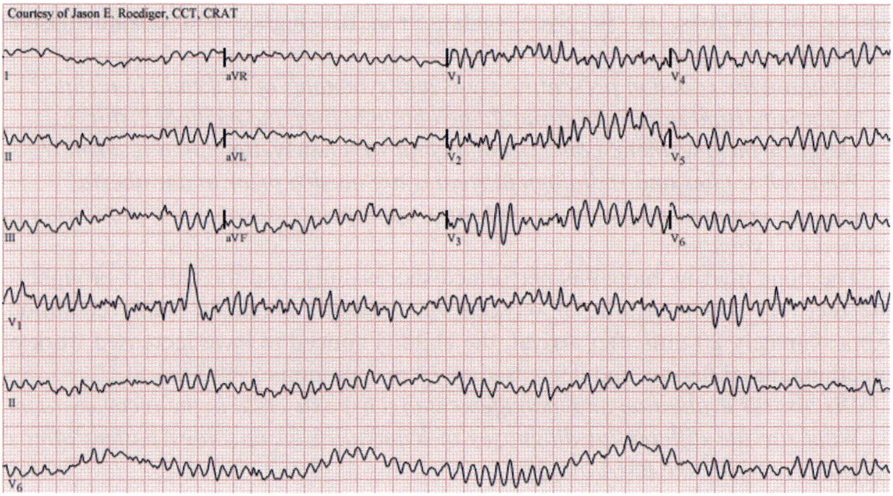

2 What Is This Rhythm and What Is the Management?

A pulse cannot be palpated, and CPR is started while intubation is being performed. Defibrillation is attempted at 2 joules per kilogram followed by 4 joules per kilogram without resolution of the dysrhythmia. After three rounds of CPR are performed and the administration of epinephrine 0.01 mg/kg, a pulse is still not palpable.

Discuss the PALS management of a pulseless arrest with a ventricular fibrillation.

During CPR a venous blood gas is obtained showing a pH of 7.01, PCO_2 of 59, PO_2 of 30, and a lactate level of 10 and is most notable for a serum potassium of 7.2 mEq/L.

3 What Is the Treatment for Hyperkalemia in This Child?

The child is administered sodium bicarbonate 2 mEq/kg and calcium gluconate 30 mg/kg. A subsequent defibrillation with 4 J/kg results in termination of the above rhythm and conversion to sinus tachycardia, and a radial pulse is palpated. CPR is continued for one more round until a blood pressure by cuff of 70/40 mmHg is measured. After return of spontaneous circulation, the child is taken to the pediatric intensive care unit in critical condition.

What is the likely cause of hyperkalemia in this child that resulted in a cardiac arrest?

The likely cause of high potassium load is secondary to the onset of tumor lysis syndrome (TLS) in this high-risk patient.

What is TLS and why is it vital for the perioperative team to become familiar with the diagnosis and treatment of this lethal clinical condition?

4 Discussion

Acute leukemias/lymphomas are the most common malignancy in children, with a peak incidence between age 2 and 5 years old. Common presenting symptoms include lymphadenopathy, organomegaly (liver and spleen), fever, and musculoskeletal pain [1]. Young children may be diagnosed after a new-onset limp is discovered. Anemia and thrombocytopenia may present as pallor and bruises or petechiae. Bleeding due to thrombocytopenia and poor platelet function and coagulopathy is very common. It is therefore important in these children to obtain a history of bleeding from the gums on brushing teeth or spontaneous epistaxis. Since children with childhood leukemias often require multiple anesthetics for diagnostic and treatment procedures, pediatric anesthesiologists should familiarize themselves with the multisystem involvement of each child's malignancy to minimize complications related to anesthesia. This includes a thorough airway evaluation for possible obstruction due to edema from chronic steroids or lymphadenopathy. Decreased pulmonary compliance and increased resistance due to disease burden or cytokine release can be present. Cardiomyopathy can occur in children treated with cardiotoxic chemotherapeutic agents such as Adriamycin. Electrolyte disturbances can result from renal dysfunction or from cellular response to chemotherapy. Most importantly, the presence of a mediastinal mass from lymphoma can rapidly lead to severe airway obstruction, cardiac compression, low cardiac output, and sudden death with the induction of anesthesia and administration of muscle relaxants. Mediastinal lymph node enlargement can clinically present with dyspnea and inability to lie flat and sometimes with superior vena caval obstruction [2]. Visceromegaly with abdominal distension can cause respiratory difficulties and oxygen desaturation on room air due to a decrease in functional residual capacity (FRC) especially when supine.

Children with new-onset rapidly dividing tumors such as non-Hodgkin's lymphoma specifically Burkitt's lymphoma and B-cell acute lymphoblastic leukemia (B-ALL) are at risk for the development of TLS which can occur spontaneously or after the initiation of cytotoxic chemotherapy. Massive tumor cell lysis will result in the release of large amounts of potassium, phosphate, and nucleic acids into the systemic circulation. This can rapidly lead to hyperuricemia, hyperkalemia, hyperphosphatemia, and hypocalcemia which can progress to acute renal failure, seizures, and cardiac arrest [3, 4]. The most common cause of acute renal failure in TLS is due to the precipitation of uric acid crystals in renal tubules which occurs when breakdown of tumor cells by chemotherapy releases uric acid and causes the formation of uric acid crystals in the renal tubules and collecting ducts [3, 4].

The diagnosis of tumor lysis syndrome requires that two or more of the metabolic abnormalities, such as hyperuricemia, hyperkalemia, hyperphosphatemia, and hypocalcemia, occur within 3 days before or up to 7 days after the initiation of therapy. Acute renal failure is initiated by precipitation of uric acid and calcium phosphate as well as renal vasoconstriction. Clinically this is accompanied by an increased serum creatinine level, seizures, cardiac dysrhythmia, or death. The rapid increase in serum potassium levels can quickly lead to cardiac dysrhythmias, including torsade de pointes. Hyperphosphatemia leads to secondary hypocalcemia, which can cause neuromuscular irritability dysrhythmia, and seizures. Large amounts of uric acid crystal precipitation can occur during TLS due to lack of an enzyme called urate oxidase which is inactive in humans. The significance of urate oxidase is that it helps in the formation of allantoin—the end product of purine oxidation—and prevents the buildup of excess uric acid which can result in acute kidney injury.

Finally, the release of large amounts of cytokines from dying cancer cells can cause a systemic inflammatory response which can cause multisystem organ failure, including acute respiratory distress syndrome (ARDS) [3–5].

5 Immediate Postanesthetic Events in PACU

In the recovery room, the child initially presented with increased work of breathing, likely due to alveolar infiltrate from ARDS related to the release of cytokines. The child was managed appropriately by increasing respiratory support and an early decision to reintubate the child due to increased work of breathing and altered mental status. A stat portable chest X-ray showed bilateral fluffy infiltrates in all lung fields. The appropriate medications for reintubation in this child would be to avoid drugs which significantly decrease systemic vascular resistance and myocardial contractility in the setting of a systemic inflammatory response syndrome. A better choice than propofol for intubation would be medications such as ketamine, etomidate, or fentanyl which have less effect than propofol on systemic vascular resistance.

6 What Are the Changes Seen in Electrocardiogram in Children with Hyperkalemia?

Electrophysiological changes in ECG are proportional directly to the absolute plasma potassium concentration as well as its rate of increase in the blood. Anesthesia provider should not only have a clear understanding of the chronological changes occurring in ECG with rising concentration of potassium but also about the urgency to initiate therapy.

Hyperkalemia may manifest in variable changes in ECG abnormalities.

Early on it may be seen as peaked T waves from cardiac action potential shortening. This is followed by the P wave widening and QRS widening.

At a serum potassium level of 6.5–8.0 mEq/L, in addition to peaked T waves, the ECG shows the following:

- Prolonged PR interval
- Decreased or disappearing P wave
- Widening of the QRS
- Amplified R wave

EKG strip of progression of hyperkalemia is shown below:

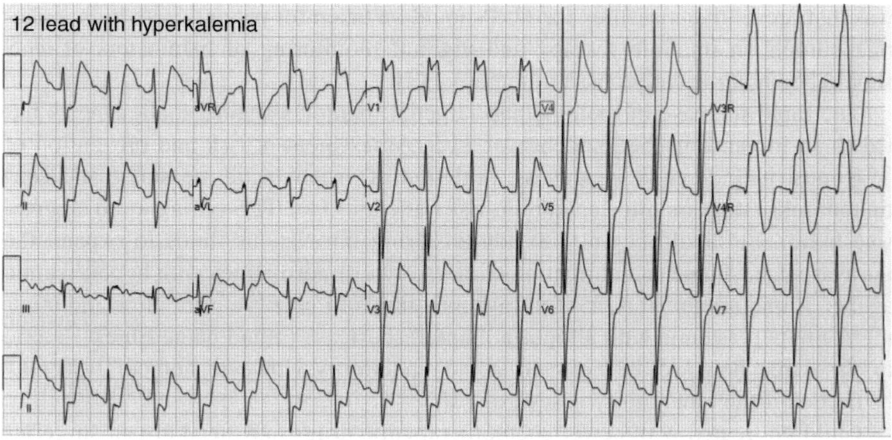

Severe hyperkalemia ($[K^+]_o > 7.0$ mmol/L) leads to heart block, asystole, and VT/VF [6, 7].

Treatment of hyperkalemia requires urgent administration of intravenous calcium which stabilizes the myocardium by lowering the action potential threshold. Sodium bicarbonate administration can move potassium intracellularly, especially in the setting of metabolic acidosis, and should also be given promptly. Administration of insulin with dextrose to prevent hypoglycemia can acutely move potassium intracellularly in addition to albuterol. Long-term management of chronic hyperkalemia involves administration of loop diuretics such as furosemide and sodium polystyrene which remove potassium from the body via the kidney and intestine, respectively [7]. This patient developed ventricular fibrillation which likely resulted from QRS widening onto the T waves, causing an R on T phenomenon. Management of ventricular fibrillation includes early initiation of CPR and defibrillation as soon as possible at 2 J/kg followed by 4 J/kg. If ventricular fibrillation persists, then amiodarone 5 mg/kg IV bolus for up to three doses should be considered [8]. If reversible causes of the cardiac arrest are present, they should be treated immediately. In this case the patient had the reversible cause of severe hyperkalemia due to tumor lysis syndrome. This should be managed as soon as possible before considering the administration of amiodarone since stabilization of the myocardium by calcium administration will increase the likelihood of a successful subsequent defibrillation.

Children with underlying malignancies are at high risk for complications with anesthesia. A case report of a child with B-cell acute lymphoblastic leukemia developing TLS after being given dexamethasone for antiemetic prophylaxis during a bone marrow biopsy is a reminder that this drug is probably best avoided in children who are at risk for developing TLS [9]. There are case reports of TLS hastened by radiation therapy, use of thalidomide, dexamethasone, and the use of newer chemotherapeutic agents like rituximab and bortezomib [10]. Studies on the use of imatinib, a selective tyrosine kinase inhibitor effective in the treatment of ALL, have shown that it can induce rapid apoptosis and TLS. The conclusion by the authors was that preventive measures for TLS should be taken for patients with high leukemia burden on imatinib therapy and vigilant monitoring of parameters of TLS should begin at the early phase of therapy [11].

The rapid increase in biologic and targeted therapies against malignancies has led to an increase in the incidence of TLS. Assessment of risk and prevention of TLS must include early awareness, initiation of prophylactic measures, and continuous laboratory monitoring in high-risk patients. Once TLS is diagnosed, aggressive treatment should begin with administering intravenous fluids to expand the intravascular volume and correction of electrolyte abnormalities with hypouricemic agents. Rapid administration of intravenous fluids to improve urine flow and treating the hyperuricemia with allopurinol and rasburicase (brand name Elitek—a uric oxidase) may help avoid the onset of acute renal injury. However, hemodialysis may be needed if the renal injury is severe [12].

Children treated with newer chemotherapeutic drugs may need urgent surgeries under anesthesia, and it is important for the anesthesiologist to have a high index of suspicion of the potential risk of TLS and knowledge on how to prevent and treat it if it occurs.

A thorough review of the medical record and detailed history and physical examination as well as an understanding of the implications of TLS by the perioperative team can minimize the risks involved in caring for these patients under anesthesia. The risk of administration of dexamethasone as an antiemetic to treat significant nausea postoperatively should be known to everyone in the perioperative team to avoid the precipitation of TLS in high-risk group of children and should be highlighted during the PACU handoff process [13].

Rapid identification and treatment of severe hyperkalemia peri-operatively can save lives. If hyperkalemia is refractory to the multiple medications available for therapy, then dialysis must be promptly initiated.

The treatment regimen for hyperkalemia before hemodialysis includes use of membrane-stabilizing agents, potassium shifters, and renal excreters [14]. Membrane stabilizers like calcium gluconate have an immediate onset and the effect lasts for 30–60 min. Shifting the potassium ions into the cell can be accomplished by intravenous insulin push with dextrose solution which has an onset of 20 min and duration over 4–6 h. Beta-agonists like albuterol also push potassium intracellularly when nebulized with normal saline with an onset of 30 min and effective duration for 2 h. Excreters of potassium ions via kidneys can be accomplished by intravenous furosemide which acts within 15 min and has a duration of 2–3 h.

The modified strategies to reduce the risk of hypoglycemia with the insulin therapy include using insulin 5 units or 0.1 unit/kg instead of 10 units and administering 50 g dextrose instead of 25 g or as a prolonged infusion instead of a rapid intravenous bolus. It is vital to monitor patient for hypoglycemia because insulin has a longer duration of action than that of dextrose [15].

Continuous insulin infusion with dextrose for 12 h has been reported to be effective in lowering severe hyperkalemia (>12 mmol/L) in a 4-month-old with pseudo hypoaldosteronism who suffered a cardiac arrest but had a successful resuscitation without implementing dialysis [16].

References

1. Clarke RT, Van den Bruel A, Bankhead C, Mitchell CD, Phillips B, Thompson MJ. Clinical presentation of childhood leukaemia: a systematic review and meta-analysis. Arch Dis Child. 2016;101(10):894–901. https://doi.org/10.1136/archdischild-2016-311251. PMID: 27647842.
2. Osborn I. Pediatric malignancies and anesthesia. Anesthesiol Clin North Am. 1998;16(3):677–89, issn:0889-8537.
3. Howard SC, Jones DP, Pui CH. The tumor lysis syndrome. N Engl J Med. 2011;364(19):1844–54. https://doi.org/10.1056/NEJMra0904569. Erratum in: N Engl J Med 2018 Sep 13;379(11):1094. PMID: 21561350; PMCID: PMC3437249.
4. Cheung WL, Hon KL, Fung CM, Leung AK. Tumor lysis syndrome in childhood malignancies. Drugs Context. 2020;9:2019-8-2. https://doi.org/10.7573/dic.2019-8-2.
5. Coiffier B, Altman A, Pui CH, Younes A, Cairo MS. Guidelines for the management of pediatric and adult tumor lysis syndrome: an evidence-based review. J Clin Oncol. 2008;26(16):2767–78. https://doi.org/10.1200/JCO.2007.15.0177. Erratum in: J Clin Oncol. 2010 Feb 1;28(4):708. PMID: 18509186.

6. Weiss JN, Qu Z, Shivkumar K. Electrophysiology of hypokalemia and hyperkalemia. Circ Arrhythm Electrophysiol. 2017;10(3):e004667. https://doi.org/10.1161/CIRCEP.116.004667. PMID: 28314851; PMCID: PMC5399982.
7. Hollander-Rodriguez JC, Calvert JF Jr. Hyperkalemia. Am Fam Physician. 2006;73(2):283–90. PMID: 16445274.
8. American Heart Association. Web-based integrated guidelines for cardiopulmonary and emergency cardiovascular care—Part 12. Pediatric advanced life support. https://eccguidelines.heart.org/index.php/circulation/cpr-ecc-guidelines-2/part-12-pediatric-advanced-life-support/. Accessed 10 Nov 2015.
9. McDonnell C, Barlow R, Campisi P, Grant R, Malkin D. Fatal peri-operative acute tumour lysis syndrome precipitated by dexamethasone. Anaesthesia. 2008;63(6):652–5. https://doi.org/10.1111/j.1365-2044.2007.05436.x. PMID: 18477278.
10. Williams SM, Killeen AA. Tumor lysis syndrome. Arch Pathol Lab Med. 2019;143(3):386–93. https://doi.org/10.5858/arpa.2017-0278-RS. Epub 2018 Nov 30. PMID: 30499695.
11. Chang H, Shih LY. Imatinib-induced tumor lysis syndrome: report of a case and review of the literature. Chang Gung Med J. 2008;31(5):510–4. PMID: 19097599.
12. McBride A, Trifilio S, Baxter N, Gregory TK, Howard SC. Managing tumor lysis syndrome in the era of novel cancer therapies. J Adv Pract Oncol. 2017;8(7):705–20. Epub 2017 Nov 1. PMID: 30333933; PMCID: PMC6188097.
13. Stephanos K, Picard L. Pediatric oncologic emergencies. Emerg Med Clin North Am. 2018;36(3):527–35. https://doi.org/10.1016/j.emc.2018.04.007. Epub 2018 Jun 11. PMID: 30037439.
14. Weisberg LS. Management of severe hyperkalemia. Crit Care Med. 2008;36(12):3246–51. https://doi.org/10.1097/CCM.0b013e31818f222b. PMID: 18936701.
15. Moussavi K, Fitter S, Gabrielson SW, Koyfman A, Long B. Management of hyperkalemia with insulin and glucose: pearls for the emergency clinician. J Emerg Med. 2019;57(1):36–42. https://doi.org/10.1016/j.jemermed.2019.03.043. Epub 2019 May 11. PMID: 31084947.
16. Awlad Thani S, Al Farsi M, Al Omrani S. Life threatening hyperkalemia treated with prolonged continuous insulin infusion. Int J Pediatr Adolesc Med. 2019;6(3):118–20. https://doi.org/10.1016/j.ijpam.2019.04.001. Epub 2019 Apr 17. PMID: 31700971; PMCID: PMC6824155

Shoulder Pain/Tachycardia After Liver Biopsy in a Teenager

Catherine Rim

1 Stem Case

A 13-year-old male weighing 105 kg was followed by his pediatrician for development of metabolic syndrome associated with obesity. He had difficulty walking because of weight gain and moderate obstructive sleep apnea which was managed with continuous positive airway pressure (CPAP). He had acanthosis nigricans and persistently elevated liver enzymes. Nonalcoholic steatohepatitis (NASH) was suspected, and he was scheduled to undergo ultrasound-guided percutaneous liver biopsy by an experienced interventional radiologist. He underwent general anesthesia with supraglottic airway device and received a total of 0.2 mcg/kg of fentanyl. The biopsy procedure was uneventful and gel foam pledgets were placed along the needle tract within the liver parenchyma and on the liver capsule. The patient was extubated awake and transferred to postanesthesia care unit (PACU).

On arrival to PACU, his vitals were heart rate of 86 beats per minute, respiratory rate 22 breaths per minute, blood pressure 101/44, temperature of 36.5, and oxygen saturation 97% on room air.

2 What Are Indications for Liver Biopsy in Pediatric Patients?

Liver diseases in pediatric patients include neonatal cholestasis, disorders of metabolism, drug-induced liver injury, viral disease, immunologic disorders, and nonalcoholic fatty liver disease (NAFLD). NAFLD is a condition where fat accumulates in the liver and there is no history of alcohol use. In pediatric patients, it is more likely

C. Rim (✉)
Division of Anesthesiology, Pain and Pediatric Medicine, Children's National Hospital and George Washington University Hospital, Washington, DC, USA

S. T. Verghese (ed.), *Anesthesia STAT! Acute Pediatric Emergencies in PACU*,
https://doi.org/10.1007/978-3-031-24396-7_8

to be diagnosed in boys 10 years and older. Both genetic and environmental factors are linked to the development of NAFLD. However, diet, exercise, and excess weight gain are significant modifiable risk factors for prevention and management.

In this teenager, the most likely etiology of transaminitis is NAFLD which is now the most common cause of chronic liver disease in obese children and adolescents. Nonalcoholic steatohepatitis (NASH) is a form of NAFLD where the fat deposition is accompanied by inflammation of liver cells and liver damage. NASH, if not diagnosed and treated, can lead to cirrhosis and ultimately live failure or cancer as an adult.

Obese children have a 38% chance of developing fatty liver disease. Other conditions of metabolic syndrome—hypertension, insulin resistance, type 2 diabetes, and high cholesterol and triglycerides—significantly increase the likelihood of NAFLD and NASH. Lifestyle modification to achieve weight loss is the initial treatment for NAFLD by reducing excess fat deposits and inflammation. However, if this fails and there is evidence of steatohepatitis, these patients may need surgical intervention to manage and prevent progression of disease.

The European and North American Societies for Pediatric Hepatology published a consensus statement paper in 2012 on the diagnosis of NAFLD. While there is no consensus on the indications for liver biopsy in the workup, it was agreed that liver biopsy should not be used as a screening procedure given its high cost and invasive nature. However, expert opinion supports liver biopsy to exclude other treatable liver pathology as well as staging the degree of fibrosis indicating a progression to nonalcoholic steatohepatitis [1].

3 What Preprocedural Workup Should Be Done Prior to Liver Biopsy for NAFLD?

Patients who are being worked up for NAFLD should have noninvasive studies performed prior to consideration for biopsy. Aspartate aminotransferase, alanine aminotransferase, gamma-glutamyl transferase, alkaline phosphatase, and bilirubin can be used as indices of hepatobiliary injury. Furthermore, noninvasive imaging such as liver ultrasounds can provide vital information for proceduralists such as significant vasculature to avoid. Recent research has been focused on identifying imaging biomarkers on modalities such as magnetic resonance imaging that help improve noninvasive forms of diagnosis and staging [2]. And yet to date, liver biopsy and histology remain the gold standard for diagnosis. Liver biopsies can be performed percutaneously, both "blind" and image-guided, via trans-jugular or from a laparoscopic or laparotomy approach. The percutaneous approach is the most common as it is the simplest and least invasive. In most suspected cases of NAFLD, the biopsy core sample obtained with a percutaneous needle will be sufficient information for diagnosis. However, in cases of more severe liver disease presenting with coagulopathy or ascites, percutaneous sampling may not be appropriate due to their increased risk for postprocedural hemorrhage. Therefore prior to percutaneous biopsy, patients should have preoperative lab work drawn including complete blood count, prothrombin time, partial thromboplastin time, and fibrinogen. And periprocedural optimization should be considered with vitamin K, fresh frozen plasma, and platelets [3].

4 What Are Postanesthetic Concerns in Obese Children?

Obesity is a well-known epidemic in the pediatric population today. We are seeing more obese patients presenting for routine pediatric surgeries as well as an increasing number of procedures in pediatric patients related to their obesity. The most well-described concern is these patients' increased risk for perioperative respiratory adverse events (PRAE). Tait et al. [4] prospectively studied the relationship between body mass index (BMI) and perioperative respiratory adverse events in children. They collected data from 2025 children undergoing elective, noncardiac surgery in a 20-month period. The obese children had a greater incidence of difficult mask ventilation, airway obstruction, bronchospasm, and significant oxygen desaturation. In developing a risk prediction tool for perioperative respiratory adverse events in pediatric ambulatory anesthesia, Subramanyam et al. [5] identified morbid obesity as one of the five significantly predictive variables. These patients' increased risk of respiratory events is also consistent with their higher rates of asthma and obstructive sleep apnea [6, 7].

Excess weight can also alter pharmacokinetics and pharmacodynamics, and the appropriate dosing of anesthetic medications is not fully understood. A general suggestion is to dose lipophilic medications by total body weight (TBW) and hydrophilic medications by ideal body weight (IBW). Yet this is an extreme oversimplification that needs to be paired with clinical judgment especially in obese patients with comorbidities such as obstructive sleep apnea [8]. Such patients with decreased respiratory compliance might be highly sensitive to a blunting of their respiratory drive, and some may require positive pressure support postoperatively. Nafiu et al. [9] and Kako et al. [10] both found increased PACU length of stays in overweight and obese children.

Other perioperative challenges with obesity include difficult vascular access, more challenging positioning, and prolonged procedural times [11]. Suboptimal positioning and inadequate padding can result in more discomfort in the recovery period.

After an hour in PACU, the patient started complaining of right shoulder pain and was tachycardic to the 130 s. He was also placed on O_2 *by NC maintaining saturations of 94%.*

5 What Are Known Complications of Liver Biopsy in Pediatric Patients?

Pain is the most common complication after a percutaneous liver biopsy. In a 2003 study by Eisenberg et al. [12], 84% of adults reported pain within the first hour post-biopsy despite oral anxiolysis and local anesthetic infiltration. Pain is typically at the incision site or referred pain to the right shoulder. Pain is categorized in the pediatric literature as a common minor complication, manageable with limited analgesia and does not prolong hospitalization. Even in a 2017 study by Hayatghaibi et al. [13] where 4 out of 198 pediatric patients returned after discharge to an emergency department for pain, none were found to have postprocedural bleeding, and all were treated with analgesics and discharged home for clinic follow-up.

This patient's anticipated postoperative pain was prophylactically treated with local anesthetic injection at the biopsy site as well as small doses of intravenous narcotics and acetaminophen intraoperatively. However due to this patient's obstructive sleep apnea, opioids were used sparingly in the postoperative period. Additional doses of intravenous acetaminophen were also limited in the setting of his liver disease. Prophylactic antiemetics should be given to help prevent pain from retching and vomiting which could worsen pain in the postoperative period.

Bleeding is a known complication of liver biopsy that can significantly increase morbidity. The incidence of post-procedure bleeding in pediatrics was initially reported at a higher rate than in adults. Based primarily on smaller single-institution studies, the incidence is reported between 1 and 12% [14–16]. However, clinically significant bleeding appears to be much rarer. Short et al. [17] reported the highest postprocedural transfusion rate of 3.3%. Since that publication, several other single-institution studies reported <1% incidence of major bleeding requiring transfusion [18–21]. To further decrease the risk of post-biopsy hemorrhage, some proceduralists inject hemostatic compounds like thrombin or collagen to the needle tract on withdrawal, and some have standardized all biopsies to be performed with image guidance. Shapira-Zaltsberg et al. [21] specifically studied the routine use of post-biopsy ultrasound but concluded that its utility was best only in cases of clinical or laboratory signs of complications.

Other rare complications reported include pneumothorax or hemothorax, organ perforation, and biliary leak. Being such rare complications, the incidence in pediatric populations is poorly described. Furthermore, the increasing use of ultrasonographic guidance is likely to significantly reduce the rates of these complications.

Infection both local and systemic is also a rare but possible complication. There is no consensus on the use of broad-spectrum prophylactic antibiotics. However, liver transplant patients with bilio-enteric anastomosis have been identified by some authors as a uniquely high-risk population for bacteremia and sepsis [22, 23].

6 What Is Kehr's Sign?

Pain at the tip of the shoulder or "Kehr's sign" is a classic example of referred pain from an irritated diaphragm. It was originally used as a harbinger of ruptured spleen more commonly with left shoulder pain [24]. However, the referred symptoms can be indicative of any peritoneal pathology including hepatic pathology such as in this patient [25]. Irritation of the diaphragm by inflammation, organ injury, or free blood is signaled by the phrenic nerve and reflected as pain in the area above the clavicle due to the shared C3–C4 origins. Spontaneous bleeding from the liver is usually seen in preeclampsia and seen rarely in healthy patients. A subcapsular hematoma of the liver is an accumulation of blood between Glisson's capsule and the liver parenchyma, and if rupture of this hematoma into the peritoneum occurs, then there is a 75% mortality rate. Spontaneous liver hemorrhage, although rare in the non-obstetrical population, should be considered in the differential diagnosis of sudden-onset abdominal pain radiating to the shoulder associated with hepatomegaly with or without signs of shock.

7 What Are Risk Factors for Complications After Percutaneous Liver Biopsy?

Appropriate patient selection is essential for optimizing the safety profile of percutaneous liver biopsies, and investigators are continuing to elicit the risk factors for complications. Uncorrected coagulopathy or thrombocytopenia that can be seen in advance liver disease is considered a contraindication to the percutaneous liver biopsy due to the increased bleeding risk. These are high-risk patients in whom trans-jugular liver biopsy or direct biopsy with laparoscopy or laparotomy is often considered. However, many have reported severe hemorrhage even in the setting of normal coagulation studies.

The use of low-molecular-weight heparin was also found to increase bleeding complications. Fortunately, though, low-dose acetylsalicylic acid (ASA), a common medication for post-liver transplant patients, did not have an increase bleeding incidence or complication rate [15].

Several authors have also tried to identify liver pathologies associated with increased risk for complications. Westheim et al. [15] noted increased risk of bleeding in patients with focal lesions as well as over increased risk of major complications in patients with acute liver failure. Older studies identified malignancy, ascites, and biliary tract dilation as additional risk factors for complications [26, 27]. Liver transplant patients did not have an increased risk for bleeding complications compared to the general population, even when suspected of rejection [15, 17, 19].

While blind percutaneous liver biopsy is still a viable and safe option in pediatric patients even when performed by trainees [3, 20, 28], since real-time ultrasound imaging is available, there is an inherent advantage of identifying and therefore avoiding injury to other structures [29, 30]. There is limited pediatric-specific data to suggest a lower complication rate with ultrasound-guided percutaneous biopsies [31]. A greater number of needle passes have also been identified as a predictor for higher incidence of minor bleeding [19]. Patients who are younger in age are also at increased risk for bleeding especially in the infants <3-month-old population [17, 32, 33]. Harwood et al. [34] reviewed 107 blind percutaneous biopsy and found no differences in number of needle passes or complication rates between obese and nonobese children. Pietrobattista et al. [35] reviewing ultrasound-guided biopsies with more than half described as obese also found no increased rates of complications with 79% of all patients needing only one needle pass.

It is worth noting that the pediatric data for many of the listed risk factors is limited by small retrospective studies. A 2019 review of predictors of bleeding complication after percutaneous liver biopsy by Midia et al., which included both adult and pediatric data, had comparable conclusions on these risk factors [36].

8 What Are Next Management Steps?

While the patient's tachycardia can be attributed to his right shoulder pain, a common complication, providers must maintain a high suspicion for less common but more severe bleeding complications. Judicious administration of analgesia may be considered as well as intravenous crystalloid resuscitation while simultaneously notifying proceduralists for workup and further evaluation. Given this patient's oxygen requirement, lung auscultation or imaging should also rule out the rare complication of pneumothorax.

Persistent indicators of hypovolemia—tachycardia and/or hypotension—or persistent pain or irritability should alert providers to possible rapid decompensation, and the workup and resuscitation are comparable to an acute penetrating trauma. Additional vascular access should be obtained, type and cross sent, and the blood bank notified. Immediate imaging should be done either with ultrasound or stat computed tomography, and an interventional radiologist or general surgeon should be contacted for further management. Morbidity and mortality are greatest when there is a delay in diagnosis and aggressive management [37].

Additional large-bore intravenous access was placed in this patient. Despite 2 L of lactated Ringer's, he remained tachycardic and was becoming increasingly somnolent and hypotensive.

Stat CT abdomen demonstrated subcapsular hemorrhage (Fig. 1a, b), and he was immediately taken to the interventional radiology suite for angiography and embolization (Fig. 2). He was further resuscitated with crystalloid as well as several units of packed red blood cells and was transferred post-embolization to pediatric intensive care unit (PICU) for observation and BiPAP support.

He was discharged home after 3 days.

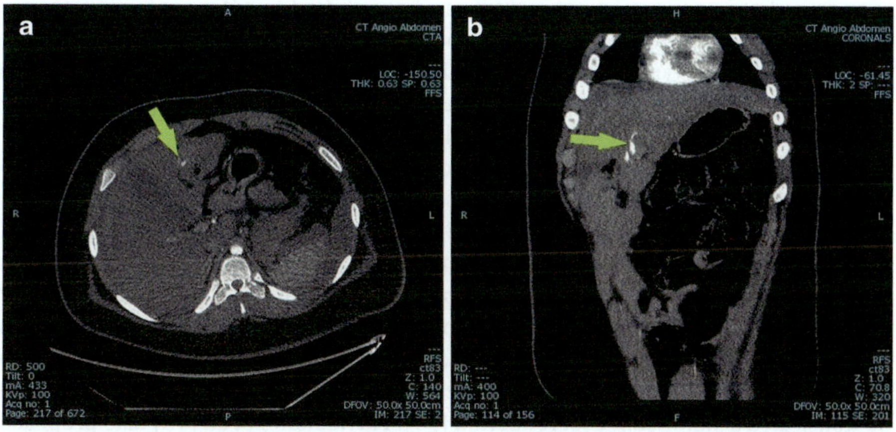

Fig. 1 (**a**, **b**) CT abdomen images (axial and coronal views) demonstrating bleeding in the liver with green arrows indicating the contrast extravasation (Courtesy of Dr. Bhupender Yadav)

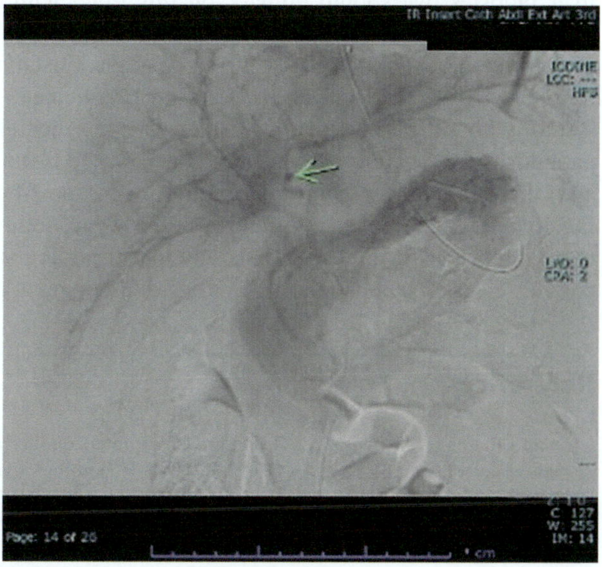

Fig. 2 IR angiography confirming post-biopsy hemorrhage (Courtesy of Dr. Bhupender Yadav)

9 What Is the Recommended Post-biopsy Observation Period?

There is currently great variability in the length of post-biopsy observation, and it is often left to the discretion of institutions or individual proceduralists. Many institutions started with an overnight observation period given the concern for the rapid decompensation that can occur in pediatric patients. With a better understanding of the risk factors for complication as well as evidence of the low rate of complications even in pediatric patients, most institutions have shifted to outpatient percutaneous liver biopsies. And several authors have published their institutions' safety and success with a shift to outpatient practices [18, 34, 38]. In the 2015 position paper on liver biopsy in children, authors recommended an initial postprocedural 2-h fasting period with at least a 6-h PACU observation [3].

Several investigators have suggested even shorter observation periods. In Govender et al.'s 2013 study, the authors reviewed their institution's policy where all patients had hematocrit levels drawn 4 h after an ultrasound-guided biopsy [33]. Those with stable hematocrits were discharged after 4 h, and the authors found no complications in these early discharge patients. Alomari and colleagues recently published their findings in 2020 paper on their quality improvement initiative to decrease the observation period from 4 to 2 h and eliminate the routine follow-up hematocrit. They likewise found no increase in complications or readmissions and demonstrated a significant cost reduction [39]. Hayatghaibi et al. [13] also proposed that a 2-h observation period after ultrasound-guided livery biopsy was sufficient for children based on their institution experience.

While there is growing excitement for the "fast-tracking" of pediatric patients for liver biopsies, we should embark on this trend with caution. At the end of this patient's procedure, the care team felt confident that he had a very routine and uneventful ultrasound-guided liver biopsy. Hemostatic agents were administered prophylactically. His anesthetic was uncomplicated, and he was transferred to PACU with no hemodynamic respiratory or other clinical concerns. Even this patient's right shoulder pain at first glance would be unremarkable as both incision and referred shoulder pain are common in the post-biopsy course. However, *this lone clinical symptom* can portend a more serious complication. It is therefore even more important for proceduralists and anesthesiologists to be vigilant in not only patient selection but also thorough clinical assessment prior to early discharge.

References

1. Vajro P, Lenta S, Socha P, et al. Diagnosis of nonalcoholic fatty liver disease in children and adolescents: position paper of the ESPGHAN Hepatology Committee. J Pediatr Gastroenterol Nutr. 2012;54(5):700–13. https://doi.org/10.1097/MPG.0b013e318252a13f.
2. Troelstra MA, Witjes JJ, van Dijk A-M, et al. Assessment of imaging modalities against liver biopsy in nonalcoholic fatty liver disease: the Amsterdam NAFLD-NASH cohort. J Magn Reson Imaging. 2021;54(6):1937–49. https://doi.org/10.1002/jmri.27703.
3. Dezsőfi A, Baumann U, Dhawan A, et al. Liver biopsy in children: position paper of the ESPGHAN Hepatology Committee. J Pediatr Gastroenterol Nutr. 2015;60(3):408–20. https://doi.org/10.1097/MPG.0000000000000632.
4. Tait AR, Voepel-Lewis T, Constance B, et al. Incidence and risk factors for perioperative adverse respiratory events in children who are obese. Anesthesiology. 2008;108:375–80.
5. Subramanyam R, Yeramaneni S, Hossain MM, Anneken AM, Varughese AM. Perioperative respiratory adverse events in pediatric ambulatory anesthesia: development and validation of a risk prediction tool. Anesth Analg. 2016;122(5):1578–85. https://doi.org/10.1213/ANE.0000000000001216.

6. Peters U, Dixon AE, Forno E. Obesity and asthma. J Allergy Clin Immunol. 2018;141(4):1169–79. https://doi.org/10.1016/j.jaci.2018.02.004.
7. Bachrach K, Danis DO 3rd, Cohen MB, Levi JR. The relationship between obstructive sleep apnea and pediatric obesity: a nationwide analysis. Ann Otol Rhinol Laryngol. 2022;131(5):520–6. https://doi.org/10.1177/00034894211028489.
8. Kyler KE, Wagner J, Hosey-Cojocari C, Watt K, Shakhnovich V. Drug dose selection in pediatric obesity: available information for the most commonly prescribed drugs to children. Paediatr Drugs. 2019;21(5):357–69. https://doi.org/10.1007/s40272-019-00352-8.
9. Nafiu OO, Reynolds PI, Bamgbade OA, Tremper KK, Welch K, Kasa-Vubu JZ. Childhood body mass index and perioperative complications. Pediatr Anesth. 2007;17(5):426–30. https://doi.org/10.1111/j.1460-9592.2006.02140.x.
10. Kako H, Tripi J, Walia H, et al. Utility of screening questionnaire and polysomnography to predict postoperative outcomes in children. Int J Pediatr Otorhinolaryngol. 2017;102:71–5. https://doi.org/10.1016/j.ijporl.2017.09.006.
11. Mpody C, Owusu-Bediako K, Raman VT, Nafiu OO. Pediatric obesity and perioperative medicine. Curr Opin Anaesthesiol. 2021;34(3):299–305. https://doi.org/10.1097/ACO.0000000000000991.
12. Eisenberg E, Konopniki M, Veitsman E, Kramskay R, Gaitini D, Baruch Y. Prevalence and characteristics of pain induced by percutaneous liver biopsy. Anesth Analg. 2003;96(5):1392–6. https://doi.org/10.1213/01.ANE.0000060453.74744.17.
13. Hayatghaibi S, Ashton D, Cleveland H, Kukreja K. Limited post-observation period in pediatric outpatient ultrasound-guided liver biopsies. Cardiovasc Intervent Radiol. 2017;40(12):1899–903. https://doi.org/10.1007/s00270-017-1720-3.
14. Gonzalez-Vallina R, Alonso EM, Rand E, Black DD, Whitington PF. Outpatient percutaneous liver biopsy in children. J Pediatr Gastroenterol Nutr. 1993;17(4):370–5. https://doi.org/10.1097/00005176-199311000-00006.
15. Westheim BH, Østensen AB, Aagenæs I, Sanengen T, Almaas R. Evaluation of risk factors for bleeding after liver biopsy in children. J Pediatr Gastroenterol Nutr. 2012;55(1):82–7. https://doi.org/10.1097/MPG.0b013e318249c12a.
16. Hoffer FA. Liver biopsy methods for pediatric oncology patients. Pediatr Radiol. 2000;30(7):481–8. https://doi.org/10.1007/s002470000244.
17. Short SS, Papillon S, Hunter CJ, et al. Percutaneous liver biopsy: pathologic diagnosis and complications in children. J Pediatr Gastroenterol Nutr. 2013;57(5):644–8. https://doi.org/10.1097/MPG.0b013e3182a0e0d8.
18. Almeida P, Schreiber RA, Liang J, Mujawar Q, Guttman OR. Clinical characteristics and complications of pediatric liver biopsy: a single centre experience. Ann Hepatol. 2017;16(5):797–801. https://doi.org/10.5604/01.3001.0010.2809.
19. Bilreiro C, Noruegas MJ, Gonçalves I, Moreira Â. Ultrasound-guided liver biopsies in children: a single-center experience and risk factors for minor bleeding. J Pediatr Gastroenterol Nutr. 2017;65(2):137–40. https://doi.org/10.1097/MPG.0000000000001601.
20. Sandy NS, Hessel G, Bellomo-Brandao MA. Major complications of pediatric percutaneous liver biopsy do not differ among physicians with different degrees of training. Am J Gastroenterol. 2020;115(5):786–9. https://doi.org/10.14309/ajg.0000000000000459.
21. Shapira-Zaltsberg G, Connolly B, Temple M, Parra DA, Amirabadi A, Amaral JG. The utility of post-biopsy ultrasonography in detecting complications after percutaneous liver biopsy in children. Pediatr Radiol. 2020;50(12):1717–23. https://doi.org/10.1007/s00247-020-04783-1.
22. Bubak ME, Porayko MK, Krom RA, Wiesner RH. Complications of liver biopsy in liver transplant patients: increased sepsis associated with choledochojejunostomy. Hepatology. 1991;14(6):1063–5. https://doi.org/10.1016/0270-9139(91)90129-J.
23. Agrawal L, Jain S, Madhusudhan KS, et al. Sepsis following liver biopsy in a liver transplant recipient: case report and review of literature. J Clin Exp Hepatol. 2021;11(2):254–9. https://doi.org/10.1016/j.jceh.2020.07.005.

24. Lowenfels AB. Kehr's sign—a neglected aid in rupture of the spleen. N Engl J Med. 1966;274(18):1019. https://doi.org/10.1056/NEJM196605052741810.
25. Ndzengue A, Hammoudeh F, Brutus P, Ajah O, Purcell R, Leadon J, Rafal RB, Balmir S, Enriquez DA, Posner GL, Jaffe EA, Chandra P. An obscure case of hepatic subcapsular hematoma. Case Rep Gastroenterol. 2011;5(1):223–6. https://doi.org/10.1159/000326998. PMID: 21552450; PMCID: PMC3088753.
26. Piccinino F, Sagnelli E, Buscarini L, et al. Complications following percutaneous liver biopsy: a multicentre retrospective study on 68 276 biopsies. J Hepatol. 1986;2(2):165–73.
27. Cohen MB, A-Kader HH, Lambers D, Heubi JE. Complications of percutaneous liver biopsy in children. Gastroenterology. 1992;102(2):629–32. https://doi.org/10.1016/0016-5085(92)90112-c.
28. Harwood J, Bishop P, Liu H, Nowicki M. Safety of blind percutaneous liver biopsy in obese children: a retrospective analysis. J Clin Gastroenterol. 2010;44(10):e253–5. https://doi.org/10.1097/MCG.0b013e3181cf8358.
29. Rockey DC, Caldwell SH, Goodman ZD, Nelson RC, Smith AD. AASLD position paper: liver biopsy. Hepatology. 2009;49(3):1017–44. https://doi.org/10.1002/hep.22786.
30. Grant A, Neuberger J. Guidelines on the use of liver biopsy in clinical practice. British Society of Gastroenterology. Gut. 1999;45 Suppl 4(Suppl 4):IV1–IV11. https://doi.org/10.1136/gut.45.2008.iv1.
31. Nobili V, Comparcola D, Sartorelli MR, et al. Blind and ultrasound-guided percutaneous liver biopsy in children. Pediatr Radiol. 2003;33(11):772–5. https://doi.org/10.1007/s00247-003-1044-0.
32. Piccinino F, Sagnelli E, Pasquale G, Giusti G. Complications following percutaneous liver biopsy. A multicentre retrospective study on 68,276 biopsies. J Hepatol. 1986;2(2):165–73. https://doi.org/10.1016/s0168-8278(86)80075-7.
33. Govender P, Jonas MM, Alomari AI, et al. Sonography-guided percutaneous liver biopsies in children. AJR Am J Roentgenol. 2013;201(3):645–50. https://doi.org/10.2214/AJR.12.9802.
34. El-Shabrawi MH, El-Karaksy HM, Okahsa SH, Kamal NM, El-Batran G, Badr KA. Outpatient blind percutaneous liver biopsy in infants and children: is it safe? Saudi J Gastroenterol. 2012;18(1):26–33. https://doi.org/10.4103/1319-3767.91735.
35. Pietrobattista A, Fruwirth R, Natali G, Monti L, Devito R, Nobili V. Is juvenile liver biopsy unsafe? Putting an end to a common misapprehension. Pediatr Radiol. 2009;39(9):959–61. https://doi.org/10.1007/s00247-009-1311-9.
36. Midia M, Odedra D, Shuster A, Midia R, Muir J. Predictors of bleeding complications following percutaneous image-guided liver biopsy: a scoping review. Diagn Interv Radiol. 2019;25(1):71–80. https://doi.org/10.5152/dir.2018.17525.
37. van Beek D, Funaki B. Hemorrhage as a complication of percutaneous liver biopsy. Semin Intervent Radiol. 2013;30(4):413–6. https://doi.org/10.1055/s-0033-1359737.
38. Kozlovich SY, Sochet AA, Son S, Wilsey MJ. Same-day versus overnight observation after outpatient pediatric percutaneous liver biopsy: a retrospective cohort study. Pediatr Gastroenterol Hepatol Nutr. 2019;22(4):377–86. https://doi.org/10.5223/pghn.2019.22.4.377.
39. Alomari MH, Kerr CL, Chewning R, et al. Two-hour observation after liver biopsy in children: clinical and economic outcome of a quality improvement intervention. J Pediatr Gastroenterol Nutr. 2020;71(4):e105–8. https://doi.org/10.1097/MPG.0000000000002821.

Teenager with Acute NPPE in PACU After Hardware Removal

Thoai An Vuong

1 Stem Case

A healthy 16-year-old, 68 kg male with ASA physical status 1 is scheduled for an elective removal of hardware. He sustained a tibial fracture 6 months prior while playing football and required fixation with orthopedic surgery. He has no other significant past medical history. Anesthesia induction is uneventful via intravenous route, and he is intubated with a 7.0 cuffed endotracheal tube (ETT) smoothly. Appropriate ETT positioning is confirmed with equal breath sounds bilaterally. He is maintained on sevoflurane 2.5% and rocuronium for paralysis and received 100 μg of fentanyl during surgery. At the end of surgery, he has two twitches on a train-of-four monitor, and he is breathing spontaneously with tidal volumes greater than 5 mL/kg. After reversal with sugammadex 2 mg/kg, the oropharynx is suctioned prior to extubation, at which point the patient coughs and desaturates after a few seconds. He suddenly bites on the endotracheal tube with both upper and lower molars on the right side where the tube is positioned. The bite block placed inside his mouth is in the midline position but is unable to prevent this occlusion. Intravenous propofol is pushed rapidly to relax the bite pressure on the tube, but because of a kinked venous catheter which required a few moments of troubleshooting, it takes a minute to get the drug into the patient. Once the jaw relaxes, the anesthesiologist is able to ventilate the patient. The patient then awakens still coughing, and the oral airway is now placed on the right side next to the endotracheal tube to prevent another occlusion of the endotracheal tube. The patient looks more awake and suddenly raises his arms and reaches toward the ETT and extubates himself while coughing.

T. A. Vuong (✉)
Division of Anesthesiology, Pain and Perioperative Medicine, Children's National Hospital, George Washington University SMHS, Washington, DC, USA
e-mail: tvuong@childrensnational.org

S. T. Verghese (ed.), *Anesthesia STAT! Acute Pediatric Emergencies in PACU*,
https://doi.org/10.1007/978-3-031-24396-7_9

He however continues to be restless and combative. The anesthesiologist applying the face mask with 10 L of 100% O_2 notices no air movement despite noticeable chest excursion with good respiratory effort. The APL valve is closed, and continuous positive airway pressure (CPAP) is applied while the nurse and surgeon are attempting to keep the patient calm and still. The pulse oximetry reading decreases to 78%, and after applying 70 cm H_2O of CPAP for 5 seconds, the patient coughs, and condensation is seen in the mask along with capnometry confirmation of air movement. The patient's respiratory pattern is regular with no further episodes of obstruction, and the saturation increases to 97% with mask support until the patient starts re-emerging and responds appropriately. His respiratory support is de-escalated, and he is placed on blow-by face mask with 6 L of O_2. He is transported to the PACU, but his work of breathing is noted to be progressively labored and tachypneic, and the patient has developed a wet cough. His saturations decline to 90%, and he complains that he cannot breathe. He continues to cough and expectorates frothy pink sputum. His oxygen support is increased to 15 L of O_2 on face mask, and his saturation does not improve. Breath sounds are decreased with crepitations bilaterally on auscultation. He is trialed on CPAP with the Jackson-Rees circuit and the APL valve slightly closed, with modest improvement of saturations to 91%. A CXR and venous blood gas are urgently obtained and shown in Fig. 1 and Table 1, respectively.

At this point the patient appears fatigued with significant work of breathing. The decision is made to induce anesthesia, reintubate, and continue care in the intensive care unit (ICU).

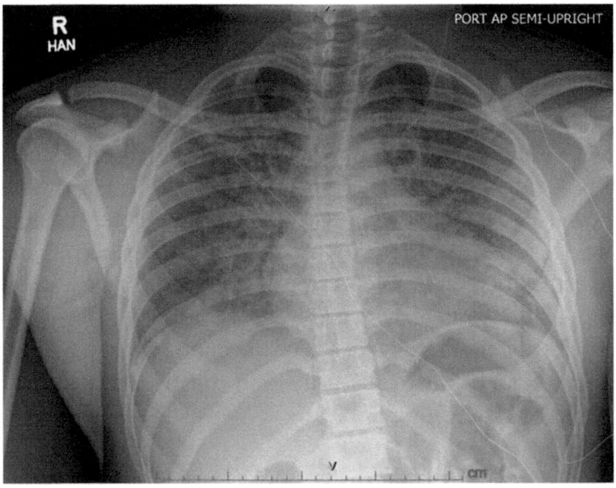

Fig. 1 Urgent portable chest radiograph. CXR report: bilateral perihilar and diffuse hazy opacities most likely reflecting edema. Otherwise, unremarkable

Table 1 Venous blood gas result

Venous blood gas	
pH	7.196
CO_2	72
O_2	43.7
HCO_3	20
Lactate	1.79

2 What Is Negative Pressure Pulmonary Edema?

Negative pressure pulmonary edema (NPPE) is defined as a form of noncardiogenic pulmonary edema (PE) that results from the generation of high negative intrathoracic pressure needed to overcome upper airway obstruction.

The phenomenon of pulmonary edema occurring after a known episode of airway obstruction has been described over the decades by several terms including negative pressure pulmonary edema, post-obstructive pulmonary edema, post-extubation pulmonary edema, and post-laryngospasm pulmonary edema. This occurrence is serious and potentially life-threatening; however if promptly identified and treated, NPPE leads to a favorable outcome.

Moore first suggested in 1927 that acute airway obstruction, particularly that prolonged inspiration against a fixed resistance, could lead to pulmonary edema based on experiments with dogs under anesthesia [1, 2].

In 1960 Swann observed pulmonary edema developing in victims of hanging at autopsy; however whether this was a pre- or post-hanging occurrence was not known at the time [3].

It was then reported in 1966 that pediatric patients with tonsillar and adenoid hypertrophy developed pulmonary edema due to changes in intrathoracic pressure caused by breathing against an obstructed airway [4].

Pulmonary edema in children following upper airway obstruction was further observed and described in 1973 by Capitanio [5]. These cases were due to obstruction from croup and epiglottitis, and within several years others reported the same phenomena in children [6, 7].

In 1977 Oswalt et al. published the first case reports of NPPE in adults, with upper airway obstruction from laryngeal tumor, strangulation, and interrupted hanging [8].

Since then, the majority of NPPE literature published have been case reports or case series.

3 How Common Is NPPE?

The estimated incidence of NPPE in adults is 0.01–0.1% during general anesthesia, although it is suggested that this is underestimated as NPPE is commonly misdiagnosed and subclinical cases are overlooked [2, 9–11].

NPPE has been observed to have a higher prevalence among otolaryngology patients, with reports of up to 11% [12, 13]. A large retrospective study of 30,000 adult patients found that of all patients who developed NPPE, 63% had ear, nose, and throat surgery [11, 13].

Although the data in pediatric patients is limited to case series and reports, the prevalence of NPPE in children appears to be similarly rare. Earlier publications in the 1980s cited an incidence of 7–12% [2, 14–16]; however more recent studies have reported much lower rates.

A retrospective cohort study published in 2014, with 216 pediatric patients undergoing adenotonsillectomy or tonsillectomy, reported 9 cases of NPPE, a prevalence of 4.3% [17]. Another cohort study in 2015 of 221 children undergoing adenotonsillectomy reported 1 case of pulmonary edema, a prevalence of 0.45% [18].

The male gender has been reported to account for the majority of NPPE cases, representing 62–80% of all cases [13, 19, 20]. In pediatric literature, the male-female ratio is 2.4–1 [2]. A retrospective, observational study, using data prospectively collected over 35 years in an ICU, showed that diffuse alveolar hemorrhage occurred commonly in young athletic males [21]. This accounts for the widely accepted theory that young healthy male patients tend to generate higher negative thoracic pressures leading to NPPE [19, 20, 22, 23].

4 What Are the Etiology, Pathophysiology, and Risk Factors of NPPE?

NPPE occurs due to an acute negative intrathoracic pressure produced during spontaneous respiration against an obstructed upper airway [23]. Two classifications have been developed over the years, Type I and Type II, and are differentiated by the inciting event [9, 13, 23, 24]. Type I NPPE is caused by an acute airway obstruction. Type II NPPE develops after chronic upper airway obstruction is relieved, typified by children with obstructive sleep apnea presenting for adenotonsillectomy. A study of NPPE in otolaryngology patients revealed Type I to be more common representing the majority (72%) of cases [13]. Examples of causes of NPPE are listed in Table 2.

In our patient from the case study, there was an airway occlusion initially caused by him biting on the endotracheal tube after muscle relaxant reversal, and it could have initiated the genesis of NPPE which worsened after the laryngospasm that occurred after extubation. Biting on the patent endotracheal tube is another factor that has been reported as the etiology of NPPE [26].

Another cause of airway obstruction that can be subtle is the occurrence of vigorous hiccups in anesthetized patients. Hiccups are spontaneous powerful inspiratory efforts albeit brief that occur when the glottis is closed, and this seemingly benign clinical effort has been reported to be the cause of NPPE [27].

Table 2 Most common NPPE causes in pediatric and adult patients [9, 10, 25]

	Type I NPPE	Type II NPPE
Pediatric	Laryngospasm	Post-tonsillectomy/ adenoidectomy
	Epiglottitis	Post-hypertrophic uvula excision
	Croup	Post-choanal stenosis surgery
	Foreign body	
	Hiccups	
Adults	Endotracheal tube obstruction, e.g., biting	Post-relief of upper airway tumor
	Laryngospasm	
	Strangulation/hanging	
	Near drowning	
	Goiter	
	Vocal paralysis	
	Migration of Foley catheter balloon for epistaxis tamponade	

Four main pathophysiological mechanisms have been proposed for Type I NPPE, as illustrated in Fig. 2, and include the following:

- Intense respiratory effort against a closed airway, usually due to laryngospasm or tube occlusion.
- Damage to capillaries with transvascular fluid shift to the lung interstitium causing alveolar edema.
- Negative inspiratory pressures (−50 to −140 cm H_2O) cause an increase in venous return to the heart. Elevated ventricular end-diastolic volumes and pressures ensue and result in pulmonary edema [29].
- Hypoxemia from airway obstruction causes increased pulmonary vascular resistance and capillary pressure. The damaged capillary bed has increased permeability leading to a transudation and pulmonary edema [23, 30].

Pulmonary edema fluid from patients with NPPE showed a low protein concentration which supports the theory that the main mechanism of its pathophysiology is hydrostatic forces exerted on the pulmonary vasculature by tremendously high negative inspiratory pressure [20]. Another study found a low pulmonary edema fluid-to-serum protein ratio with normal alveolar fluid clearance, further supporting a hydrostatic mechanism for edema fluid formation [29].

The pathogenesis of NPPE is multifactorial, ranging from transudative to high-permeability edema when a very high transmural pulmonary capillary pressure has been produced [28].

A clear understanding of the normal pulmonary fluid homeostasis helps one to identify the pathophysiological mechanisms for NPPE formation [28].

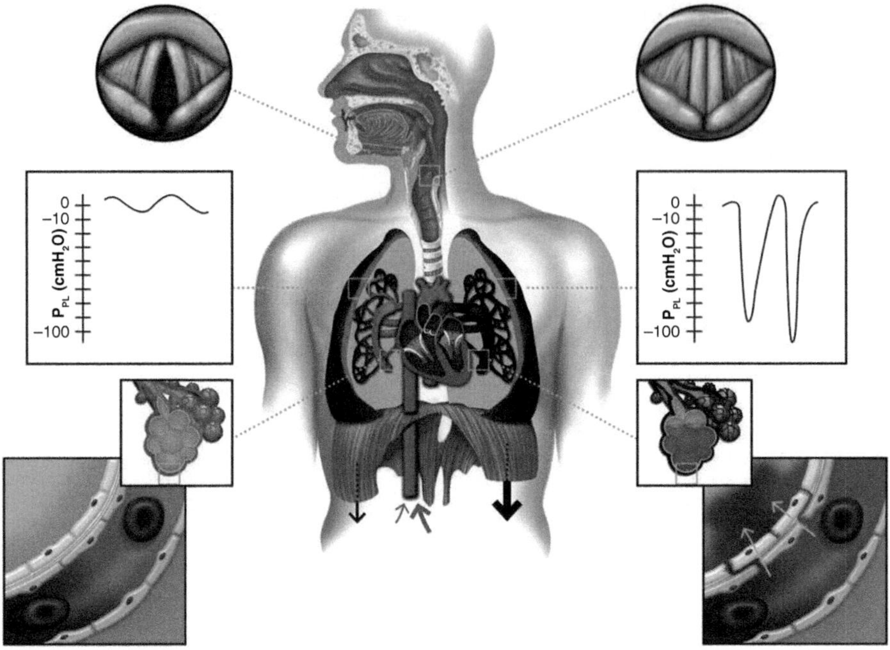

Fig. 2 Normal airway mechanics and NPPE mechanics[28]

The left side of the illustration depicts normal breathing, as the glottis is open and minimal diaphragmatic muscle exertion leads to minor changes in negative pleural pressure during inspiration. This creates a small alveolar-capillary pressure gradient, and any hydrostatic pressures driving fluid into the pulmonary capillary bed can be compensated by lymphatic drainage [28].

The right side illustrates breathing against a closed glottis. Mechanical stress generated by muscular forces (negative intrathoracic pressures up to −140 cm H_2O) trying to inspire against a closed glottis can produce tears in both alveolar epithelial and pulmonary microvascular membranes causing increased pulmonary capillary permeability and pulmonary edema [28].

Chronic airway obstruction, however, leads to a different mechanism to NPPE as it provides an auto-positive end-expiratory pressure (PEEP). Once this chronic airway obstruction is relieved, the auto-PEEP is absent, and this leads to a relative negative intrapulmonary pressure, resulting in transudation of fluids [23, 31]. The pathophysiology of Type II NPPE is shown in Fig. 3.

Although rare, the presence of one or more risk factors increases the probability of NPPE occurrence in patients. These include patient age less than 3 years, otolaryngologic surgery, asthma, history of prematurity or chronic lung disease, obstructive sleep apnea (OSA), trisomy 21, and craniofacial malformations [13, 24].

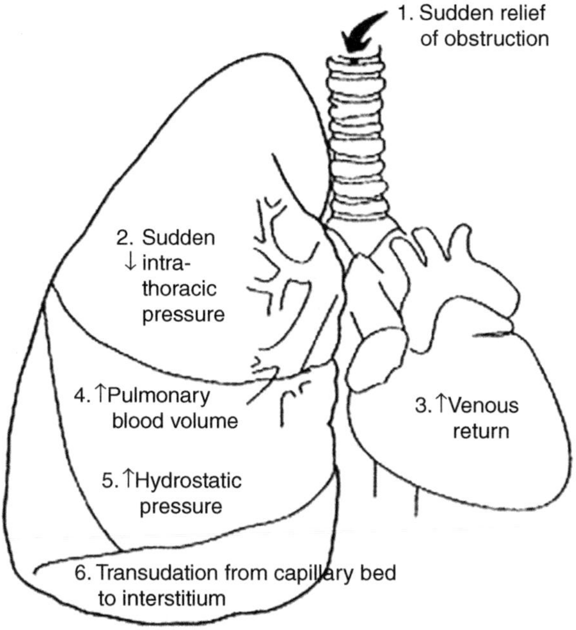

Fig. 3 Pathophysiology of NPPE Type II [25]

5 How Does NPPE Present?

The clinical features of NPPE can be grouped into two stages [30]. The first stage portends to airway obstruction. In the setting of emergence from anesthesia, this is usually manifested as biting on the endotracheal tube before extubation, or after extubation with laryngospasm or stridor with retractions of the suprasternal and supraclavicular muscles due to the obstruction.

The second stage relates to the relief of obstruction and the development of pulmonary edema. The work of breathing is increased with tachypnea, tachycardia, and use of accessory muscles of respiration. The respiratory distress is accompanied by hypoxia and coughing of pink frothy secretions [2, 9, 13, 19, 20, 23, 30, 32]. On auscultation crackles and wheezing may be heard. These signs and symptoms typically follow soon after extubation; however the onset of pulmonary edema may not occur until several hours into the postoperative period [9, 24].

For adenotonsillectomy patients with OSA that develop Type II NPPE, the onset of pulmonary edema may be rapid and immediately following intubation or extubation due to the loss of auto-PEEP [33].

A chest radiograph reveals diffuse interstitial and alveolar infiltrates bilaterally. A computed tomography of the chest shows ground glass attenuation in the central and nondependent lung fields. [23, 32, 34] This is in contrast to other forms of pulmonary edema, which preferentially are located in the dependent and peripheral lung regions [9].

6 What Is the Differential Diagnosis?

Important differentials must include aspiration pneumonitis, volume overload, cardiogenic or neurogenic pulmonary edema, acute respiratory distress syndrome (ARDS), pulmonary embolism, and anaphylaxis [2, 23, 25].

Although more likely in adults, cardiogenic pulmonary edema should be considered in pediatric patients with a history of congenital cardiac disease. Neurogenic pulmonary edema, resulting from an autonomic dysfunction and sympathetic overdrive that increases pulmonary capillary pressure and fluid transudation, should be considered in patients with acute neurological injuries such as head or spine trauma, metabolic encephalopathy, as well as pheochromocytomas [23]. Multiple etiologies may account for an acute lung injury that may lead to ARDS such as trauma, burns, sepsis, and blood transfusion reaction. While also a diagnosis of exclusion, anaphylactic pulmonary edema is often precipitated by the administration of commonly implicated drugs such as muscle relaxants and antibiotics and then immediately followed by multi-organ manifestations including tachycardia, hypotension, bronchospasm, urticaria, or skin rash.

7 Which Tests Will Be Helpful in Making the Diagnosis?

NPPE is a clinical diagnosis made when other etiologies have been ruled out. The typical appearance of a chest radiograph, depicted in Fig. 1, is confirmatory and helps differentiate NPPE from aspiration pneumonitis, volume overload, and other causes of pulmonary edema. In addition to the appearance of the chest radiograph, the timing of resolution as shown on imaging is also unique to NPPE. Studies indicate that radiologic changes due to NPPE rapidly resolve within 24 h; however radiologic changes due to aspiration pneumonitis were much slower to resolve with only half normalizing after 3 days [10, 25, 35]. An arterial blood gas is also commonly employed. If cardiogenic etiology is a concern, an electrocardiogram, echocardiogram, and cardiac enzymes should be obtained. Levels of histamine and tryptase may help to rule out anaphylaxis.

8 How Should NPPE Be Treated?

The mainstay of therapy for patients with NPPE should be supportive care and close monitoring of patients in an intensive care unit or subacute care unit.

The airway should be free of obstruction, and if laryngospasm or endotracheal tube biting is observed, an anesthetic agent (such as propofol) or paralytic agent (such as succinylcholine) should be administered [24]. Hypoxemia should be corrected with oxygenation and an escalation of oxygen delivery should be employed as necessary.

In mild cases, where the airway is stable without further obstruction and oxygen saturations are reliably maintained with supplemental oxygen, these patients may be closely observed in the step-down unit.

Persistent airway obstruction or acute respiratory failure requires mechanical ventilation with PEEP and monitoring in the ICU. The use of noninvasive respiratory support with continuous positive airway pressure (CPAP) or bi-level positive airway pressure (BiPAP) in these patients decreases work of breathing, improves gas exchange, and improves hemodynamics by reducing left ventricular preload and afterload [9]. Thus the use of CPAP and BiPAP has been an effective means to reduce intubation rates, ICU length of stay, hospital length of stay, and overall morbidity and mortality [36, 37].

In severe cases, invasive mechanical ventilation should be provided with PEEP. PEEP is required to maintain functional residual capacity and lung inflation. It is also thought to lessen the transudation from capillaries into the interstitium and redistribute alveolar fluid into the interstitial spaces, thereby improving pulmonary edema [12, 31, 32]. A review of pediatric NPPE cases indicated that the majority of these patients (85%) required reintubation [2, 11, 31].

The use of diuretics and steroids has been frequently employed previously; however the evidence to support this practice is lacking, and clinicians must pay attention to the patient's fluid status, renal function, and hemodynamics when considering diuretic therapy [2, 9, 10, 23–25, 32, 33].

In the rare and catastrophic event of failed mechanical ventilation, successful resolution of NPPE with venovenous extracorporeal membrane oxygenation has been reported in adults [38].

9 What Is the Typical Course of NPPE?

NPPE has an excellent prognosis if identified and treated early. As long as the alveolar fluid clearance mechanisms are intact, the resolution of NPPE is rapid. [20] The literature overwhelmingly indicates the resolution of pulmonary edema typically within 24 h with appropriate management [2, 20, 22, 23, 30–33]. Historically significant morbidity and mortality have been associated with NPPE with mortality rates up to 40%; however this is thought to be due to a delay in diagnosis and management [9, 12, 13, 32]. A more recent literature review estimates the mortality rate of NPPE to be 2–4% [13].

10 Conclusion

NPPE is a serious respiratory complication associated with upper airway obstruction in the postanesthetic period. Although rare, it may be more common in children receiving otolaryngologic surgeries, age less than 3, and with history of asthma, trisomy 21, OSA, and craniofacial abnormalities. NPPE should be considered in any patient with a witnessed airway obstruction followed by respiratory distress and coughing pink frothy sputum. The inciting airway obstructing event is commonly laryngospasm, ETT biting, epiglottitis, or croup. Although a clinical diagnosis of exclusion, a chest radiography is useful to differentiate from other causes as well as monitor the progression and resolution of NPPE. Therapy should include relief of airway obstruction, oxygenation, and mechanical ventilation with PEEP as necessary. The institution of CPAP or BiPAP has been shown to be an extremely effective therapy for NPPE. Prompt identification and management of NPPE provide an excellent prognosis and resolution within 24 h.

References

1. Moore R. The response to respiratory resistance: a comparison of the effects produced by partial obstruction in the inspiratory and expiratory phases of respiration. J Exp Med. 1927;45:1065–80.
2. Ringold S, Klein EJ, Del Beccaro MA. Postobstructive pulmonary edema in children. Pediatr Emerg Care. 2004;20(6):391–5.
3. Swann HJ. Occurrence of pulmonary oedema in sudden asphyxial death. Arch Pathol Lab Med. 1960;69:557–70.
4. Luke MJ, Mehrizi A, Folger GM, Rowe RD. Chronic nasopharyngeal obstruction as a cause of cardiomegaly, cor pulmonale, and pulmonary edema. Pediatrics. 1966;37(5):762–8.
5. Capitanio MA, Kirkpatrick JA. Obstruction of the upper airway in children as reflected on the chest radiograph. Pediatr Radiol. 1973;107:159–61.
6. Travis KW, Todres ID, Shannon DC. Pulmonary edema associated with croup and epiglottitis. Pediatrics. 1977;59(5):695–8.
7. Soliman MG, Richer P. Epiglottitis and pulmonary oedema in children. Can Anaesth Soc J. 1978;25(4):270–5.
8. Oswalt CE, Gates GA, Holmstrom MG. Pulmonary edema as a complication of acute airway obstruction. JAMA. 1977;238:1833–5.
9. Bhaskar B, Fraser JF. Negative pressure pulmonary edema revisited: pathophysiology and review of management. Saudi J Anaesth. 2011;5(3):308–13.
10. McConkey P. Postobstructive pulmonary oedema—a case series and review. Anaesth Intensive Care. 2000;28(1):72–6.
11. Deepika K, Kenaan CA, Barrocas AM, Fonseca JJ, Bikazi GB. Negative pressure pulmonary edema after acute upper airway obstruction. J Clin Anesth. 1997;9:403–8.
12. Goldenberg JD, Portugal LG, Wenig BL, Weingarten RT. Negative-pressure pulmonary edema in the otolaryngology patient. Otolaryngol Head Neck Surg. 1997;117(1):62–6.
13. Din-Lovinescu C, Trivedi U, Zhang K, Barinsky GL, Grube JG, Eloy JA, Hsueh WD. Systematic review of negative pressure pulmonary edema in otolaryngology procedures. Ann Otol Rhinol Laryngol. 2021;130(3):245–53.
14. Davis HW, Gartner JC, Galvis AG, Michaels RH, Mestad PH. Acute upper airway obstruction: croup and epiglottitis. Pediatr Clin North Am. 1981;28(4):859–80.
15. Galvis AG. Pulmonary edema complicating relief of upper airway obstruction. Am J Emerg Med. 1987;5(4):294–7.
16. Kanter RK, Watchko JF. Pulmonary edema associated with upper airway obstruction. Am J Dis Child. 1984;138(4):356–8.
17. Sonsuwan N, Pornlert A, Sawanyawisuth K. Risk factors for acute pulmonary edema after adenotonsillectomy in children. Auris Nasus Larynx. 2014;41(4):373–5.
18. Konstantinopoulou S, Gallagher P, Elden L, Garetz SL, Mitchell RB, Redline S, Rosen CL, Katz ES, Chervin RD, Amin R, Arens R, Paruthi S, Marcus CL. Complications of

adenotonsillectomy for obstructive sleep apnea in school-aged children. Int J Pediatr Otorhinolaryngol. 2015;79(2):240–5.
19. Tsai PH, Wang JH, Huang SC, Lin YK, Lam CF. Characterizing post-extubation negative pressure pulmonary edema in the operating room—a retrospective matched case-control study. Perioper Med (Lond). 2018;7:28.
20. Bhattacharya M, Kallet RH, Ware LB, Matthay MA. Negative-pressure pulmonary edema. Chest. 2016;150(4):927–33.
21. Contou D, Voiriot G, Djibré M, Labbé V, Fartoukh M, Parrot A. Clinical features of patients with diffuse alveolar hemorrhage due to negative-pressure pulmonary edema. Lung. 2017;195(4):477–87.
22. Liu RZ, Wang J, Zhao GQ, Su ZB. Negative pressure pulmonary edema after general anesthesia. Medicine. 2019;98(17):e15389.
23. Singh BS, Kulshrestha A. Diagnosis, prevention and management of postoperative pulmonary edema. Ann Med Health Sci Res. 2012;2(2):180–5.
24. Ahmed E, Almutairi NK. Pulmonary edema post-adenotonsillectomy in children. Saudi Med J. 2018;39(6):551–7.
25. Udeshi A, Cantie SM, Pierre E. Postobstructive pulmonary edema. J Crit Care. 2010;25(3):508.e1–5.
26. Dicpinigaitis PV, Mehta DC. Postobstructive pulmonary edema induced by endotracheal tube occlusion. Intensive Care Med. 1995;21(12):1048–50.
27. Stuth EAE, Stucke AG, Berens RJ. Negative-pressure pulmonary edema in a child with hiccups during induction. Anesthesiology. 2000;93:282–4.
28. Lemyze M, Mallat J. Understanding negative pressure pulmonary edema. Intensive Care Med. 2014;40(8):1140–3.
29. Fremont RD, Kallet RH, Matthay MA, Ware LB. Postobstructive pulmonary edema: a case for hydrostatic mechanisms. Chest. 2007;131:1742–6.
30. Scarbrough FE, Wittenberg JM, Smith BR, Adcock DK. Pulmonary edema following postoperative laryngospasm: case reports and review of the literature. Anesth Prog. 1997;44(3):110–6.
31. Lang SA, Duncan PG, Shephard DA, Ha HC. Pulmonary oedema associated with airway obstruction. Can J Anaesth. 1990;37:210–8.
32. Thiagarajan RR, Laussen PC. Negative pressure pulmonary edema in children—pathogenesis and clinical management. Paediatr Anaesth. 2007;17(4):307–10.
33. Austin AL, Kon A, Matteucci MJ. Respiratory failure in a child due to type 2 postobstructive pulmonary edema. Pediatr Emerg Care. 2016;32(1):23–4.
34. Cascade PN, Alexander GD, Mackie DS. Negative-pressure pulmonary edema after endotracheal intubation. Radiology. 1993;186:671–5.
35. Landay MJ, Christensen EE, Bynum LJ. Pulmonary manifestations of acute aspiration of gastric contents. Am J Roentgenol. 1978;131:587–92.
36. Jaber S, Chanques G, Jung B. Postoperative noninvasive ventilation. J Am Soc Anesthesiol. 2010;112:453–61.
37. Pelosi P, Jaber S. Noninvasive respiratory support in the perioperative period. Curr Opin Anaesthesiol. 2010;23:233–8.
38. Matsumura K, Toyoda Y, Matsumoto S, Funabiki T. Near-fatal negative pressure pulmonary oedema successfully treated with venovenous extracorporeal membrane oxygenation performed in the hybrid emergency room. BMJ Case Rep. 2020;13(9):e234651.

Latex Allergy Developing in PACU in a Child with Spina Bifida After Suprapubic Catheter Placement

Mingfei Wang

Objectives
- Define spina bifida and its different forms.
- Describe the pathophysiology of latex allergy.
- Understand the correlation between spina bifida and latex allergy.
- Recognize the symptoms of an allergic reaction and anaphylaxis.
- Assess and manage patients with anaphylaxis.

1 Case Presentation

A 2-year-old, 16 kg boy with past medical history of a VP shunt for hydrocephalus, repaired myelomeningocele, and neurogenic bladder presents at our children's hospital for a suprapubic catheter placement. Patient is well known to the preoperative team because he has had more than ten surgeries and procedures in the past year due to various comorbidities and complications associated with his myelomeningocele. The only other significant history from the parent was the tendency for the patient to develop croup during certain seasons. Previous anesthetics have been reviewed and were uneventful.

1. What is spina bifida?
2. What are the different types of spina bifida?
3. What other organ system abnormalities are often associated with spina bifida?
4. What are some of the associated physiological problems in children with spina bifida?

M. Wang (✉)
Children's National Medical Center, Washington, DC, USA
e-mail: mwang2@childrensnational.org

S. T. Verghese (ed.), *Anesthesia STAT! Acute Pediatric Emergencies in PACU*,
https://doi.org/10.1007/978-3-031-24396-7_10

Patient was given PO midazolam as the anxiolytic before induction. He was induced with inhaled nitrous oxide and sevoflurane. An intravenous catheter was placed in the upper extremity. At first, a laryngeal mask airway was attempted; however due to airway obstruction and improper seating, patient was eventually intubated with rocuronium. Before the start of surgery, vancomycin was requested by the surgeon as antibiotic prophylaxis. After a test dose, the drug was infused slowly and vital signs were monitored closely. The rest of the surgery was uneventful, and patient was extubated awake without any issue. He presents to the PACU still recovering from his anesthetic. His breathing is a bit noisy with an occasional mild croupy cough. The croupy cough worsens after he wakes up and now, he is crying inconsolably. He is tachycardic and tachypneic and seems to have developed a red rash over his face, trunk, and limbs and as well as the erythema around his newly placed suprapubic catheter. On auscultation of his lungs, diffuse wheezes are heard bilaterally.

5. What is your differential diagnosis for the croupy cough and body rash and what is your plan of management?
6. Could this be the red man syndrome (RMS) due to vancomycin being flushed inadvertently into the patient at the end of surgery?
7. Could this be from the neuromuscular blocker that was used?
8. What other medications are commonly associated with allergic reactions and anaphylaxis?

Upon further questioning, it was determined that the circulating nurse had mistakenly given the surgeon a latex-containing suprapubic catheter which was not supposed to be in the OR. The suprapubic catheter is promptly removed. Patient is now profoundly hypotensive with a blood pressure of 43/23.

Multiple large-bore IVs are obtained. After aggressive fluid resuscitation and multiple doses of IM epinephrine, patient remains profoundly hypotensive.

9. Do these new findings change your differential and management?
10. What is latex and where is it commonly found in the hospital setting?
11. What is the pathophysiology of latex allergy?
12. Why do patients with spina bifida especially myelomeningocele have increased risk for latex allergy?
13. What is anaphylaxis?
14. What are the signs and symptoms of anaphylaxis?
15. What are the diagnostic criteria for anaphylaxis?
16. What laboratory test should be sent for suspected anaphylaxis?
17. How do you manage a patient with anaphylaxis?
18. What is your next step in the management of this patient?
19. Which patients should be admitted or discharged after an anaphylactic reaction?
20. What can be done to prevent latex allergy in high-risk patients?

2 Discussion

2.1 Spina Bifida

Spina bifida, which encompasses a range of malformations, is a congenital defect caused by the failure of the neural tube to close by the fourth week postconception. This leads to deformities of the spinal cord and vertebral column. Most occurrences of neural tube defect are isolated and multifactorial; however they can be associated with certain genetic syndromes, chromosomal abnormalities, nutritional deficiencies, or environmental exposures. The incidence of spina bifida is highly variable across ethnicities, geographical locations, and genders. In the United States, the rate is approximately 0.2 per 1000 births and is more common in boys than girls. Across ethnicities, the highest rates are found in the Caucasian and Hispanic population [1]. Folic acid deficiency during the first trimester has been linked to neural tube defects and spina bifida. The rates of neural tube defects have dramatically decreased since folic acid supplementation and food fortification were implemented in the 1990s [2].

Spina bifida can be classified into three categories: occulta, meningocele, and myelomeningocele (Fig. 1).

In spina bifida occulta, there is a defect to one or more vertebrae; however the neural tissue and meninges are unaffected, and the patients are usually asymptomatic. As much 10–20% of the general population may have spina bifida occulta.

Meningocele is the rarest form of spina bifida characterized by the protrusion of a spinal fluid-filled sac or meninges without neural tissue through a vertebral defect. Meningocele accounts for about 5% of patients with spina bifida.

Myelomeningocele, the most common and severe form, accounts for 75% or more of all spina bifida cases [3]. In myelomeningocele, the spinal cord, neural tissue, and meninges protrude through the vertebral arch. The most common location is in the lumbosacral region; however it can occur anywhere along the spine.

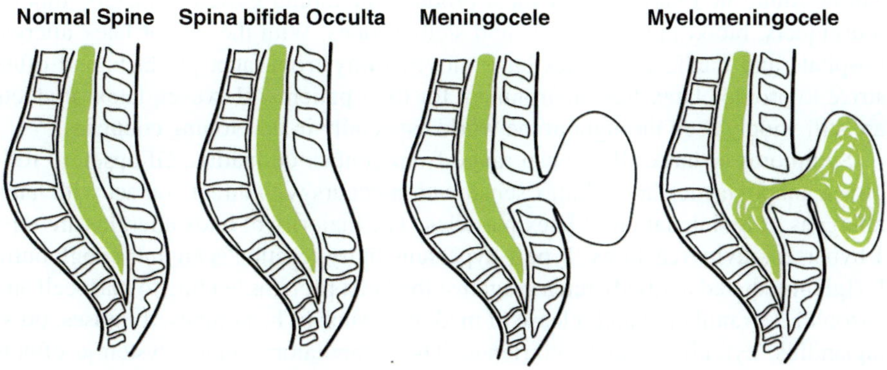

Fig. 1 Types of spina bifida

Although some patients with spina bifida are symptoms-free, the majority of patients especially those with myelomeningocele have neurologic, musculoskeletal, gastrointestinal, and urologic abnormalities. Common neurologic complications include Arnold Chiari II malformation, obstructive hydrocephalus, and tethered cord. Intellectual disability occurs infrequently but can affect up to 20–25% of spina bifida patients. Patients with spina bifida usually have normal kidney functions; however sacral nerves S2–4 are almost always affected leading to neurogenic bladder, frequent urinary tract infections, vesicoureteral reflux, and hydronephrosis. Similarly, intestinal motility and rectal sphincter tone are affected in almost 90% of patients with spina bifida leading to constipation and fecal incontinence [4]. The degree of musculoskeletal derangement depends on the level of the spinal defect. The higher the level, the greater the effect, ranging from minor mobility difficulties to complete paraplegia.

2.2 Latex

Latex is derived from the sap of the plant, *Hevea brasiliensis*. Natural rubber latex undergoes extensive manufacturing processes resulting in the final commercial and consumer product. Natural latex contains more than 240 polypeptides with at least 15 known allergenic proteins (Hev b 1 to 15). Spina bifida patients are primarily sensitized against Hev b 1 and b 3, while healthcare workers are primarily sensitized against Hev b 5 and b 6 [5]. Latex allergy was first documented in the 1930s; however incidence peaked in the 1980s to 1990s when high protein content latex gloves were mass-produced to combat the HIV and hepatitis C epidemic [6]. Latex proteins have also been found to have high cross-reactivity with certain fruits such as avocado, banana, kiwi, and chestnut. Patients with allergies to these fruits should be considered high risk for latex allergy as well [7].

Latex has many beneficial properties such as tear resistance, strong tensile, and elongation abilities making it ideal for many medical and household products. Latex can be found in a variety of medical products including gloves, catheters, tubing, tourniquets, blood pressure cuffs, and stethoscopes. With the rise of latex allergy, hospitals and medical facilities have moved away from latex products and often strive to provide latex-free environment for their patients. However, latex products are still widely used throughout the world especially in developing countries.

Symptoms of latex allergy can range from contact dermatitis, GI upset, to full-blown anaphylactic shock. Latex sensitization occurs with direct contact with latex allergens or by inhalation of latex particles. The majority of latex allergies are type 1 hypersensitivity reactions. Type 1 hypersensitivity reaction is an immunoglobulin E (IgE)-mediated antibody release against the latex proteins leading to mast cell and basophil degranulation and release of mediators such as histamines, tryptases, prostaglandins, cytokine, and leukotrienes. These mediators induce systemic effects such as vasodilation, bronchospasm, nausea/vomiting, mucosal edema, and tachycardia. This reaction is almost immediate and occurs usually within minutes of exposure. Very rarely patients may develop a delayed type 4 hypersensitivity reaction to latex. Type 4 hypersensitivity reaction typically occurs 24–48 h postexposure and is mediated by activated T cells or macrophages leading to tissue inflammation and damage. Most of the delayed reactions are not due to latex proteins but due to other components and preservatives added during the manufacturing process.

Children with spina bifida often have orthopedic, urologic, gastrointestinal, and neurologic abnormalities requiring multiple surgeries and procedures during their first few years of life. The repeated hospitalizations and exposure to latex allergens during surgeries and procedures increase the risk for latex allergy. The prevalence of latex allergy in patients with spina bifida has been documented to be as high as 70% compared to just 1–2% in the general population [8, 9].

2.3 Anaphylaxis

Anaphylaxis is a severe systemic hypersensitivity reaction characterized by rapid onset with life- threatening airway, breathing, and circulatory collapse with or without cutaneous or mucosal changes. The most common allergens to cause anaphylaxis in the perioperative settings are antibiotics, neuromuscular blocking agents, and latex. It can be difficult to identify the symptoms of anaphylaxis under general anesthesia, and there are a multitude of reactions that can mimic anaphylaxis. Vancomycin is a glycopeptide antibiotic and is the most prescribed parenteral antimicrobial for treating methicillin-resistant ***Staphylococcus aureus*** (MRSA) infections. Adverse effects of vancomycin include nephrotoxicity, ototoxicity, and red man syndrome (RMS). RMS is secondary to histamine release and not due to a true IgE- mediated allergic reaction and therefore not a true allergy [10]. True anaphylaxis can affect almost every system in the body. The symptoms of anaphylaxis are summarized in Table 1.

The diagnostic criteria for anaphylaxis according to the National Institute of Allergy and Infectious Diseases are summarized in Table 2.

Confirmatory test for anaphylaxis should not delay treatment. The primary mediator of anaphylaxis is histamine; however the half-life of plasma histamine is only 15–20 min which limits its usefulness. Serum tryptase in comparison has a plasma

Table 1 Symptoms of anaphylaxis

Systems	Signs and symptoms
Mucocutaneous	Warmth, erythema, pruritus, urticaria, angioedema, piloerection, cyanosis
Upper airway	Angioedema of lips, tongue, uvula, and palate, rhinorrhea, congestion, hoarseness, voice changes, stridor, cough
Lower airway	Dyspnea, bronchospasm, tachypnea, respiratory arrest
Gastrointestinal	Nausea, vomiting, dysphagia, abdominal pain or cramping, diarrhea, urine/fecal incontinence
Cardiovascular	Hypotension, tachycardia, bradycardia, dysrhythmia, dizziness, syncope, chest pain, cardiac arrest
Neurologic	Fussiness, anxiety, altered mental status, headache, seizure, sense of impending doom, behavioral changes

Adopted from ref. [11]

Table 2 Diagnostic criteria for anaphylaxis

Anaphylaxis is highly likely when any *one* of the three following criteria is fulfilled:	
Criteria 1	Sudden onset of an illness (minutes to several hours), with involvement of the skin, mucosal tissue, or both (e.g., generalized hives, itching or flushing, swollen lips-tongue-uvula)
	<u>*And*</u> at least one of the following:
	1. Sudden respiratory symptoms and signs (e.g., shortness of breath, wheeze, cough, stridor, hypoxemia)
	2. Sudden hypotension or symptoms of end-organ dysfunction (e.g., hypotonia, collapse, incontinence)
Criteria 2	Two or more of the following that occur suddenly after exposure to a likely allergen or other trigger for that patient (minutes to several hours):
	1. Sudden skin or mucosal symptoms and signs (e.g., generalized hives, itch-flush, swollen lips-tongue-uvula)
	2. Sudden respiratory symptoms and signs (e.g., shortness of breath, wheeze, cough, stridor, hypoxemia)
	3. Sudden hypotension or symptoms of end-organ dysfunction (e.g., hypotonia, collapse, incontinence)
	4. Sudden gastrointestinal symptoms (e.g., crampy abdominal pain, vomiting)
Criteria 3	Reduced blood pressure after exposure to a known allergen for that patient (minutes to several hours)
	Infants and children: low systolic BP (age specific)[a] or greater than 30% decrease in systolic BP
	Adults: systolic BP less than 90 mmHg or greater than 30% decrease from that person's baseline

Adapted with permission from ref. [12]

[a] Low systolic BP in children is defined as systolic BP less than 70 mmHg from 1 month to 1 year, less than 70 mmHg + [2 × age] from 1 to 10 years, and less than 90 mmHg from 11 to 17 years

half-life of 90–120 min and can be elevated up to 6 h after the event. The positive predictive value for an elevated tryptase can be as high as 93%; however, a negative tryptase level does not rule out anaphylaxis [13]. Obtaining serial tryptase levels improves the sensitivity and specificity of the test compared to a single measurement [14, 15]. There are currently ongoing research in developing a more rapid and sensitive laboratory test to confirm anaphylaxis by looking at potential markers such as mast cell and basophil degranulation, chymase, and platelet-activating factors.

2.4 Assessment and Management of Anaphylaxis

Clinical history is crucial in aiding in the diagnosis of anaphylaxis and determining the potential triggering agent. There are many disorders that can mimic anaphylaxis in children. These include acute generalized urticarial or angioedema, asthma exacerbation, vasovagal syncope, panic or anxiety attack, foreign body aspiration, croup or epiglottitis, and other forms of shock. Once an allergic reaction or anaphylaxis is suspected, the first step is to remove the allergen from the patient if possible. Immediate assessment of airway, breathing, and circulation should be performed as death from anaphylaxis can occur within minutes after onset.

Epinephrine is the medication of choice for the treatment of anaphylaxis. There are no absolute contraindications to the use of epinephrine in the setting of anaphylaxis. Epinephrine is a nonselective agonist to all adrenergic receptors and counteracts all the deleterious effects of anaphylaxis. It increases peripheral vascular resistance and decreases mucosal edema by stimulating the $\alpha 1$ receptors, improves cardiac output via activation of the $\beta 1$ receptors, and reverses bronchoconstriction and stabilizes mast cells and basophils via the $\beta 2$ receptors. Early epinephrine administration is vital in avoiding clinical progression toward cardiovascular collapse. Epinephrine can be administered intravascularly (IV) or intramuscularly (IM) in the anterolateral thigh. IM is preferred due to increased cardiovascular complications associated with IV dosing [16]. There are currently three IM epinephrine auto-injectors available on the market with different dosing (0.1, 0.15, and 0.3 mg).

Dosage for IM epinephrine is 0.01 mg/kg with a maximum of 0.5 mg. For infants less than 10 kg, 0.01 mg/kg is preferred. However, if it is not available, then 0.1 or 0.15 mg IM can be used. For children between 10 and 25 kg, 0.15 mg IM should be used. For children between 25 and 50 kg, 0.3 mg IM is indicated. For children greater than 50 kg, 0.5 mg IM should be used and if not available, then 0.3 mg IM can be used. However, there are instances where IV epinephrine is indicated such as when a patient is presenting with cardiovascular collapse or when the patient is refractory to IM epinephrine. IV epinephrine for anaphylaxis is dosed at one-tenth or less the dosing for cardiac arrest or 1 mcg/kg which may be repeated or titrated to restore blood pressure. Epinephrine dosing for children with anaphylaxis is summarized in Table 3.

For selected patients who do not respond to multiple doses of IM or IV epinephrine and aggressive fluid resuscitation, IV epinephrine infusion may be indicated. For infants and children, epinephrine infusion dosing is 0.02–0.2 mcg/kg/min titrated to target blood pressure. A central line is preferred when administering epinephrine infusion; however its placement should not delay the initiation of the infusion. In rare cases where refractory hypotension does not respond to epinephrine, other vasopressors such as vasopressin, dopamine, and norepinephrine may be considered. If the patient is in cardiovascular collapse with no pulse, begin cardiopulmonary resuscitation, and follow the Pediatric Advanced Life Support (PALS) algorithm.

Table 3 Epinephrine dosing in children with anaphylaxis

Route	Weight	Preferred dosing	Alternative option
IM	<10 kg	0.01 mg/kg	0.1 or 0.15 mg auto-injector
	10–25 kg	0.15 mg auto-injector	
	25–50 kg	0.3 mg auto-injector	
	>50 kg	0.5 mg	0.3 mg auto-injector
IV	All weights	Slow bolus 1 mcg/kg or one-tenth the dosing for cardiac arrest	

Adopted from ref. [17]

Large-bore IV access should be obtained in all cases of anaphylaxis. Anaphylaxis can cause massive fluid shift via vasodilation and increased vascular permeability. IV fluid resuscitation should be started immediately for hypotensive patients and those not responding to IM epinephrine. Balanced crystalloids are preferred as the first-line resuscitation fluid. Children should receive 10–20 mL/kg initial bolus which can be repeated as needed while monitoring for signs of volume overload.

Initial airway assessment should include signs of angioedema to the face, lips, tongue, and uvula, listening for airway stridor, and evaluating for signs of respiratory distress. To assess for peri-glottic edema, patients should be asked to phonate and observed for hoarseness or changes in their voice. Supplemental oxygen should be started on all patients suspected of anaphylaxis. Airway assessment is crucial in determining if the patient requires emergent intubation as angioedema and upper airway compromise can deteriorate rapidly. Intubation may be difficult due to the severity of the upper airway edema and distortion of normal anatomy and landmarks. Difficult airway cart along with video laryngoscopes and fiber-optic scope should be immediately available. For older patients, awake fiber-optic intubation could be tried; however for younger patients it may not be a feasible option. If difficult airway is suspected, maintaining spontaneous ventilation during induction of anesthesia is important to prevent complete airway collapse. In severe cases of angioedema, otolaryngologist should be consulted and present during intubation in the event rigid bronchoscopy or emergent cricothyroidotomy is needed to secure the airway.

Adjunct treatments for anaphylaxis include H1 antihistamines, H2 antihistamines, beta 2 adrenergic agonist, and glucocorticoids. These medications can be used to treat specific symptoms of anaphylaxis but should not be used as first-line, sole therapy, or replacement for epinephrine. H1 antihistamines such as diphenhydramine may be used to treat cutaneous symptoms such as flushing and pruritus and improve patient comfort. The dosing for diphenhydramine is 1 mg/kg IV with a maximum single dose of 50 mg which may be repeated up to daily maximum of 200 mg or 5 mg/kg. H2 antihistamines such as famotidine can be used to treat pruritus and GI symptoms. The dosing for famotidine is 0.25 mg/kg with a maximum of single dose of 20 mg. However, H2 antihistamines play a minor role in the treatment of anaphylaxis [18]. Beta 2 agonist such as albuterol can be used to treat bronchospasm and mild respiratory symptoms via metered dose inhaler or nebulizer. Glucocorticoids such as methylprednisolone are commonly given during allergic reactions or anaphylaxis; however their onset of actions may take 4–6 h. The dosing for methylprednisolone is 1 mg/kg with a maximum single dose of 125 mg. They may be beneficial to patients with history of asthma, significant bronchospasm, or airway edema. However, they are nonspecific and slow acting with many adverse side effects and should not be used to treat acute anaphylactic reactions.

All patients with anaphylaxis should be monitored until all related symptoms have resolved. There is currently no consensus on how long these patients must be observed for. The observation period should be individualized and tailored to the severity of the allergic reaction. Some studies recommend at least 4–8 h observation after resolution of symptoms [19]. Anaphylaxis can be biphasic in which there is a recurrence of symptoms after apparent resolution of the initial episode. The incidence of biphasic anaphylaxis can be as high as 14.7% in pediatric anaphylaxis and is associated with more severe initial presentation and those requiring more than one dose of epinephrine. Recurrences usually develop within 12 h of initial onset; however up to 72 h have been reported [20, 21]. Patients with severe anaphylaxis or those requiring multiple doses or infusion of epinephrine should be admitted and observed in the intensive care setting for an extended period. For patients to be discharged, there should be an emergency action plan in place, epinephrine autoinjector dispensed with instructions, and follow-up with an allergist or primary care physician.

2.5 Prevention of Latex Allergy

Primary prevention is aimed at avoiding or decreasing exposure to latex allergenic proteins and preventing sensitization. Since the 1990s and the rise of latex allergy, governmental agencies and medical establishments have been moving away from latex-containing products and providing latex-free environment for patients. Latex gloves particularly high protein powdered latex gloves were targeted and replaced by powder-free low protein latex gloves, ultimately leading to the ban by the FDA on all powdered gloves in 2016. There has also been a push for novel manufacturing protocols and chemical processes to reduce the allergenic proteins in natural latex products. Other synthetic materials such as nitrile, neoprene, and polyvinyl are now widely used in the manufacturing of surgical and examination gloves. These changes have dramatically decreased the incidence of latex sensitization. In addition, the development of latex awareness, education, protocols, and policies have been crucial in the fight against latex allergy. Intra-op management includes assuring a latex-free environment. Even a needle entry via the rubber cap of a vial to draw medication can lead to an allergic response in sensitized patients.

Personnel taking care of the patient should be aware of personal items such as watches, necklaces, and bracelets which may have potential to contain latex allergen.

Secondary prevention focuses on eliminating latex exposure to high-risk or known patients with latex sensitization and avoiding the development of an allergic reaction or anaphylaxis. Screening of the general population for latex sensitization is not cost-effective as the prevalence is only 1–2%. However, screening for high-risk patients may be indicated. There are several tests used to identify latex sensitization, the most common test being the skin prick test. Serum IgE levels can also be measured to confirm suspected latex allergy with no risk for anaphylaxis. The disadvantages of IgE testing are the increased cost and prolonged waiting period. Provocation testing or challenge test involves exposing a patient to suspected allergen under controlled setting to determine the severity of the reaction. For patients sensitized to latex, the best prevention is to provide a latex-free environment during their hospital stay.

When patients with latex allergy are inadvertently exposed to latex, there should be a root cause analysis to determine the cause. Root cause analysis is used to review the events in chronological order and discover systemic failures leading to the event. Failures may include improper identification of at-risk patients, unclear labels on products containing latex, or miscommunication between healthcare professionals. Once the issue is found, there should be discussion between the stakeholders in rectifying the cause by ensuring latex allergies are clearly documented and displayed, labeling equipment with latex components, educating stakeholders on latex allergy, developing a checklist, and finally providing reporting tools for near misses and adverse events. In addition to spina bifida patients, it is important to recognize the possibility of latex sensitization in other pediatric patients with congenital malformations who had undergone multiple corrective surgeries soon after birth. Prophylactic measures should be taken in these children as well to avoid perioperative latex anaphylaxis [22].

3 Conclusion

Although the incidence of latex allergy has declined in the recent years, it remains an important allergen especially in spina bifida patients. Latex products are continuously being replaced by alternatives; however due to its availability and cheaper cost, it remains widely used worldwide. In the event a sensitized patient comes into contact with latex, it is imperative to be able to recognize the signs and symptoms of latex allergy and successfully manage patients with anaphylaxis.

References

1. Centers for Disease Control and Prevention (CDC). Racial/ethnic differences in the birth prevalence of spina bifida—United States, 1995–2005. MMWR Morb Mortal Wkly Rep. 2009;57(53):1409–13. Erratum in: MMWR Morb Mortal Wkly Rep. 2009 Jan 30;58(3):61.
2. Middleton JC, Coker-Schwimmer EJ, Nicholson WK. Folic acid supplementation for the prevention of neural tube defects: an updated evidence report and systematic review for the US preventive services task force. JAMA. 2017;317(2):190–203.
3. Stern A, et al. Spina bifida. In: Avani C, Driscoll K, editors. Adherence and self-management in pediatric populations. Elsevier; 2020. pp. 235–261.
4. Krogh K, Christensen P. Neurogenic colorectal and pelvic floor dysfunction. Best Pract Res Clin Gastroenterol. 2009;23(4):531–43.
5. Kelly KJ, Sussman G. Latex allergy: where are we now and how did we get there? J Allergy Clin Immunol Pract. 2017;5(5):1212–6.
6. Weido AJ, Sim TC. The burgeoning problem of latex sensitivity. Postgrad Med. 1995;98(3):173–84.
7. Brehler R, Theissen U, Mohr C, Luger T. "Latex-fruit syndrome": frequency of cross-reacting IgE antibodies. Allergy. 1997;52(4):404–10.
8. Bernardini R, et al. Prevalence of and risk factors for latex sensitization in patients with spina bifida. J Urol. 1998;160:1775–8.
9. Taylor JS, Erkek E. Latex allergy: diagnosis and management. Dermatol Ther. 2004;17:289–301.
10. Huang V, Clayton NA, Welker KH. Glycopeptide hypersensitivity and adverse reactions. Pharmacy (Basel). 2020;8(2):70. https://doi.org/10.3390/pharmacy8020070. PMID: 32326261; PMCID: PMC7357119.

11. Simons FE. Anaphylaxis. J Allergy Clin Immunol. 2010;125(2 Suppl 2):S161–81. https://doi.org/10.1016/j.jaci.2009.12.981. Erratum in: J Allergy Clin Immunol 2010 Oct;126(4):885.
12. Sampson HA, et al. Second symposium on the definition and management of anaphylaxis: summary report—Second National Institute of Allergy and Infectious Disease/Food Allergy and Anaphylaxis Network symposium. J Allergy Clin Immunol. 2006;117(2):391–7.
13. Schwartz LB, Yunginger JW, Miller J, Bokhari R, Dull D. Time course of appearance and disappearance of human mast cell tryptase in the circulation after anaphylaxis. J Clin Invest. 1989;83(5):1551–5.
14. Buka RJ, Knibb RC, Crossman RJ, Melchior CL, Huissoon AP, Hackett S, Dorrian S, Cooke MW, Krishna MT. Anaphylaxis and clinical utility of real-world measurement of acute serum tryptase in UK emergency departments. J Allergy Clin Immunol Pract. 2017;5(5):1280–7.
15. Sala-Cunill A, Cardona V, Labrador-Horrillo M, Luengo O, Esteso O, Garriga T, Vicario M, Guilarte M. Usefulness and limitations of sequential serum tryptase for the diagnosis of anaphylaxis in 102 patients. Int Arch Allergy Immunol. 2013;160(2):192–9.
16. Campbell RL, Bellolio MF, Knutson BD, Bellamkonda VR, Fedko MG, Nestler DM, Hess EP. Epinephrine in anaphylaxis: higher risk of cardiovascular complications and overdose after administration of intravenous bolus epinephrine compared with intramuscular epinephrine. J Allergy Clin Immunol Pract. 2015;3(1):76–80.
17. Sicherer SH, Simons FER, Section on Allergy and Immunology. Epinephrine for first-aid management of anaphylaxis. Pediatrics. 2017;139(3):e20164006.
18. Lin RY, Curry A, Pesola GR, Knight RJ, Lee HS, Bakalchuk L, Tenenbaum C, Westfal RE. Improved outcomes in patients with acute allergic syndromes who are treated with combined H1 and H2 antagonists. Ann Emerg Med. 2000;36(5):462–8.
19. Campell RL, Li JT, Nicklas RA, et al. Emergency department diagnosis and treatment of anaphylaxis: a practice parameter. Ann Allergy Asthma Immunol. 2014;113:599–608.
20. Alqurashi W, Stiell I, Chan K, Neto G, Alsadoon A, Wells G. Epidemiology and clinical predictors of biphasic reactions in children with anaphylaxis. Ann Allergy Asthma Immunol. 2015;115(3):217–223.e2.
21. Lee S, Bellolio MF, Hess EP, Erwin P, Murad MH, Campbell RL. Time of onset and predictors of biphasic anaphylactic reactions: a systematic review and meta-analysis. J Allergy Clin Immunol Pract. 2015;3(3):408–16.e1–2.
22. Cremer R, Lorbacher M, Hering F, Engelskirchen R. Natural rubber latex sensitization and allergy in patients with spina bifida, urogenital disorders and oesophageal atresia compared with a normal paediatric population. Eur J Pediatr Surg. 2007;17(3):194–8. https://doi.org/10.1055/s-2007-965144. PMID: 17638159.

O_2 Desaturation in a Teenager After Esophagoscopy, Dilatation and Biopsy

David A. Rico Mora

1 Stem

A 13-year-old male is scheduled for esophagoscopy, dilatation, and biopsy for a recurrent esophageal stricture. His past medical history includes tracheoesophageal fistula (TEF) type C repaired at birth, intermittent asthma (last asthma exacerbation 2 years ago), gastric esophageal reflux disease (GERD), and failure to thrive. He has undergone numerous esophagoscopies, dilatations for residual strictures, and biopsies as well as T&A for obstructive sleep apnea (OSA) under general anesthesia in the past with no complications. Patient has been treated with omeprazole, multivitamins, and albuterol at home. Patient's vital signs in the preoperative area were unremarkable and nil per os (NPO) status was adequate. He underwent an esophagoscopy under general anesthesia with esophageal balloon dilatation and biopsy. Rapid sequence induction with propofol and rocuronium was performed; an oral endotracheal tube (6.5 mm) was placed without any complications. Maintenance of anesthesia was achieved with sevoflurane. Sugammadex was given at the end as a reversal agent and an uneventful awake extubation was performed after completion of the procedure. Patient was taken to the PACU, and his vital signs were the following: blood pressure 95/55, heart rate 98/min, oxygen saturation 99% on 4 Liters of O_2 blowby, respiratory rate 19/min, and temperature 36.4 °C.

Fifteen minutes after arrival to the PACU, the PACU nurse calls you urgently because the patient's oxygen saturation has acutely dropped to 82–84%. He is retching; coughing; breathing rapidly; complaining of neck, chest, and abdominal pain; and tossing around in his bed. His BP is now 76/43, his heart rate is 120/min, and his respirations are shallow and rapid.

D. A. Rico Mora (✉)
Department of Anesthesiology, Pain, and Perioperative Medicine, Children's National Medical Center, Washington, DC, USA
e-mail: dricomora@childrensnational.org

S. T. Verghese (ed.), *Anesthesia STAT! Acute Pediatric Emergencies in PACU*,
https://doi.org/10.1007/978-3-031-24396-7_11

2 What Is the Differential Diagnosis for the Abrupt Desaturation?

A sudden exacerbation of his asthma problem?

Bout of coughing due to aspiration of stomach contents into his lungs because of an esophageal motility problem?

Inadequate muscle strength from residual paralysis and inability to cough out blood or secretions?

Is this all due to an inadvertent injury to the esophagus during surgery?

Perioperative respiratory adverse events (PRAE) are not uncommon in pediatric patients and can be rapidly managed if successfully identified and addressed by trained personnel. Neonates and younger infants are the most susceptible age group affected by these complications. Data has shown that pediatric patients with PRAE and cardiopulmonary arrest had better outcomes whenever their care was supervised by trained pediatric anesthesiologists in pediatric centers when compared with the care provided by general anesthesiologists in mixed practices. In addition, these events are most seen on induction and recovery from anesthesia, and the main pathologic processes involved in the origin of PRAE are laryngospasm, bronchospasm, severe persistent coughing, partial/complete airway obstruction, apnea, desaturation, and stridor among others. Severe persistent coughing and desaturation are the two most common etiologies [1].

The potential complications of PRAE can compromise different organ systems, respiratory system (negative pressure pulmonary edema and prolonged oxygen requirements), cardiovascular system (cardiac arrest), and neurologic system (permanent brain damage), and in the worst-case scenario can be a cause of death. Furthermore, PRAE are associated with most reintubations, prolonged hospital stays, and unplanned admissions to the intensive care unit (ICU) which can negatively impact the healthcare revenue and increase medical expenditure. For instance, postoperative hypoxemia can be caused by medications utilized perioperatively: respiratory depressants (narcotics and opioids), volatile agents and neuromuscular blocking agents (depolarizing and non-depolarizing muscle relaxants), as well as respiratory pathologies (atelectasis) [1].

This patient is high risk for PRAE due to the past medical history of intermittent asthma (increased risk of laryngospasm and bronchospasm) and OSA (increased risk of partial or complete airway). It is important to consider not only the patient's risk factors for desaturation but also the possible procedural risk factors that could be intimately involved with his current clinical presentation.

3 What Would You Do in This Clinical Scenario?

First, airway patency assessment should be prioritized. It is necessary to look for airway secretions or foreign bodies to rule out possible aspiration or laryngospasm. If secretions are found in the airway, rapid oropharyngeal suction needs to be initiated, and simultaneously, 100% inspired oxygen needs to be administered. At this time, if airflow obstruction is witnessed, continuous positive airway pressure (CPAP) should be applied, and the placement of an oropharyngeal airway should be considered. Additionally, if laryngospasm is the possible diagnosis, forced jaw thrust and intravenous propofol should be given to deepen the level of anesthesia to break the laryngospasm. However, if these maneuvers are unsuccessful, intravenous succinylcholine must be given as soon as possible, and endotracheal intubation should follow if the clinical scenario abruptly deteriorates [1, 2].

Lung auscultation should be rapidly performed, being the main goal to guarantee adequate air exchange and identify the presence of wheezes which can be associated with bronchospasm and aspiration. If bronchospasm is high on the differential, inhaled beta 2 agonists (albuterol) should be given rapidly. For the most part if this treatment is unsuccessful, titratable doses of intravenous epinephrine should follow. Magnesium sulfate and ketamine are treatment alternatives described in the literature as well [1].

Upper airway obstruction against a close glottis could produce an overwhelming elevation of the negative intrathoracic pressures increasing hydrostatic pressures and capillary permeability with ensuing leaking that will trigger the formation of negative pressure pulmonary edema. Therefore, this complication needs to be addressed acutely with measures to maintain airway patency and oxygenation, mechanical ventilation needs to be started in severe cases, and fluid restriction and diuretics should be considered as possible treatment options if improvement is not achieved [2].

In case respiratory depression is high on the differential diagnosis, it is important to perform a pupil exam to rule out miosis that is a common finding in opioid overdose, and residual neuromuscular blockade should be assessed as well. If opioid overdose is suspected, intravenous naloxone needs to be given. If residual neuromuscular blockade is present, the use of reversal agents needs to be considered when these agents have not been given to the patient beforehand. In most cases if the airway is patent, and the lung auscultation is normal, other possible etiologies like atelectasis should be ruled out and rapidly addressed with the use of pulmonary toilet maneuvers and incentive spirometry. Additionally, postoperative atelectasis can be prevented with the use of positive end expiratory pressure intraoperatively [1, 2].

Alternatively, if the patient is presenting with stridor following endotracheal extubation, humidified mist, racemic epinephrine, and dexamethasone should be considered as treatment options for the possible diagnosis of postintubation croup [2]. It is paramount to look for acute changes in the patient's vital signs and rapid deterioration of the clinical status which is commonly associated with medical emergencies like tension pneumothorax, massive pulmonary embolism (PE), pericardial tamponade, or iatrogenic esophageal rupture that will require emergent surgical consultation and management.

4 Which Pediatric Patients Are at Higher Risk of Cardiopulmonary Arrest? What Is the Commonest Cause of Cardiopulmonary Arrest in Kids?

Patients who are younger than 5 years old are at higher risk of cardiopulmonary arrest compared with older patients. Infants are the highest-risk group and the population less likely to survive these events [3].

The most common cause of cardiopulmonary arrest events in pediatric patients is associated with respiratory complications (respiratory insufficiency, inadequate invasive and natural airways, invasive airway displacement, acute pneumothorax, and pulmonary edema). On the other hand, cardiac/hemodynamic causes occupy the second place (active myocardial infarction, arrhythmias, and hypotension/hypoperfusion as main etiologies) [3]. Interestingly, respiratory complications are directly linked to one third of known perioperative cardiac arrests, 20% of these events occur while emerging from anesthesia or in the PACU and 50% of these events that were witnessed in the PACU were associated with the presence of PRAE [1].

5 What Are Well-Known Risk Factors for PRAE in Pediatric Patients?

Airway comorbidities (airway sensitivity, reactive airway disease, upper respiratory infection (URI) symptoms, and eczema) are known risk factors. These comorbidities could be associated with the presence of bronchospasm and/or laryngospasm on emergence from anesthesia. Pediatric patients who are second-hand smokers are also at risk for PRAE. In addition, there are other known airway comorbidities that could increase the risk: genetic defects (cystic fibrosis), congenital abnormalities (skeletal dysplasia with tracheomalacia), genetic syndromes (trisomy 21 and Alport syndrome), and craniofacial abnormalities (micrognathia and glossoptosis) [4].

Common respiratory comorbidities that increase the risk for PRAE are the following: asthma (leading cause of chronic disease in kids), obstructive sleep apnea, pulmonary dysplasia, and cystic fibrosis. Likewise, other known respiratory risk factors are obesity (restrictive airway disease) and genetic, hormonal, or neurogenic factors [4].

The main neurologic factors known for increasing the risk for PRAE are the following: seizures, arteriovenous malformation, brain tumors, and neuromuscular diseases (Duchenne muscular dystrophy, cerebral palsy, and myasthenia gravis) [4].

The cardiac comorbidities that increase the risk for PRAE are the following: significant heart murmurs, congenital heart disease, arrhythmias, and hemodynamic unstable cardiac disease requiring ongoing vasoactive agents. Moreover, research have shown that African American kids have higher risk for PRAE compared to other races [4].

The surgical procedures associated with increased risk of respiratory complications in the PACU are the following: upper airway procedures with expected blood/secretions, shared airway procedures (ear, nose, throat, dental, and pulmonary medicine), sudden surgical stimulation, and emergency surgery [1].

The main anesthesia/recovery management factors associated with increased risk for respiratory complications in the PACU are the following: use of invasive airway, repeated attempts at airway placement, use of desflurane as maintenance anesthetic agent, less experienced anesthesiologist and PACU staff, inadequate patient ratio in the PACU, inadequate opioid titration and dosing, administration of neuromuscular blocking agents, inadequate timing for the removal of airway devices, use of topical lidocaine, premedication with midazolam, emergence (versus induction of anesthesia), and mixed population hospitals (versus pediatric hospitals) [1].

6 What Are Some Prevention Strategies for Respiratory Complications in the PACU?

It has been described in the literature some prevention strategies to decrease the respiratory complication in pediatric patients in the PACU. It is paramount to optimize children with known risk factors preoperatively, and listed below are the several preventive strategies [1]:

1. Use of inhaled beta-agonists in children with known respiratory risk factors
2. Following age-appropriate fasting guidelines
3. Avoidance of the use of midazolam as a premedication agent (use clonidine if necessary)
4. Use of noninvasive airways instead of invasive airways if possible
5. Use of cuffed endotracheal tubes over uncuffed endotracheal tubes
6. Total intravenous anesthesia (TIVA) and regional anesthesia instead of volatile anesthesia
7. Avoidance of desflurane for maintenance of anesthesia
8. Appropriate opioid dosing by titration
9. Careful flushing of intravenous lines
10. Monitoring of neuromuscular function after the use of neuromuscular blocking agents
11. Supervision of patient by pediatric anesthesiologists over general anesthesiologists
12. Pediatric hospital PACU management over mixed population hospitals
13. Oxygen administration during transport of patients from the OR to the PACU
14. Adequate patient/nurse ratio in the PACU 1:1
15. Use of continuous SaO2 and CO2 monitoring in the perioperative setting [1]

Patient's oxygen saturation improved after starting oxygen delivery via high-flow nasal cannula at 15 L/min, but BP drops to 68/34, and HR is now 146 per minute. Patient is complaining of worsening of chest pain and chest crepitus was found on palpation.

The presence of tachycardia, hypotension, and acute chest pain associated with chest crepitus on examination can be caused by a variety of pathologic processes.

Patient's clinical status is deteriorating rapidly, and immediate treatment to improve the hemodynamic derangement must be prioritized. The differential diagnosis is broad, and detrimental complications such as tension pneumothorax, hemothorax, pericardial tamponade, and massive PE need to be swiftly ruled out. The history of recent EGD with esophageal dilatation and biopsy makes esophageal perforation as the most probable diagnosis. Confirmation of the diagnosis and treatment should be undertaken promptly to prevent further deterioration.

7 What Is the *Incidence* of Esophageal Perforation?

The incidence of esophageal injury is 0.018–0.003% in flexible endoscopies, 0.11% in rigid endoscopies, and up to 10–15% in therapeutic interventions [5]. The immediate mortality rate is 9.86%, and the surgical management of this complication has been associated with higher death rates when compared with conservative treatments in some studies. More importantly, the pooled mortality was higher before the year 2010 which could be related to the improvement in the diagnosis and management of this feared complication in recent times [6]. The thoracic esophageal rupture is associated with the highest mortality rate followed closely by the abdominal esophageal rupture (second) and the cervical esophageal rupture (third) [7]. The mortality of iatrogenic esophageal perforation in pediatric patients has been as high as 28% in some studies [8].

8 What Is the *Etiology* of Esophageal Perforation?

The etiology of esophageal perforation is divided into four main groups:

1. Instrumental or iatrogenic (endoscopy/trauma)
2. Pressure induced or spontaneous (Boerhaave syndrome and barotrauma)
3. Ingestion of foreign bodies (coins/detergents)
4. Previous esophageal pathology (diverticula, stricture, Bochdalek hernia) [8]

The etiology of esophageal perforation can also be classified into two types: intraluminal and extraluminal—the intraluminal injuries are caused by instruments, caustics, barotrauma, and foreign bodies, and the extraluminal injuries occur after blunt or penetrating injury and operative trauma [5].

9 What Is the *Most Common Etiology* of Esophageal Perforation?

In the pediatric population, the iatrogenic esophageal perforation occurrence has been shown to be as high as 71–84%. The most common etiology of iatrogenic esophageal perforation in pediatric patients is associated with the dilatation of esophageal strictures and in neonates after the placement of nasogastric tubes. Furthermore, the number one complication seen postoperatively after undergoing an esophageal dilatation is the iatrogenic perforation of the esophagus [8]. However, iatrogenic esophageal perforation occurs more frequently in complex, malignant, radiation-induced strictures from caustic agents, compared with benign, simple ring, peptic, or anastomotic strictures [9].

There are different factors that could be responsible for the genesis of iatrogenic esophageal perforation in pediatric patients; the first is the extreme force used during esophageal intubation during EGD, and the second one is the use of inappropriate excessive neck extension while performing it. For instance, the procedures with the highest risk of iatrogenic esophageal perforation are the following: transendoscopic surgery, variceal injection, foreign body removal, peroral endoscopic myotomy (POEM), submucosal dissection, mucosal resection, and dilatation of stricture like in the case of our patient [10].

It is paramount for the anesthesiologist to recognize the risk of iatrogenic esophageal perforation while performing common procedures such as endotracheal intubations and the placement of suction catheters and nasogastric/orogastric tubes in inpatient and outpatient settings [11].

10 What Is the Most Common Cause of Esophageal Stenosis in Children and Infants?

The most common cause of esophageal stenosis in children and infants is the presence of anastomotic strictures following esophageal atresia repair which is a very common complication (18–50%). In addition, the principal etiologies that are involved in the pathophysiology of esophageal strictures are the presence of tension anastomosis, two-layer anastomosis, anastomotic leak, and gastroesophageal reflux [12].

Fifty percent of patients with esophageal stenosis (status post-esophageal atresia repair) who underwent esophageal dilatation will have substantial improvement of symptoms within 6 months of the intervention; however, 30% of these patients will have recurrence of the esophageal strictures that will require multiple interventions in the future. Despite all this, after a patient has undergone esophageal atresia repair, the diagnosis of gastroesophageal reflux is very prevalent becoming one of the main reasons why these patients suffer from persistent postoperative strictures; then it is paramount to treat gastroesophageal reflux symptoms in this population either by using medical treatment or laparoscopic surgical treatment to prevent further complications [12].

11 Why Is Esophageal Perforation Life-Threatening?

The esophagus has a unique anatomical structure that makes it more susceptible to infections and inflammatory processes when perforated due to the lack of protective barriers (serosa and loose areolar connective tissue). For instance, the diagnosis of esophageal perforation allows polymicrobial flora and digestive enzymes to spread into the mediastinum or subphrenic space leading to mediastinitis, empyema, abscesses, and sepsis which could be life-threatening if prompt diagnosis is missed and treatment therefore delayed.

12 What Are the Most Common Anatomical Areas Affected by Esophageal Perforation?

Killian's triangle (Fig. 1) is the most common anatomical zone affected by esophageal perforation in a normal esophagus (union of constrictor pharyngeal and cricopharyngeus muscles). Nevertheless, the most common zone compromised by esophageal perforation after esophageal instrumentation occurs in anatomical areas of narrowing (gastroesophageal junction, the impingement of the aortic arch, and the left main stem bronchus). Biopsy sites or areas proximal to strictures are also at risk for esophageal perforation. In contrast, the spontaneous perforation of the esophagus occurs mainly in the left wall of the supradiaphragmatic esophagus [7].

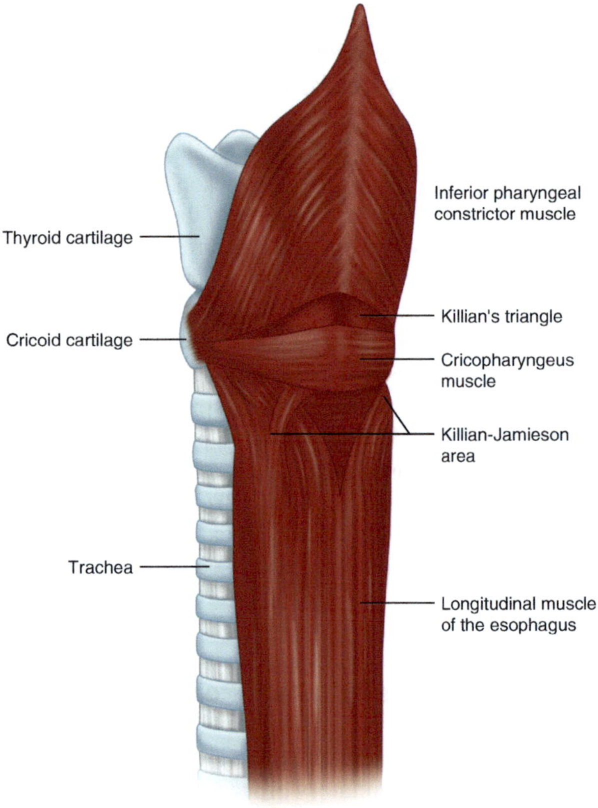

Fig. 1 Drawing of Killian's triangle: union of the constrictor pharyngeal muscles and cricopharyngeus muscles

When the esophageal perforation is produced by impaction of foreign bodies, the most common areas affected are zones of anatomical narrowing (cricopharynx, mid-esophagus at the level of the aortic arch, gastroesophageal junction, gastric outlet, and terminal ileum) like the zones affected by iatrogenic esophageal perforation. Furthermore, most foreign bodies are found proximal to the cricopharynx, and in case of impaction, the thoracic esophagus is the most common portion of the esophagus affected [10]. Spontaneous perforation without surgical instrumentation can occur after forceful retching and prolonged vomiting. Ingestion of chicken or fish bones can also produce esophageal perforation at any site in the esophagus including neck, chest, and upper abdomen.

13 What Area of the Esophagus Is Affected in Neonates?

The most common zone affected in neonates is the pharyngoesophageal junction, proximal to the cricopharyngeal muscle. This is the narrowest zone of the esophagus that after being stimulated with esophageal instrumentation will produce an esophageal muscular constriction with subsequent esophageal closure producing esophageal perforation. Additionally, neck hyperextension after repeated intubation attempts could produce significant collapse of the posterior pharyngeal wall against the cervical vertebrae causing esophageal perforation as well [11].

14 What Is the Clinical Presentation of Esophageal Perforation?

The accurate diagnosis of esophageal perforation is challenging because the clinical presentation is easily confounded with other pathologies (pneumothorax, pancreatitis, myocardial infarction, peptic ulcer perforation, pneumonia, and aortic dissection) [13]. For this reason, the diagnosis is usually delayed for more than 24 h due to the presence of signs and symptoms that are nonspecific. The clinical presentation will also depend on the etiology that caused the esophageal perforation; for instance, if the esophageal perforation was spontaneous, the clinical presentation is usually more severe and abrupt compared with the clinical presentation and complications expected from an iatrogenic esophageal perforation [5].

In the early stages of perforation, the absence of signs and symptoms is characteristic which makes its diagnosis even more complicated and confusing. The area of the esophagus affected will also play an important role in the diagnosis because the severity and onset of symptoms may differ from one esophageal zone to the other. Most often chest pain is seen in 70% of patients and dysphagia in 60% followed by dyspnea and fever [8, 13]. On the other hand, the presence of tachycardia, fever, and chills is associated with mediastinitis, sepsis, and toxic progression of the disease [10].

Cervical esophageal perforation is associated with dysphagia, dysphonia, hoarseness, localized neck pain odynophagia, bloody regurgitation, and subcutaneous emphysema.

The *thoracic esophageal perforation* is characterized by chest pain radiated to the back, dyspnea, tachypnea, tachycardia, fever, leukocytosis, and subcutaneous emphysema.

Abdominal esophageal perforation is associated with the presence of peritonitis with abdominal (retrosternal/epigastric) pain, nausea, and vomiting, and the onset of systemic signs tends to occur more rapidly (within few hours) [8, 9].

15 What Are the Main Symptoms of Esophageal Perforation in Neonates and Infants?

The clinical presentation of esophageal perforation in neonates and infants is atypical compared with adults and older kids. This is characterized by the presence of hypersalivation, choking, coughing, and cyanosis and is associated with difficult/repeated endotracheal intubation attempts and the placement of orogastric/nasogastric tubes [11]. Furthermore, esophageal perforation should be suspected if blood-tinged or coffee ground aspirates are found in nasogastric/orogastric tubes in a neonate. By contrast, rapid deterioration associated with acute respiratory distress is common in neonates or infants whenever free perforation of the pleural cavity occurs, giving rise to pneumothorax or pleural effusions that are not well-tolerated by this population [8].

16 What Is the Mackler Triad?

The Mackler triad is characterized by the presence of vomiting, chest pain, and subcutaneous emphysema which are the three cardinal signs described in esophageal perforations [14].

17 Patient Starts Complaining of Left Shoulder Pain and Is Tachypneic and Febrile. What Is the Possible Pathophysiology?

There is a high suspicion that the patient is presenting with an intra-abdominal esophageal perforation due to his rapid clinical deterioration. This intra-abdominal esophageal perforation is generating a systemic response that could end up in sepsis and shock if not managed judiciously. Subsequently, a diaphragmatic irritation is produced secondary to this ongoing intra-abdominal esophageal perforation which could be responsible for referred pain to the left shoulder that the patient is reporting [7].

18 Complete Blood Count Was Ordered, and Hematocrit Is 33%, and White Blood Count Is 22,000 and Platelet Count 440,000. What Other Labs Would You Order?

Patients with esophageal perforation are at higher risk for acute clinical deterioration, sepsis, and shock. Therefore, it is important to order pertinent blood work like hematologic studies (complete blood count), renal profile (electrolytes, blood urea nitrogen, and creatinine), liver profile, and acid-base status as an initial assessment tool to track the progression of the illness and to look for multiorgan failure. However, lab work is not the gold standard for the diagnosis of esophageal perforation in patients because most changes may appear several hours after symptoms have appeared and the findings are nonspecific [15].

19 A Portable Posterior-Anterior Chest Radiograph Was Ordered at Bedside and Showed Subcutaneous Emphysema with No Other Findings. Is This Radiographic Change Expected in an Esophageal Perforation? What Are the Main Radiographic Changes Expected on a Chest Radiograph in a Patient with Esophageal Perforation?

A plain chest radiograph can be ordered as part of the radiologic workup for esophageal perforation. This simple radiologic study provides important diagnostic information in 70–90% of suspected cases. Mediastinal emphysema is present in 50% of patients and hydropneumothorax in 25% of cases [5]. However, the presence of normal findings in a plain chest radiograph will not rule out the presence of esophageal perforation because during the early stages of the disease, no radiographic changes will be encountered in 33% of affected patients [14].

The main radiographic changes in patients with esophageal perforation are the following: presence of pleural effusions, pneumomediastinum, subcutaneous emphysema, hydrothorax, pneumothorax, subdiaphragmatic air, mediastinal dilation, foreign matter, retro-tracheal dilation, and misplacement of enterogastric tubes. Moreover, soft tissue and mediastinal emphysema are the first radiographic changes that appear, whereas pleural effusions and mediastinal widening will appear in a delayed fashion [5].

20 Would You Order Any Other Imaging Study if the Chest Radiograph Is Normal? What Is the Gold Standard for Diagnosing Esophageal Rupture?

Water-soluble contrast esophagography is the gold standard for the diagnosis of esophageal perforation (Fig. 2) [7]. The main diagnostic finding for esophageal perforation will be the extravasation of contrast to the pleura or mediastinum [5].

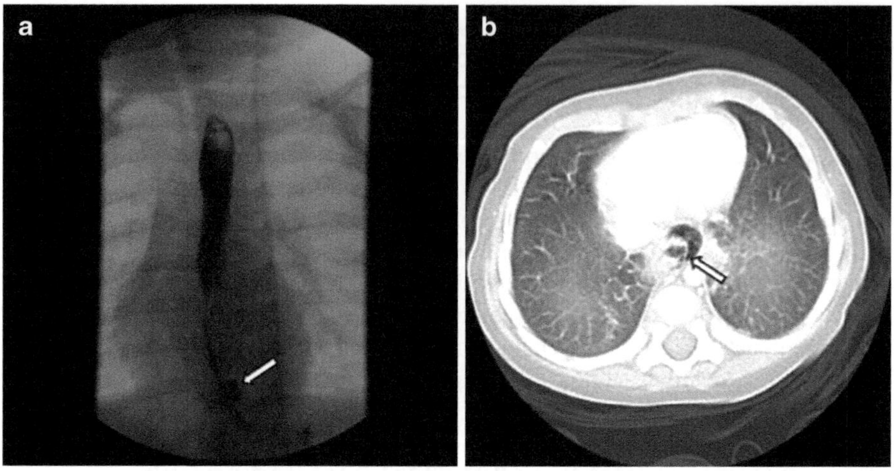

Fig. 2 (**a**) Water-soluble contrast esophagram demonstrating a mid-esophageal perforation (arrow) with extravasation of contrast material into the mediastinum and no extravasation into the pleural space [8]. (**b**) Computed tomography of the chest demonstrating the esophageal wall with perforation (arrow) in the axial view. There is no contrast that was administered. There is no contamination of the pleural space [8]

Interestingly, water-soluble contrast esophagogram can diagnose 75% of esophageal ruptures, and some studies have shown to have a sensitivity as high as 100%. In most cases Gastrografin has been the most common contrast used. If no extravasation is noted and there is high clinical suspicion of esophageal perforation, a serial barium contrast esophagography should be performed, but this study could produce an inflammatory response in the pleural space increasing the radiation exposure received by the patient [7, 8]. In conclusion, esophagography is necessary to confirm diagnosis, localization, and treatment of the esophageal perforation [5].

The three main types of injuries identified by esophagography are the following: (1) collection of contrast in the retropharyngeal pocket from a localized cervical leak, (2) submucosal perforation parallel and posterior to the esophagus, and (3) free perforation into the pleural space [8, 9].

Computed tomography has been shown to be useful as a diagnostic tool in perforations that are difficult to be found by other diagnostic methods (Fig. 2). The other remarkable use of the computed tomography is the placement of image-guided catheters to drain pleural effusions [7, 8]. In addition to this, the computed tomography is also useful for diagnosing pneumothorax, pneumomediastinum, subcutaneous emphysema, mediastinal dilation, abscess cavities, lesion level, and foreign matter and detection of small extravasation of contrast and the presence of vertical invasion of infectious processes in the mediastinum [5].

The use of endoscopy is controversial mainly because small perforations could be missed by experienced endoscopists and the endoscope could easily produce enlargement of an existing perforation increasing the risk for additional contamination; apart from this, its accuracy is also inferior when compared with other contrast studies [8]. Nevertheless, the use of flexible endoscopy is a valuable diagnostic tool that provides direct visualization of esophageal perforations and helps with the assessment of perforations produced by external perforating trauma [7].

21 What Are Important Factors to Consider When Deciding How to Treat an Esophageal Perforation?

The most important factors to consider when treating an esophageal perforation are the time between the rupture and the established diagnosis, the zone affected, the size, the extent of contamination, and the general health status of the patient [7]. It should be noted that the main treatment goal is to achieve the restoration of the esophageal lumen and the second one is the control of extraluminal contamination to prevent sepsis [5].

The prognostic factors for esophageal perforation are the following: early diagnosis and management achieved within 24 h of clinical onset, etiology (iatrogenic causes), absence of patient's comorbidities, absence of esophageal disease, hemodynamic stability, preserved nutritional status, cervical location compared with thoracic and abdominal injury, and sharp injury compared with blunt injury [10].

The prognostic factors when the presentation/diagnosis is early are the following: presence of localized perforation, absence of mediastinitis, no contamination by solid food, and demonstration of free contrast flow into the distal gastrointestinal tract. In contrast, the prognosis factors when the presentation/diagnosis is late are the following: well-contained contamination, minimal sepsis, no other comorbidities or risk factors, and initiation of enteral/parenteral nutrition [10].

22 What Patients Might Benefit from a Surgical Approach?

The surgical management might be beneficial in patients who have large perforations, peritonitis, sepsis, and ongoing deterioration of the clinical status. The other important conditions to consider are the following: failure of previous percutaneous treatments, presence of active leaks, and the presence of free fluid unable to be drained percutaneously [9].

23 What Is the Pittsburg Perforation Severity Score?

The Pittsburg perforation severity score (PPS) is a clinical score based on preexisting esophageal pathology and clinical findings at the time of the esophageal perforation presentation. All variables are assigned points (range 1–3) for a possible maximum total score of 18. Points are given to each variable according to the following scale: 1 point, age >75 years, tachycardia (>100 bpm), leukocytosis (>10,000 white blood cells/mL), or pleural effusion (on chest radiograph, computed tomography, or barium swallow); 2 points, fever (>38.5 °C), non-contained leak (on barium swallow or computed tomography), respiratory compromise (respiratory rate >30, increasing oxygen requirement, or need of mechanical ventilation), or time to diagnosis >24 h; and 3 points, presence of cancer or hypotension [16].

The Pittsburg perforation severity score is divided into three groups. The group 1 has a low PPS (0–2 points), the group 2 has a medium PSS (3–5 points), and group 3 (>5 points) has a high PSS. The group 1 is managed with nonoperative treatment. In case of contained leaks, a simple conservative management is recommended, and in non-contained esophageal perforations, the use of endoscopic stenting is advised, and as an alternative management, a primary surgical repair or repair over drain can be performed. In contrast, the surgical intervention is the preferred management for patients in the group 2 with non-contained leaks and endoscopic stenting as an alternative option. In case of contained perforations, the conservative treatment is the preferred one. On the other hand, group 3 has the worst outcome of the three groups, and aggressive treatment is the preferred management option in all cases. Perforated esophageal cancer requires individualized treatment [16].

24 What Is the Nonsurgical or Nonoperative Treatment of Esophageal Perforations?

The two main treatment options for esophageal perforations are operative and nonoperative management. Furthermore, it is always imperative to ask for surgical consultation even if the nonoperative treatment is the one selected for the patient to prevent further clinical deterioration [7]. The nonoperative management starts with intravenous broad-spectrum antibiotics, nil per mouth orders, nasogastric suction, pain control, gastric acid suppression, enteral nutrition, hemodynamic monitoring, and supportive treatment [9]. Finally, the nonoperative treatment is preferred in patients with well-contained, small perforations and minimal mediastinal/pleural contamination [7].

The antibiotic coverage chosen is usually against gram-negative bacteria and anaerobes and should be extended for 7–14 days from the time of the injury. Alternatively, if the follow-up image shows persistence of the perforation, the antibiotic regime needs to be extended for one more week. The preferred antibiotic choice consists of piperacillin/tazobactam alone or combined with vancomycin and gentamicin. However, depending on the clinical presentation, on some occasions an antifungal regime needs to be added to the therapy [8].

It is important to consider the timing of the esophageal perforation because when the injury is detected early, there is a better chance that the esophageal perforation will be treated successfully with nonoperative options. It is also paramount to consider the location of the perforation when treating esophageal perforations. For instance, cervical esophageal perforations have less mediastinal contamination; therefore, there is a high probability that the nonoperative treatment will be successful at managing these perforations. At the same time, when the perforation is iatrogenic, and the patient has minimal symptoms, the likelihood that the implementation of conservative options will be successful is higher [7].

There are other important circumstances where the nonoperative treatment can be considered: when the drainage occurs into the esophageal lumen, the injury is not proximal to neoplastic tissue, the abdomen, or obstructions and when there is confirmed availability of a thoracic surgeon and imaging studies [7, 11]. Meanwhile, it is paramount to initiate nothing by mouth orders for 48–72 h and start the placement of chest tubes, drains, and suctions guided by transluminal endoscopy. The placement of thoracostomy tubes is vital to control the leak from pneumothorax and pleural effusions [7]. Furthermore, in the case scenario where collections are drained, a sample of fluid should be collected and sent for bacteriological analysis [9].

Currently, the management of esophageal perforation in the pediatric population has shifted toward the conservative management if the closure of the perforation occurs automatically. If there is absence of downstream obstruction, the contamination is addressed successfully, and the nutritional status is preserved [10].

25 What Is the Surgical Treatment of Esophageal Perforations?

The most important factor that needs to be addressed prior to performing an endoscopic closure of an iatrogenic esophageal perforation is the size of the perforation. For instance, if the perforation is <10 mm, the preferred method to achieve closure is the use of through-the-scope clips. On the other hand, the use of over-the-scope clips deems necessary whenever perforations are >10 mm but <20 mm. In the case scenario where the esophageal perforation is larger than 20 mm, the use of self-expandable stents for diversion of enteral contents is preferred. Endoscopic vacuum therapy (EVT) is a modern technique that uses negative pressure with the main goal of decreasing secretions. This technique has become an effective treatment strategy with better outcomes and less complications compared with stents. Nevertheless, new data has shown that even larger perforations >30 mm have been successfully closed with over-the-scope clips and suturing systems [9].

Stenting has been unsuccessful at treating larger perforations (60 mm) and cervical and gastroesophageal junction esophageal perforations. Above all, surgical repair should be performed when tracheoesophageal fistula is present, the defect is large, and thoracic esophageal perforation is accompanied with signs of sepsis [10]. The most common complications associated with placement of stents are migration (most common one), mispositioning, and obstruction. Therefore, the surveillance endoscopy needs to be performed 2 weeks after stent placement, and the removal of the stent should be performed 3–4 weeks after placement with a repeat esophagogram when removed [8].

Small or well-contained cervical esophageal perforations down to the level of the carina can be managed with drainage alone with cervical incision (left neck) along with the lower third of the sternocleidomastoid muscle. Conversely, perforation in the middle third of the esophagus is approached with right thoracotomy in the sixth intercostal space, and perforations in the lower third of the esophagus are approached through a left thoracotomy in the seventh/eighth intercostal space. On the other hand, the abdominal esophagus with no underlying pathology or long-term inflammation is approached with an upper midline laparotomy [7, 8]. The surgical repair can be accomplished with a primary repair which is the treatment of choice in an otherwise healthy esophagus, exclusion and diversion, controlled fistula, or resection [7].

Decompression and diversion of gastrointestinal fluids with nasogastric or nasoduodenal tubes are paramount. Decompression should be performed emergently in cases of hemodynamic instability and respiratory failure. Moreover, tension pneumoperitoneum needs to be acutely treated to prevent the development of compartment syndrome. Meanwhile, the use of CO_2 in gastrointestinal endoscopy is currently a standard practice for most procedures but most importantly for those procedures with a higher risk for iatrogenic esophageal perforation or when the perforation has already occurred [9].

Esophageal perforation due to caustic ingestion with complete esophageal necrosis should be rapidly managed with an esophagectomy with immediate or delayed reconstruction always evaluating the magnitude of the damage and the severity of the pathologic process. However, if the esophagus is too fragile, patient is hemodynamically unstable, surgical repair is not an option, or there is widespread infection (mediastinitis); the best management would be to perform an esophageal diversion with cervical esophagostomy. Nevertheless, patients with esophageal perforation with mediastinitis will require thoracic drainage using minimally invasive thoracoscopic approach [8].

The successful management of esophageal perforation is multidisciplinary where radiologists, endoscopists, and surgeons are involved in the decision-making. In summary, the most common operative treatment options known are the following: drainage alone, decortication and drainage, primary repair with or without tissue aid, controlled tissue aid, controlled fistula formation with T-tube, esophageal resection, and esophageal exclusion [7].

26 What Is the Rule of 3?

This is an expert opinion released in 1977 which recommended the avoidance of boogie and balloon dilations greater than 3 mm to decrease the risk of esophageal perforation. However, new studies have shown that esophageal dilatations less than 5 mm are still safe and do not increase the risk of esophageal perforation in pediatric patients with esophageal strictures, but additional prospective randomized studies are necessary to confirm this hypothesis [17].

27 When Would You Start Diet After Repair and How Long Would You Expect to Be the Length of Stay at the Hospital?

A liquid diet can be allowed 48 h after repair only if water-soluble contrast radiological tests show no leakage. However, if a mediastinal or pleural collection is noticed, a surgical or radiological drainage is mandatory [5]. Patients who had uncomplicated and asymptomatic esophageal perforation have been released from the hospital the same day, but in more involved and severe cases, the length of stay goes from 18 to 44 days [9, 18].

28 What Surveillance Should Be Done After Stent Placement?

After stent placement, a chest radiograph should be performed every 2 days to rule out stent migration. A gastroscopy should be performed 4 weeks after the repair to examine the site of perforation and replace or reposition the stent [18].

29 Summary

Clinical signs and manifestations of esophageal rupture include difficulty swallowing, vomiting, rapid breathing, fever and chills, low BP and rapid heart rate, rapid or labored breathing, pain at the site of perforation (neck, chest, abdomen, or referred to shoulder), crepitus, or presence of air under the skin.

29.1 Rapid Diagnosis

1. Esophagography with water-soluble contrast agent minimizes irritation of mediastinum which can occur with barium.
2. Chest X-ray and CT of the thorax detect mediastinal air and fluid but do not localize the perforation site.
3. Endoscopy under general endotracheal anesthesia may be useful to locate the site of perforation unless the lesion is very small.

Occurrence of esophageal perforation can be a life-threatening condition that requires prompt diagnosis and surgical repair in addition to intravenous fluids and antibiotic.

Procedures that are undertaken to treat are dependent on the severity of the perforation.

Drainage of the spilled fluid and food with chest tubes, endoscopy, and stent placement.

Minimally invasive repair of the perforation site or open repair of the perforation.

Esophagectomy only in extreme cases when the esophagus cannot be repaired.

References

1. Von Ungern-Sternberg B. Respiratory complications in the pediatric postanesthesia care unit. Anesthesiol Clin. 2014;32(1):45–61.
2. Pawar D. Common post-operative complications in children. Indian J Anaesth. 2012;56(5):496–501.
3. Christensen R, Voepel-Lewis T, Lewis I, Ramachandran SK, Malviya S. Pediatric cardiopulmonary arrest in the postanesthesia care unit: analysis of data from the American Heart Association get with the guidelines-resuscitation registry. Pediatr Anesth. 2013;201:517–23.
4. Mamaril ME. Preoperative risk factors associated with PACU pediatric respiratory complications: an integrative review. J Perianesth Nurs. 2020;35(2):125–34.
5. Eroğlu A, Aydın Y, Yılmaz O. Minimally invasive management of esophageal perforation. Turk J Thorac Cardiovasc Surg. 2018;26(3):496–503.
6. Deng Y, Hou L, Qin D, Huang T, Yuan T. Current treatment and outcome of esophageal perforation a single-center experience and a pooled analysis. Medicine. 2021;100(16):e25600.
7. Brinster CJ, Singhal S, Lee L, Marshall MB, Kaiser LR, Kucharczuk JC. Evolving options in the management of esophageal perforation. Ann Thorac Surg. 2004;77:1475–83.
8. Rentea RM, St Peter SD. Neonatal and pediatric esophageal perforation. Semin Pediatr Surg. 2017;26(2):87–94.
9. Paspatis GA, Arvanitakis M, Dumonceau JM, Barthet M, Saunders B, Turino SY, Dhillon A, Fragaki M, Gonzalez JM, Repici A, Van Wanrooij RLJ, Van Hooft JE. Diagnosis and management of iatrogenic endoscopic perforations: European Society of Gastrointestinal Endoscopy (ESGE) position statement—update 2020. Endoscopy. 2020;52(9):792–810.
10. Govindarajan KK. Esophageal perforation in children: etiology and management, with special reference to endoscopic esophageal perforation. Korean J Pediatr. 2018;61(6):175–9.
11. Gander JW, Berdon WE, Cowles RA. Iatrogenic esophageal perforation in children. Pediatr Surg Int. 2009;25(5):395–401.
12. Antoniou D, Soutis M, Christopoulus-Geroulanos G. Anastomotic strictures following esophageal atresia repair: a 20-year experience with endoscopic balloon dilation. J Pediatr Gastroenterol Nutr. 2010;51(4):464–7.
13. Hasimoto CN, Cataneo C, Eldib R, Thomazi R, Pereira RS, Minossi JG, Cataneo AJ. Efficacy of surgical versus conservative treatment in esophageal perforation. a systematic review of case series studies. Acta Cir Bras. 2013;28(4):266–71.
14. Søreide JA, Viste A. Esophageal perforation: diagnostic work-up and clinical decision-making in the first 24 hours. Scand J Trauma Resusc Emerg Med. 2011;19:66.
15. Chirica M, Kelly MD, Siboni S, Aiolfi A, Riva CG, Asti E, Ferrari D, Leppaniemi A, Ten Broek RPG, Brichon PY, Kluger Y, Pereira Fraga GP, Frey G, Andreollo NA, Coccolini F, Frattini C, Moore EE, Chiara O, Di Saverio S, Sartello M, Webwe D, Ansaloni L, Biffl W, Corte H, Wani I, Baiocchi G, Cattan P, Catena F, Bonavina L. Esophageal emergencies: WSES guidelines. World Journal of Emergency Surgery. 2019;14:26.
16. Schweigert M, Sousa HS, Solymosi N, Yankulov A, Fernandez MJ, Beattie R, Dubecz A, Rabl C, Law S, Tong D, Petrov D, Schabitz A, Stadlhuber RJ, Gumpp J, Ofner D, Mcguigan J, Costa-Maia J, Witzigmann H, Stein HJ. Spotlight of esophageal perforation: a multinational study using the Pittsburg esophageal perforation severity score. J Thorac Cardiovasc Surg. 2016;151(4):1002–9.
17. Clark SJ, Staffa SJ, Ngo PD, Yasuda JL, Zendejas B, Hamilton TE, Jennings RW, Manfredi MA. Rules are meant to be broken: examining the "Rule of 3" for esophageal dilations in pediatric stricture patients. J Pediatr Gastroenterol Nutr. 2020;71(1):e1–5.
18. Al Ghossaini N, Lucidarme D, Bulois P. Endoscopic treatment of iatrogenic gastrointestinal perforations: an overview. Dig Liver Dis. 2014;46(3):195–203.

Respiratory Arrest in an Obese Teenager in PACU After Cardiac Catheterization

Daniela Perez-Velasco

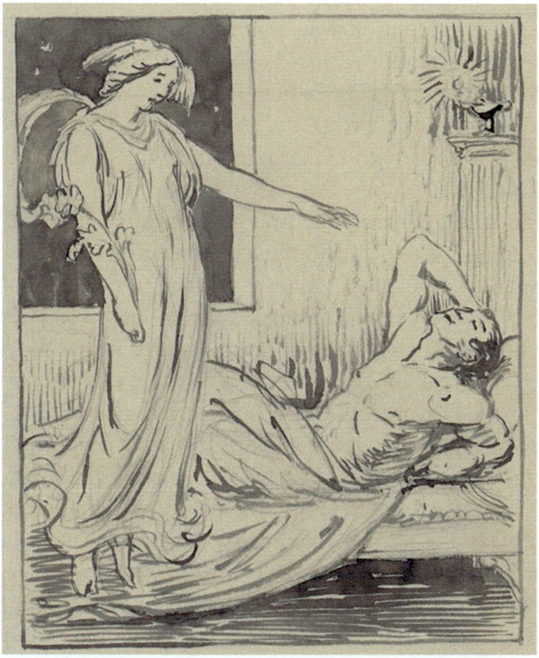

"'The Blessing of Sleep,' Study for a Poster for Paine's Celery Compound" by Kenyon Cox, American, 1856–1919 is marked with CC0 1.0

D. Perez-Velasco (✉)
Division of Pediatric Cardiac Anesthesiology, George Washington University, Washington, DC, USA

Division Anesthesiology, Pain and Perioperative Medicine, Children's National Hospital, Washington, DC, USA
e-mail: dperezvel2@childrensnational.org

S. T. Verghese (ed.), *Anesthesia STAT! Acute Pediatric Emergencies in PACU*,
https://doi.org/10.1007/978-3-031-24396-7_12

1 Case Presentation

A 16-year-old, 90 kg weight, obese male with history of congenital heart disease presented to the cardiac catheterization laboratory for a diagnostic examination under general anesthesia. Significant medical history includes: 22q.11 deletion syndrome (DiGeorge syndrome), postsurgical complete heart block with pacemaker, seasonal allergies, and hypothyroidism. Details of the patient's congenital heart defect are described as: double outlet right ventricle, ventricular septal defect, and interrupted aortic arch type B which was repaired in infancy at an international hospital outside. This repair involved combining the aorta and pulmonary artery into a new aorta and then using a graft to form a new connection between the right ventricle and the pulmonary arteries. Prior to this routine cardiac catheterization, the patient reported no symptoms, and the procedure was elective.

The family lives a far distance from the hospital and has limited English proficiency. The preoperative evaluation was conducted with video-enhanced language interpretive services (an example of this is the MARTTI or My Accessible Real-Time Trusted Interpreter system). The patient states he was told in the past that there was something wrong with his thyroid, but he currently takes no medications, and has no drug allergies. He lives with his grandmother, and she reports that he is sedentary, mainly playing video games several hours per day.

The patient underwent general endotracheal anesthesia after an intravenous induction with etomidate 0.2 mg/kg and rocuronium and for his cardiac catheterization. The volatile agent used for maintenance of anesthesia was isoflurane. He was easily extubated deep after reversal of muscle relaxant at the end of the catheterization and transferred to the postanesthesia care unit (PACU) in the supine position. The patient received midazolam 2 mg, fentanyl 25 mcg, and approximately 1 mcg/kg of dexmedetomidine. For prevention of postoperative nausea and vomiting, the patient received ondansetron intravenously. Shortly after arriving to the PACU, the patient began obstructing his airway, and his oxygen saturation showed an abrupt drop to the low 50s on pulse oximetry. An oral airway was immediately placed, and his breathing was assisted with 100% oxygen via bag mask ventilation to provide positive end expiratory pressure. Post-catheterization patients are required to remain supine for 4–6 hours to decrease risk of bleeding from vascular access sites in the groin since heparin is routinely given, but not reversed with protamine. This supine positioning worsened his airway obstruction. Therefore, bi-level positive airway pressure (BiPAP) was started until the patient was sufficiently awake to maintain his airway without support.

Upon questioning his grandmother further, she reported a history of loud nighttime snoring, periods of apnea, and daytime sleepiness. She also reported that he jerks his arms and legs sporadically while sleeping. Since she considered these movements were related to nightmares, she had not taken him to a doctor.

The patient was closely observed in postanesthesia care unit overnight and an endocrine consultation was made for follow-up. His pediatrician was notified of the events, and a sleep study was ordered which confirmed the diagnosis of severe obstructive sleep apnea and periodic limb movement disorder. The endocrine assessment showed that he had moderate hypothyroidism and started him on levothyroxine.

In reviewing this patient's acute respiratory depression after general anesthesia combined with his undiagnosed obstructive sleep apnea and occult hypothyroidism, the following questions need answers to elucidate how this problem could have been averted:

1. *Were the language barrier and absence of a thorough preoperative history contributory to this outcome?*
2. *Was there a need for the patient to be assessed preoperatively by a dedicated preoperative screening clinic because of his comorbidities?*
3. *Was the lack of complete assessment of this young obese man with congenital cardiac disease with occult OSA and hypothyroidism the reason for his respiratory failure in PACU?*
4. *Could management of his postoperative course have been improved by obtaining expert consultation by the sleep medicine physicians regarding his OSA or by completing some preoperative labs to evaluate the status of his thyroid function by an endocrinologist?*
5. *Should this case have been postponed to a later date if the anesthesiologist felt that the patient was not properly screened or optimally prepared for a general anesthesia for cardiac catheterization followed by supine position?*

2 Discussion

2.1 What Is Obstructive Sleep Apnea (OSA)?

Functions of the upper airway (anatomy as illustrated in Fig. 1) include air warming and humidification, pathways for olfaction, coordination of ventilation with swallowing and protection from aspiration of food, primary defense of infection, and, especially for humans, speech [1]. During sleep, however, maintenance of upper airway patency is a primary physiologic objective, failure of which can lead to obstructive sleep apnea (OSA) and its sequelae. During sleep protective upper airway reflexes are attenuated, leaving the upper airway susceptible to collapse [1].

OSA is disordered breathing during sleep which disturbs sleep and ventilation in children and/or adults. It is characterized by periods of periodic cessation of air exchange (apnea), with apneic episodes lasting longer than 10 s. These episodes occur more frequently during rapid eye movement (REM) sleep and increase in frequency as more time is spent in REM sleep periods as the night progresses [2]. Once thought to only be an isolated disorder of pharyngeal muscle mechanical dysfunction leading to intermittent airway obstruction, we know now that it is more complicated [3].

Because of the multisystem implications, it can also be referred to as obstructive sleep apnea syndrome (OSAS) since it involves the central nervous, cardiovascular, metabolic, and immune systems [3]. Sleep apnea may be defined as central (absent gas flow, lack of respiratory effort), obstructive (absent gas flow, upper airway obstruction, and paradoxical movement of rib cage and abdominal muscles), or mixed (due to both CNS defect and obstructive problems) [2].

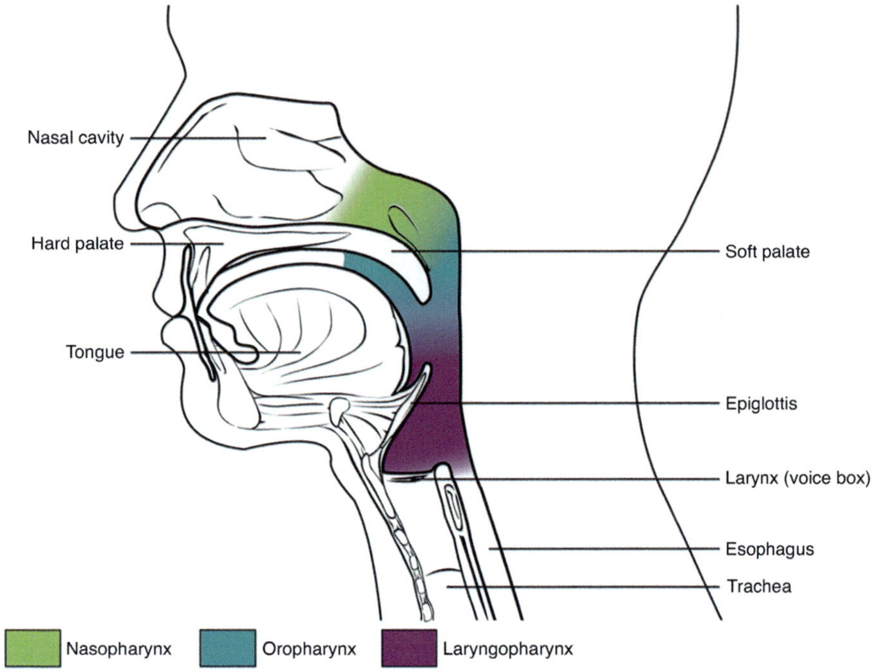

Fig. 1 Anatomy of the head and neck. (*Image credit: OpenStax CNX* via *OpenStaxCollege*. http://cnx.org/contents/t2sgkCQ-@8/Organs-and-Structures-of-the-R.. *License:* CC BY: Attribution)

The estimated prevalence of OSA is between 1 and 5% making it a common childhood disorder [4]. OSA occurs in children of all ages (about 1.2% of all children) but is more common in children 3–7 years of age. In a large study looking at over 5000 children, Bixler et al. [5] found the prevalence of AHI ≥ 5 was 1.2% in a representative sample of elementary school children. Risk factors for sleep-disordered breathing (SDB) included waist circumference and nasal abnormalities (e.g., chronic sinusitis/rhinitis). Black or Latino heritage was also a risk factor for OSA, and this could be attributed to recent studies that show that predominately Black and Latino neighborhoods have increased air pollution. A 2019 study published in the *Annals of the American Thoracic Society* showed a relationship between chronic air pollution exposure and sleep apnea [6]. Since air pollution exposures differ geographically, for example, in the United States due to racial and ethnicity discrimination in housing which lead to geographic segregation of people, this may partially explain difference in lung and sleep health by demographics such as socioeconomic status, race and ethnicity [6]. The strong linear relationship between waist circumference and BMI across all degrees of severity of SDB suggests that, as in adults, metabolic factors may be among the most important risk factors for SDB in children [5].

2.2 How Is OSA Diagnosed?

Diagnosis is made by clinical assessment and nocturnal pulse oximetry, but the gold standard is an overnight polysomnography study in a laboratory. The disadvantage is that this diagnostic test is time intensive and costly and requires the child to sleep in a laboratory with multiple monitors placed to assess hemoglobin oxygenation levels, apneas, and hypoxic events. Therefore, obtaining a formal diagnosis with polysomnography is not a simple task and may not be accessible to all persons needing the study.

Periodic limb movement disorder is also diagnosed during polysomnography (1) by visualizing movements (periodic limb movement in sleep (PLMS)); (2) PLMS exceeding norms for age ($\geq$ 5/h for children); (3) clinical sleep disturbance or daytime fatigue; and (4) the absence of another primary sleep disorder or reason for the PLMS, including restless leg syndrome (RLS) and OSA [7].

2.3 What Are Risk Factors for OSA?

OSA is associated with many other diagnoses. Obesity and tonsillar hypertrophy increase incidence of OSA in children. The strongest risk factors for OSA in adolescence are obesity (measured by age-corrected BMI or abdominal waist circumference), male sex, and history of tonsillectomy and adenoidectomy.

Signs and Symptoms Suggesting Possible OSA:

Physical Risk Factors:	History of Airway Obstruction during Sleep	Other
•Weight 95% or greater for age and sex •Craniofacial Abnormailities •Tonsillar Hypertrophy	•Two or More Observed: •Loud Snoring •Frequent snoring •Frequent arousal from sleep •Parentaly report of: •Difficult Breathing •Struggling respiratory efforts during sleep	•Child with: • history of night terrors •New enuresis •Sleeps in unsual position •Parent/caregiver/teacher report daytime sleepiness

Practice Guidelines for the Perioperative Management of Patients with Obstructive Sleep Apnea: An Updated Report by the American Society of Anesthesiologists Task Force on Perioperative Management of Patients with Obstructive Sleep Apnea [8]

2.4 What Determines the Severity of Obstructive Sleep Apnea?

If a child has signs or symptoms in two or more of the above categories from Table 1, there is a significant probability that he or she has OSA. The severity of OSA may be determined by sleep study. An apnea-hypopnea index (AHI) was created to measure the total number of obstructive episodes per hour of sleep. This allows the

Table 1 Practice guidelines for the perioperative management of patients with obstructive sleep apnea: an updated report by the American Society of Anesthesiologists task force on perioperative management of patients with obstructive sleep apnea [8]

Determination of OSA severity		
	Adult AHI	Pediatric AHI
None	0–5	0
Mild	6–20	1–5
Moderate	21–40	6–10
Severe	>40	>10

severity to be categorized as mild, moderate, or severe. There are different parameters used for adults as compared to children as noted in Table 1.

If a sleep study is not available, such patients should be treated as though they have moderate sleep apnea unless one or more of the signs of symptoms above are severely abnormal (e.g., weight ≥95th percentile for age and gender, respiratory pauses that are frightening to the observer, child regularly falls asleep within minutes after being left unstimulated without another explanation), in which cases patients should be treated as though they have severe sleep apnea. If a sleep study is completed, then you can use the results to guide the perioperative anesthetic management of a child. The severity of OSA can be categorized by the chart in Table 1:

It is important to note that because sleep laboratories differ in their criteria for detecting episodes of apnea and hypoxemia, the sleep laboratory's report (none, mild, moderate, or severe) takes precedence over the actual apnea-hypopnea index (AHI, the number of episodes of sleep-disordered breathing per hour).

2.5 Does Obstructive Sleep Apnea Affect Anesthetic Management?

Yes. Nocturnal desaturation to less than 85% upregulates the genes responsible for control of opioid receptors, resulting in an increased sensitivity to opioids; opioid requirement is reduced by approximately 50%, making standard doses of opioids a relative overdose in children with severe OSA [2].

If the patient uses a device (such as a CPAP machine) to assist with breathing while sleeping, then that should be available for use postoperatively. There should be judicious use of sedatives. All non-opioid medications should be used as first-line pain regimen including acetaminophen and ibuprofen.

2.6 Does the Presence of 22q11 Deletion Syndrome Affect the Probability of OSA?

Otolaryngologic problems are common in the 22q11.2 deletion syndrome population. Structural anomalies and retrognathia may predispose these patients to obstructive sleep apnea (OSA). Prevalence of OSA in this population of 22q11.2 DS patients is higher than expected in the general population. OSA risk is highest after VPI surgery and may be decreased by adenotonsillectomy. Providers should have awareness of increased prevalence of OSA in patients with 22q11.2 deletion syndrome [9].

2.7 Does Hypothyroidism Contribute to Worsening of OSA?

There is a complex relationship between body mass index (BMI), thyroid function, and its effects on OSA—raising the question "should all patients with suspected OSA should be screened?". Some studies have described an association between thyroid disorders and OSA. Whether this is a direct effect of thyroid disorders or it is indirectly related to BMI values is an important point to ponder. A recent study by Sharma et al. evaluated the prevalence of thyroid disorders in relation to BMI in newly diagnosed patients with OSA confirmed by polysomnography. This study found that the prevalence of hypothyroidism was common among patients with OSA and the severity of OSA correlated with thyroid function tests and BMI [10].

Hypothyroidism can also contribute to OSA because of its impact on metabolic syndrome. In a 2018 study, Bruyneel et al. [11] showed that TSH levels did not correlate to AHI, but they did to BMI. Thyroid function parameters were associated with BMI but not with the severity of OSA. The one factor that is consistently a strong risk factor for OSA is obesity. There is a two-pronged association between thyroid dysfunction and obesity. The prevalence of thyroid dysfunction is higher in obese people, and patients with overt hypothyroidism (OH) are more prone to gain weight compared to euthyroid patients. Therefore, there is a natural link between hypothyroidism, obesity, and OSA.

Nocturnal breathing abnormalities, such as snoring, choking, and, in severe cases, apnea/hypopnea events, occur in 25–35% of patients with hypothyroidism [12]. The effects of hypothyroidism treatment on OSA have been mixed [13]. Although many studies support the hypothesis that OSA is associated with thyroid dysfunction, the level of thyroid dysfunction does not appear to predict OSA severity, and the severity of the OSA may have subtle effects on the thyroid hormone levels [13]. The indirect effects of hypothyroidism such as increased weight gain and metabolic syndrome can increase risk of developing OSA.

A meta-analysis of patients with euthyroid and hypothyroid status and OSA showed that AHI, duration oxygen desaturation <90%, and Epworth sleepiness scale (scale for daytime sleepiness) were higher in patients with OSA and hypothyroidism. BMI increase was positively associated with AHI increase in these patients with OSA and hypothyroidism [14].

2.8 What Is the Postoperative Management?

If a patient carries a diagnosis of OSA, anesthesiologists are cautioned that the administration of sedative agents (e.g., benzodiazepines) increases the risk of respiratory depression and airway obstruction [8]. The most common surgical intervention these patients present for is tonsillectomy and/or adenoidectomy. Opioids and benzodiazepines should be minimized or avoided completely. Dexmedetomidine is an alternative sedative that does not impair respiratory drive.

Several studies have looked at using local anesthetics to help with postoperative pain, but the results have been mixed. A 2022 meta-analysis published in the *International Journal of Pediatric Otorhinolaryngology* showed the injection of local anesthetic did improve postoperative pain on days 0 and 1; however, this is not a widely accepted technique due to concerns of postoperative bleeding and possibility of intravascular injection of local anesthetic leading to local anesthetic systemic toxicity [15].

Supplemental oxygen should be administered continuously to all patients who are at increased perioperative risk from OSA until they are able to maintain their baseline oxygen saturation while breathing room air. However, it should be cautioned that supplemental oxygen may increase the duration of apneic episodes and may hinder detection of atelectasis, transient apnea, and hypoventilation by pulse oximetry.

If a patient is using a CPAP or noninvasive positive pressure ventilation (with or without supplemental oxygen) at home, this should be continued, unless contraindicated by the surgical procedure. Compliance with CPAP or noninvasive positive pressure ventilation may be improved if patients bring their own equipment to the hospital. If possible, patients at increased perioperative risk from OSA should be placed in a non-supine position throughout the recovery process.

Hospitalized patients who are at increased risk of respiratory compromise from OSA should have continuous pulse oximetry monitoring after discharge from the recovery room. If frequent or severe airway obstruction or hypoxemia occurs during postoperative monitoring, initiation of nasal CPAP or noninvasive positive pressure ventilation should be considered.

Patients at increased perioperative risk from OSA should not be discharged from the recovery area to an unmonitored setting (i.e., home or unmonitored hospital bed) until they are no longer at risk of postoperative respiratory depression. Because of their propensity to develop airway obstruction or central respiratory depression, this may require a longer stay as compared with non-OSA patients undergoing similar procedures. To establish that patients can maintain adequate oxygen saturation levels while breathing room air, respiratory function may be determined by observing patients in an unstimulated environment, preferably while asleep. The preferred patient positioning is lateral and prone, with the least preferred positioning being the supine position.

2.9 What Could Have Been Done Differently if the Diagnosis of OSA Was Made Beforehand?

Assuming that the diagnosis of OSA was made prior to this procedure and that the patient would have been issued a CPAP or other noninvasive breathing assistance device, then we would have extubated the patient and transitioned to his home breathing device. If the data from his sleep study showed that his OSA was severe, then he should have recovered in an intensive care setting that could easily escalate breathing support if necessary. We would have also avoided benzodiazepines and minimized opioids and sedatives.

2.10 What Is the Effect of Using Dexmedetomidine in Cardiac Patients Undergoing Catheterization?

In an electrophysiological study in children, the researchers showed that dexmedetomidine produced depression in both sinus and atrioventricular nodal function with a decrease in heart rate with concomitant increase in blood pressure in them. Their conclusion was that dexmedetomidine must be used with caution in patients with bradycardia or atrioventricular block [16, 17]. Although dexmedetomidine can be safely used to decrease narcotics given, it can still produce bradycardia in patients and must be used with caution. In this case the patient has a pacemaker, and assuming it is functioning well, this would not be a contraindication to using dexmedetomidine.

Whenever a patient with a pacemaker is presenting for surgery, the pacemaker should be interrogated by electrophysiologists. Ideally there should be a report completed within 6 months from the date of surgery or procedure to ensure it is functional and has adequate battery life.

2.11 How Does Oral Premedication with Midazolam Affect Respiration in Healthy Children?

In a study by von Ungern-Sternberg et al. [18], in children with normal lungs, premedication with a relatively small dose of midazolam led to mild changes in respiratory variables shortly after its administration. However, the anesthesiologist should be aware that using midazolam in children at high risk of respiratory complications under anesthesia might lead to a greater decrease in respiratory function.

2.12 What Else Can You Use if You Do Not Have Access to a CPAP?

If the patient is obstructing their airway, you can try an oral airway or nasal airway to open the passage for ventilation. If the patient will not tolerate placement of an oral or nasal airway device, utilize a strap which interlocks to the mask to make a seal around the nose and mouth, and connect it to a Jackson-Rees. You can also connect it to a ventilator machine that has a CPAP setting. This will not be as comfortable as a custom-fit CPAP device but can work to facilitate ventilation.

In this case of a cardiac catheterization, you can incline the bed in reverse Trendelenburg to maintain the patient supine. If the case does not require the patient to lay supine in the bed, elevating the head of the bed 30° can help decrease obstruction. You can also try to place a shoulder roll under the patient. Alternative positioning such as placing the patient in a lateral decubitus position can help alleviate airway obstruction.

A recent article published as a front page in the journal *Anesthesiology* discussed the use of alternative methods when CPAP is not available. They found that elevating the head of the bed 30 degrees and using high-flow nasal cannula at 20 L/min helped decrease AHI [19].

2.13 Are There Any Serum Biomarkers Available to Evaluate the Degree of OSA in Our Patient if He Did Not Have Any Polysomnography Studies in the Past?

Yes, there are biomarkers which have been identified; however, this is not routinely used as a screening tool. In adult patients with OSA, high serum levels of erythropoietin have been associated with higher AHI. A prospective study in children aged 4–12 years old who underwent polysomnography (PSG) study overnight showed positive correlation with serum erythropoietin levels and the degree of OSA [20].

2.14 What Is the Etiology for Impaired Respiratory Function in Obese Patients Under Anesthesia?

Functional residual capacity in normal patients decreases by 20% under general anesthesia in the supine position. When a normal healthy patient assumes supine position and anesthesia is induced, there is a change in the configuration of the thoracic and abdominal cavity which can decrease efficient oxygenation due to atelectasis, airway closure, and increased ventilation/perfusion mismatching in the dependent zones of the lung. Increasing tidal volume and vital capacity breaths can help re-expand atelectatic areas in the lung.

In obese patients, reduction of FRC is much greater due to the loss of inspiratory muscle tone of the muscles acting on the rib cage and from gas trapping when anesthetized.

Obesity alters the mechanical properties of both chest wall and lungs because of excess fat deposition in the abdominal and thoracic cavities. The net effect of these results in poor compliance of the lungs causing alteration in the pattern of breathing. The reduction in diaphragmatic movement downward due to intra-abdominal fat results in compression atelectasis of the lung bases and reduction in expiratory reserve volume and functional residual capacity. Distribution of ventilation in obese patients is toward the upper lobes which have lesser perfusion, thus increasing ventilation perfusion mismatch and existing intrapulmonary shunting. The reduction of FRC is directly proportional to the severity of obesity. Airway closure in obese patients can occur at normal resting breathing because of reduction of FRC to levels at or even below closing capacity.

General anesthesia worsens lung atelectasis in morbidly obese patients for 24 h after surgery compared to non-obese patients. Application of CPAP will improve postoperative pulmonary function in these patients at risk for persistent atelectasis. Another strategy that reportedly can improve ventilation is placing them in reverse Trendelenburg position [21].

3 Summary

Obesity is a significant risk factor in children and a modifier of disease conditions like asthma, OSA, and pulmonary hypertension. In obese teenagers, a thorough preoperative evaluation of their cardiac and pulmonary function and comorbid conditions (OSA, hypertension, hypothyroidism, metabolic syndrome) should be obtained prior to scheduling the patient for elective surgery. During anesthesia, careful titration of drugs that can affect respiratory drive and vigilant intraoperative and postoperative monitoring of oxygenation are important. Applying CPAP or BIPAP to improve oxygenation and ventilation in patients with OSA and continuously monitoring the adequacy of ventilation can help optimize their perioperative stability and safety.

In patients who need to be supine after a catheterization procedure, a reverse Trendelenburg position in the postoperative period may be helpful to improve ventilation. Waist circumference and not BMI should be used to estimate the impairment of lung function in obese patients because it is considered as a marker of metabolic disease from obesity. Ideally this patient should have been seen in a preoperative clinic to facilitate time to discuss his complex medical history with appropriate interpreter services, to gather records from previous surgeries, and to investigate his snoring and excess somnolence as well as his thyroid function. Preoperative knowledge that this obese patient was hypothyroid with significant OSA would have enabled the anesthesiologist to choose a technique to avoid postoperative respiratory complications. It is important for the anesthesiologist to have a team discussion with the operative service to delay the case if the patient is not optimized preoperatively—preparing for success can prevent adverse events.

References

1. Strohl KP, Butler JP, Malhotra A. Mechanical properties of the upper airway. Compr Physiol. 2012;2(3):1853–72. https://doi.org/10.1002/cphy.c110053.
2. Coté CJ, Lerman J, Anderson BJ. Coté and Lerman's a practice of anesthesia for infants and children. 6th ed. Elsevier; 2018.
3. Schwengel DA, Dalesio NM, Stierer TL. Pediatric obstructive sleep apnea. Anesthesiol Clin. 2014;32(1):237–61. https://doi.org/10.1016/j.anclin.2013.10.012.
4. Marcus CL, Brooks LJ, Draper KA, et al. Diagnosis and management of childhood obstructive sleep apnea syndrome. Pediatrics. 2012;130(3):e714–55. https://doi.org/10.1542/peds.2012-1672.
5. Bixler EO, Vgontzas AN, Lin HM, et al. Sleep disordered breathing in children in a general population sample: prevalence and risk factors. Sleep. 2009;32(6):731–6. https://doi.org/10.1093/sleep/32.6.731.
6. Billings ME, Gold D, Szpiro A, et al. The Association of Ambient Air Pollution with Sleep Apnea: The Multi-Ethnic Study of Atherosclerosis. Annals of the American Thoracic Society. 2019;16(3):363–370. https://doi.org/10.1513/AnnalsATS.201804-248OC.
7. Gingras JL, Gaultney JF, Picchietti DL. Pediatric periodic limb movement disorder: sleep symptom and polysomnographic correlates compared to obstructive sleep apnea. J Clin Sleep Med. 2011;7(6):603–609A. https://doi.org/10.5664/jcsm.1460.
8. Practice guidelines for the perioperative management of patients with obstructive sleep apnea: an updated report by the American Society of Anesthesiologists task force on

perioperative management of patients with obstructive sleep apnea. Anesthesiology (Philadelphia). 2014;120(2):268–86. https://doi.org/10.1097/ALN.0000000000000053.
9. Kennedy WP, Mudd PA, Maguire MA, et al. 22q11.2 deletion syndrome and obstructive sleep apnea. Int J Pediatr Otorhinolaryngol. 2014;78(8):1360–4. https://doi.org/10.1016/j.ijporl.2014.05.031.
10. Sharma R, Sharma BB, Sharma R, Suthar N R, Jain R, Mathur S. Obesity, thyroid and OSA: an intriguing triangle. J Assoc Physicians India. 2022;70(4):11–2. PMID: 35443334.
11. Bruyneel M, Veltri F, Poppe K. Prevalence of newly established thyroid disorders in patients with moderate-to-severe obstructive sleep apnea syndrome. Sleep Breath. 2018;23(2):567–73. https://doi.org/10.1007/s11325-018-1746-z.
12. Sorensen JR, Winther KH, Bonnema SJ, Godballe C, Hegedüs L. Respiratory manifestations of hypothyroidism: a systematic review. Thyroid. 2016;26(11):1519–27. https://doi.org/10.1089/thy.2015.0642.
13. Green ME, Bernet V, Cheung J. Thyroid dysfunction and sleep disorders. Front Endocrinol (Lausanne). 2021;12:725829. https://doi.org/10.3389/fendo.2021.725829.
14. Zhang M, Zhang W, Tan J, Zhao M, Zhang Q, Lei P. Role of hypothyroidism in obstructive sleep apnea: a meta-analysis. Curr Med Res Opin. 2016;32(6):1059–64.
15. Ortega B, Stramiello JA, Brigger M, Nation J. Anesthetic injections and analgesia use in pediatric post-tonsillectomy patients: a meta-analysis and systematic review. Int J Pediatr Otorhinolaryngol. 2022;152:110976. https://doi.org/10.1016/j.ijporl.2021.110976.
16. Ergul Y, Unsal S, Ozyilmaz I, Ozturk E, Carus H, Guzeltas A. Electrocardiographic and electrophysiologic effects of dexmedetomidine on children. Pacing Clin Electrophysiol. 2015;38(6):682–7. https://doi.org/10.1111/pace.12623. Epub 2015 Apr 11. PMID: 25753681.
17. Hammer GB, Drover DR, Cao H, Jackson E, Williams GD, Ramamoorthy C, Van Hare GF, Niksch A, Dubin AM. The effects of dexmedetomidine on cardiac electrophysiology in children. Anesth Analg. 2008;106(1):79–83, table of contents. PMID: 18165557. https://doi.org/10.1213/01.ane.0000297421.92857.4e.
18. von Ungern-Sternberg BS, Erb TO, Habre W, Sly PD, Hantos Z. The impact of oral premedication with midazolam on respiratory function in children. Anesth Analg. 2009;108(6):1771–6. https://doi.org/10.1213/ane.0b013e3181a324c3.
19. Sakaguchi Y, Nozaki-Taguchi N, Hasegawa M, Ishibashi K, Sato Y, Isono S. Combination therapy of high-flow nasal cannula and upper-body elevation for postoperative sleep-disordered breathing: randomized crossover trial. Anesthesiology. 2022;137(1):15–27. https://doi.org/10.1097/ALN.0000000000004254.
20. Kalogritsas ND, Lachanas VA, Liakos P, Alexopoulos EI, Beka D, Petinaki E, Hajiioannou J, Simos G, Skoulakis CE. Erythropoietin levels in children with obstructive sleep apnea. Int J Pediatr Otorhinolaryngol. 2021;151:110932. https://doi.org/10.1016/j.ijporl.2021.110932. Epub 2021 Oct 1. PMID: 34619581.
21. Dixon AE, Peters U. The effect of obesity on lung function. Expert Rev Respir Med. 2018;12(9):755–67. https://doi.org/10.1080/17476348.2018.1506331. Epub 2018 Aug 14. PMID: 30056777; PMCID: PMC6311385.

Inability to Walk After Caudal Anesthesia in a Toddler

Elisha Peterson

Objectives

1. Identify complications following caudal approach to an epidural.
2. Recognize the unique considerations for regional anesthesia in children.
3. Describe the diagnostic workup for the motor block following caudal epidural.
4. Describe current methods to achieve successful caudal block including the use of ultrasound technology.

1 Case and Questions

A 15-month-old 11-kg boy presents to the recovery unit following an uncomplicated right orchiopexy under general anesthesia. He had an uneventful inhalational anesthetic induction with oxygen nitrous oxide and sevoflurane by mask followed by an intravenous line placement on his left hand and easy placement of LMA. A caudal block was placed with the patient positioned with knees bent and legs flexed upward in the left lateral position using a sterile technique. He received an epidural single shot via caudal approach of 11 mL of 0.2% ropivacaine administered in slow incremental doses. The surgery proceeded smoothly with the patient breathing spontaneously via an LMA, 60% oxygen 40% air and less than 2.7% sevoflurane, requiring no narcotics or intravenous agents. Having confirmed the success of the caudal block, the LMA was removed deep, and he was transferred to the PACU lying on his side with an oral airway in place. Vital signs on arrival to PACU were stable, and during the hand off to the PACU nurse, the anesthesiologist emphasized that the caudal block was easy to perform and was assessed to be successful during the intraoperative period. Upon waking up after 10 min, he cried and moved his right

E. Peterson (✉)
Children's National Medical Center, Washington, DC, USA
e-mail: epeterson@childrensnational.org

S. T. Verghese (ed.), *Anesthesia STAT! Acute Pediatric Emergencies in PACU*,
https://doi.org/10.1007/978-3-031-24396-7_13

leg as he spat out the oral airway but did not appear to move his left leg at all. He appeared agitated when his left leg was lifted off the bed and cried until he was reunited with his parents. The parents were allowed to hold him and notices that he is not moving his left leg at all. The PACU nurse calls the PACU attending saying that the parents are with the child and want to know the reason for this left foot weakness. You arrive at the bedside and evaluate the clinical situation. He appears comfortable, drinking his bottle, and his vital signs are stable. On examination, the right leg is held normal and responds to tickling but he shows no response to tickling his left foot.

2 What Are the Complications Following a Caudal Block? What Additional Information Would Be Helpful?

He is a healthy full-term boy on no medications with a normal perinatal history. This physical exam in the preoperative bay was a normal neuromuscular exam; he ambulated independently. The surgeon did not perform any additional block. The anesthesiologist who performed the caudal block reported use of the "whoosh" test prior to administration of local anesthetic to confirm epidural placement.

3 What Is the Whoosh Test? What Are Other Ways to Confirm Epidural Placement Via Caudal Approach?

After observation in the recovery room for 4 h, the patient continues to move his right leg but not his left leg. Family appears more anxious and wants some answers.

4 What Is Next in the Diagnostic Work Up for This Motor Block?

After discussion with radiology and neurosurgery, the decision was made to acquire a lumbar CT scan. CT scan revealed a 0.5 mm collection consistent with air at the left lumbar nerve root. CBC was normal.

5 Should This Patient Be Discharged with Close Follow-Up or Admitted?

The patient was admitted for serial neurologic exams. CBC continued to be normal. Ten hours after the procedure, the child moved his toes on his left leg and bent his knee. Fourteen hours after the procedure, he walks without any issue. Parents are relieved but also very upset about the events that happened requiring emergency CT scan and prolonged stay in the hospital with uncertainty.

6 Discussion

Caudal blocks are simple and easy to perform, and they have a lower learning curve than other regional anesthesia techniques [1]. Caudal approach to epidural is the most common regional block in pediatric anesthesiology [1–4]. For surgical procedures inferior to the umbilicus, caudal approach provides targeted dense analgesia which decreases the amount of volatile anesthetic and systemic analgesics needed throughout the perioperative period which results in decreased time in the hospital [3].

Caudal blocks are also safe to perform with a complication rate of 3% in children for single caudal shots. The most common problem during single-shot caudal is the technical challenge to identify the epidural space resulting in block failure [5]. Other complications from caudal approach to epidural include violation of dura, blood vessel, rectum, seizure, cardiac arrest, urinary retention and/or incontinence, pain, paresthesia, or transient neurologic deficit and extremely rare possibility of permanent neurologic damage [4–7]. In a cohort of over 18,000 children, rate of seizures and cardiac arrest occurred in 2/10,000 cases [4]. No complication lasted longer than 3 months [5].

Most caudal blocks are performed as a single shot, where a dose of local anesthetic is deposited in the epidural space [2]. Catheters can be left in the epidural space through the caudal approach, but this clinical practice is less common. Contraindications to caudal block are spinal dysraphism, pilonidal cyst, localized infection, spinal anomalies, bleeding disorders, or coagulation disorders [2].

Pediatric caudal blocks can be conducted via a palpation technique based purely on landmarks or a technique based on ultrasound guidance. The ultrasound is easy to use and radiation-free and can provide real-time images in guiding the needle entry into the caudal space. This technique however has not gained popularity perhaps due to the current high success of caudal blocks accomplished by using landmarks in children with low complications.

In adults with chronic pain, fluoroscopic guidance is used for definitive confirmation during placement of specific drugs for blocking pain fibers arising from the lower lumbar and sacral segments.

A technique based on anatomic landmarks is the most common technique for performing a caudal epidural block in children. Caudal blocks in children are mainly performed after the patient has undergone a general anesthetic with an airway device and an intravenous line in place [8]. Patients are positioned on their side with knees, hips, and neck in a flexed position to facilitate palpation of anatomical landmarks and to decrease risk dural sac puncture [2].

The anatomic landmarks form an inverted triangle with the posterior superior iliac spines as the base and the sacral hiatus forming the apex (Fig. 1a, b). Needle should be positioned at a 45-degree angle to the horizontal plane in between the sacral cornua into the sacral hiatus [2]. A distinct "pop" or "sudden give" sensed by the proceduralist's hand while advancing the needle often indicates the entry into the caudal epidural space. The loss of resistance thus sensed is an important sign

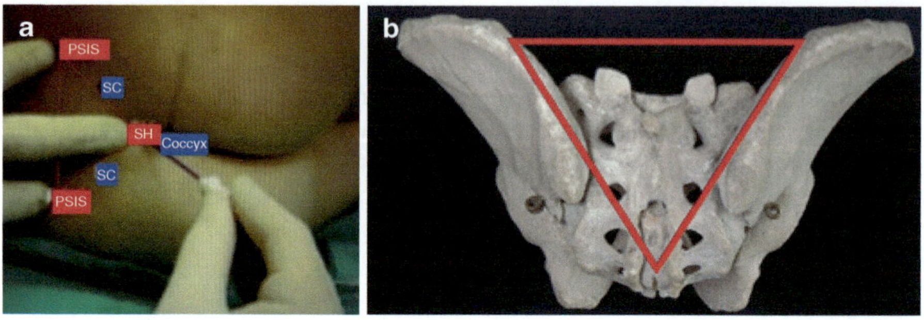

Fig. 1 (**a**, **b**) Sacral triangle shown on the anesthetized child. (**a**) With red triangle. *PSIS* posterior superior iliac spine, *SC* sacral cornua, *SH* sacral hiatus. (**b**) Skeletal landmarks of sacral triangle. https://commons.wikimedia.org/wiki/File:Pelvis_-_os_coxae,_os_sacrum_%28posterior_view%29.jpg#filelinks. Red triangle added by author

sought in confirming successful needle entry in the landmark technique to caudal block. The epidural space is encountered by piercing the sacrococcygeal ligament which lies between the sacral cornua [2]. The angle of the beveled needle is then flattened once the sacrococcygeal ligament is perforated in the sacral hiatus. A common mistake is directing the needle, deep perpendicularly, without flattening and hitting the bone beneath instead of entering the sacrococcygeal ligament. The termination of the spinal cord in adults is at L1–2 and the dural sac at S1–2. In children the spinal cord terminates much lower at L3–4 and the dural sac at S3–4. Therefore, there is a possibility of inadvertent needle entry into the dural sac during the performance of a caudal block in young infants. If heme or spinal fluid is encountered during needle puncture, then the needle is removed, and a decision can be made to try again with the use of imaging guidance or abort the procedure. If subcutaneous injection is encountered, reattempt can be made with a steeper needle angle. The administration of the desired volume of the local anesthetic is usually done in 2 mL aliquots with the needle held steady with the operator's left hand and a negative aspiration of blood or spinal fluid confirmed by the right hand before administering the next 2 mL bolus.

Although the use of ultrasound was not found to decrease the complications of caudal block [4] for infants and neonates, real-time use of ultrasound can be invaluable in decreasing the likelihood of block failure and dural puncture [2].

The type of needles recommended for use for caudal block is 22–25 g Tuohy or short 20–22 g angiocath, and the needle is inserted into the caudal space using a sterile technique. A short beveled blunt needle is often used for caudal block since sharp long needles can cause injury to the pelvic and retroperitoneal structures.

A timeout is performed after confirmation of the identification of the patient under anesthesia by repeating the patient's name, MR number, and birth date on the wristband with the chart with the same identification parameters. The planned local anesthetic drugs are drawn up by the proceduralist performing the caudal block a few minutes before the time of caudal block procedure. A nonsterile assistant holds the local anesthetic vial allowing needle entry into it in a sterile manner at the proceduralist's request, to ensure correct medication and appropriate expiration date and amount of local anesthetic to be delivered into the epidural space to ensure correct dosing.

Bupivacaine and ropivacaine are the most common local anesthetics used for the caudal block at 1 mL/kg volume in children [2].

6.1 Concentration Vs Volume of the Local Anesthetic Drug Dose

The sensory level blockade and the success of the caudal blockade are dependent on the dose, volume, and concentration of the injected local anesthetic drug. A low-concentration high-volume injectate strategy is more efficacious than a high-concentration low-volume strategy for caudal blocks in children if a higher-level sensory block is required [9]. In a single-center study in children undergoing orchiopexy, the researchers found that a higher volume (1 mL/kg) of a 0.20% bupivacaine decreased reactivity to spermatic cord traction intraoperatively than 0.8 mL/kg of 0.25% bupivacaine without any change in the quality of postop analgesia [8].

Additives can be included with the local anesthetic to prolong block duration such as sodium bicarbonate, epinephrine, morphine, clonidine, dexmedetomidine, midazolam, ketamine, neostigmine, and dexamethasone. A meta-analysis of 15 studies concluded that alpha 2 agonists prolong block duration with less side effects than other adjuvants but could not offer an ideal dose for alpha 2 agonist due to mixed results of these studies and publication bias [10]. When it comes to method of delivery, caudal alpha 2 agonists were found to be superior to IV agonists for analgesia [11]; however, use of IV dexamethasone 0.5 mg/kg at the time of regional blockade prolongs block duration to the same extent as 0.1 mg/kg caudal dexamethasone [12]. Caution should be exercised when considering the use of additives such as dexamethasone in the epidural space in children due to the lack of safety data of additives and concern for potential neurotoxicity [12].

6.2 Test Dose for Confirmation of Correct Needle Placement in Caudal Space

To confirm the needle is in the epidural space, a test dose of epinephrine 0.5 μg/kg can be provided with saline or 1 mg/kg of lidocaine with attention to heart rate, blood pressure, and T wave changes on the EKG. Of the vital signs to monitor, T wave changes were found to be the most sensitive indicator of an intravascular injection [13]. Changes in heart rate and/or blood pressure changes do not always occur in the face of an intravascular injection [13]. The injectate should be provided incrementally to watch for these changes and vitals observed 90 s after test dose is administered [13].

6.3 Auditory Tests for Correct Needle Placement Confirmation

6.3.1 Whoosh (Air) Vs Swoosh (Saline)

Other methods to ensure the needle's presence in the epidural space is use of the **whoosh** test. The use of the whoosh test was described in 1992 in adult patients [14]. A "whoosh" sound is heard through a stethoscope over the lumbar region when 2 mL of air is placed in the epidural space. If the air is not in the epidural space, no sound is heard [14]. This technique has fallen out of favor due to neurologic complications from residual gas in the epidural space. Motor weakness and sciatica have been described from gas compressing a nerve root [6, 15].

A modified "whoosh" test is the "swoosh" test which is the use of liquid instead of air [16]. 1 mL of saline or local anesthetic is injected into the caudal space while the lumbar spine is auscultated to listen for a "swoosh" sound. No sound is heard if the injectate is not in the caudal space.

In a cohort of 60 children, no significant difference was found in identifying the epidural space between the whoosh and swoosh tests. Currently, the swoosh test is recommended to avoid complications due to placing air in the epidural space [16]. A contention of these tests is the lack of clarity surrounding sounds of whoosh and swoosh [2].

6.4 Ultrasound Use for Caudal Block in Children (Fig. 2)

Ultrasound imaging at the midline using both longitudinal and transverse alignments of the probe is helpful to identify the sacrococcygeal ligament, dural sac, and caudal space and to view the anatomical structures around them.

The use of real-time ultrasound is superior to these tests as the presence of a color Doppler signal during injection can identify the epidural space, but the absence of a signal suggests that the injectate is not in the epidural space and that it could be in the intrathecal or subcutaneous space [17]. Placement of the curved ultrasound probe transversely at the lumbar level while injecting a volume of at least 0.1 mL/kg at a rate of 0.5–1 mL/s helps identify the deposition of the injectate [17]. Ultrasound can be used for caudal injections under real time by placing a linear probe ultrasound in a long axis along the lumbar spine. The sacrococcygeal ligament can be seen between the sacral cornua in a transverse view. The transverse view shows hyperechoic structures of sacrococcygeal ligament lying in between the sacral cornua and the sacral bone beneath. The Target for the needle is the hypoechoic part between the sacrococcygeal ligament and the sacral bone. In the longitudinal view, obtained by turning the probe 90°, the needle can be advanced "in-plane" into the sacral hiatus (Fig. 2). Since only the tip of the needle is visible in the caudal space, it is important not to advance the needle further than 3–5 mm upon entry but to obtain visualization of the unidirectional flow by color Doppler to identify successful placement of drug into the caudal space.

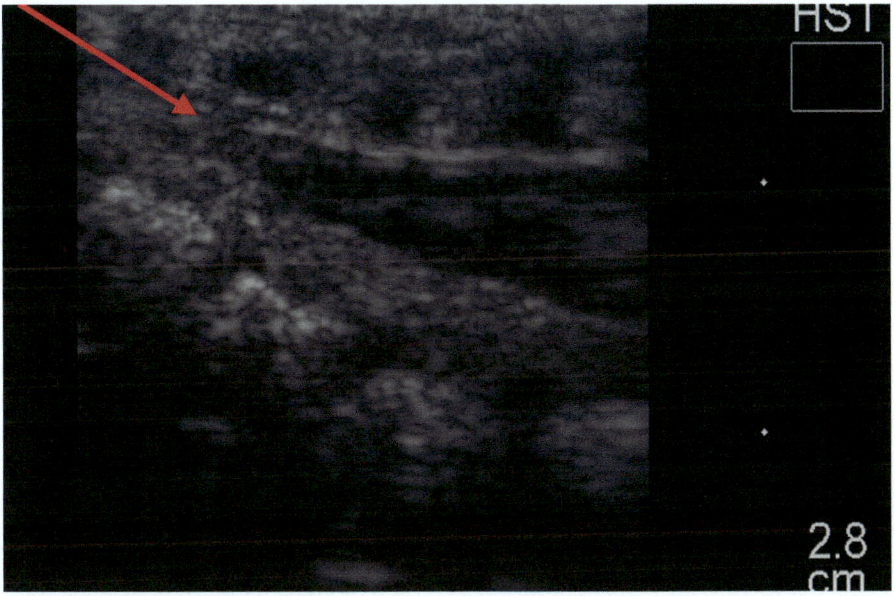

Fig. 2 Ultrasound image of caudal space in a 6-month-old. Arrow pointing to sacral hiatus position. (Ultrasound image courtesy of Dr. Adrian Bösenberg (Bosie))

6.5 Efficacy of Caudal Block Evaluation

Once the caudal block is delivered, observing response to surgical incision and manipulation can provide clues as to the efficacy of the block. A single-center study identified the assessment of anal sphincter tone before emergence from anesthesia as a tool to check for caudal efficacy in children undergoing inguinal and penile surgery. A lax anal sphincter tone at the end of surgery suggested a functional caudal block and correlated with reduced narcotic administration intraoperatively. A tight anal sphincter may therefore suggest the need for a repeat caudal block or use alternate ways to provide postoperative analgesia [18].

In another study in 223 children already under anesthesia, the researchers showed that the anal sphincter tone test was the best predictor for a successful caudal block when compared to swoosh test or the heart rate response to injection [19].

Following the procedure, the recovery room team should be provided a detailed hand off regarding the type of regional block, number of attempts, local anesthetic and amount provided, as well as the presence of any relevant medical history such as baseline neurologic deficits. Patient should be monitored for sensory and motor function in addition to the standard post-anesthesia care. Motor block in caudal blocks of 6 h has been reported, but asymmetric motor exam should raise suspicion and prompt further investigation. Neurosurgical evaluation and imaging should be obtained [20].

CT or MRI can detect the presence of epidural gas [6, 15]. Epidural gas is usually absorbed by the body over time, although large pockets of epidural gas may need to be evacuated through needle aspiration [6]. Serial neurologic exams to document and track resolution are warranted.

The parents are both lawyers and expressed dissatisfaction with the occurrence of this rare postoperative problem and would like to know why this was not mentioned before surgery during the preoperative interview. They both state that there was no mention of injecting air or possible neurologic sequelae with the caudal block. In fact, they emphasize that they recall only the part that the trainee who introduced the caudal block said that it will be done to decrease pain and that it is done usually without any problems in children.

Is there a need for written informed consent before performing pediatric regional technique?

Is there a need for an information leaflet available for parents to review and sign off to prevent future legal malpractice claims?

Caudal approach has continued to be regarded as a safe technique in anesthetized children but can occasionally result in an unexpected complication as in the case described. Obtaining written consent for caudal spinal or epidural in children is currently not in existence although its need is debated often. The volume of same-day surgeries is increasing, leading to shorter time for preoperative interview in most surgical centers. The anesthetic consent is often included in the surgical consent, and therefore a separate signed consent is currently not necessary before proceeding to the administration of general anesthesia. Informing parents about the specific regional technique planned, including its complications and side effects, is done during the preoperative visit. In turn, the parents usually express their willingness to go ahead with the plan for their child and ask questions related to the type of anesthetic procedure and the reason for the choice of regional block if they are knowledgeable or familiar with these blocks. It is important to document this preoperative discussion and verbal consent in the electronic chart of the patient with a witness if necessary.

Most parents and caregivers have poor recall of verbally detailed discussion, and there is always a possibility of saying that they were uninformed about the specific complication that occurred in their child. The quality of information regarding adjunct procedures and regional blocks can be improved by providing parents with information leaflets and documenting that a valid informed consent was obtained. This time-consuming yet legally necessary documentation can be helpful in preventing parental dissatisfaction and escalation to a legal malpractice claim [21].

7 Conclusion

Caudal block in children is a versatile regional block that provides both intraoperative and postoperative analgesia in young, anesthetized children for surgeries below the umbilicus. It is the most utilized, easy to learn regional technique currently performed with a single-needle entry into the caudal space if landmarks are clear on palpation. There are other tests to assure correct needle entry if anatomical difficulty is encountered and additives to prolong the duration of the local anesthetics. Real-time ultrasound use is useful in allowing the proceduralist to visualize the entry of the needle and the injected drug into the caudal space, but the setup and its use may prolong the caudal block procedure.

References

1. Silvani P, Camporesi A, Agostino MR, Salvo I. Caudal anesthesia in pediatrics: an update. Minerva Anestesiol. 2006;72:453–9.
2. Wiegele M, Marhofer P, Lönnqvist P-A. Caudal epidural blocks in paediatric patients: a review and practical considerations. Br J Anaesth. 2019;122:509–17.
3. Beyaz SG, Tokgöz O, Tüfek A. Caudal epidural block in children and infants: retrospective analysis of 2088 cases. Ann Saudi Med. 2011;31:494–7.
4. Suresh S, Long J, Birmingham PK, de Oliveira GS. Are caudal blocks for pain control safe in children? An analysis of 18,650 caudal blocks from the Pediatric Regional Anesthesia Network (PRAN) database. Anesth Analg. 2015;120:151–6.
5. Polaner DM, Taenzer AH, Walker BJ, Bosenberg A, Krane EJ, Suresh S, Wolf C, Martin LD. Pediatric Regional Anesthesia Network (PRAN). Anesth Analg. 2012;115:1353–64.
6. Lee MH, Han CS, Lee SH, Lee JH, Choi EM, Choi YR, Chung MH. Motor weakness after caudal epidural injection using the air-acceptance test. Korean J Pain. 2013;26:286–90.
7. Abdullayev R, Sabuncu U, Uludağ Ö, et al. Caudal anesthesia for pediatric subumbilical surgery, less load on the postoperative recovery unit. Cureus. 2019;11:e4348.
8. Verghese ST, Hannallah RS, Rice LJ, Belman AB, Patel KM. Caudal anesthesia in children: effect of volume versus concentration of bupivacaine on blocking spermatic cord traction response during orchidopexy. Anesth Analg. 2002;95:1219–23.
9. Hong J-Y, Han SW, Kim WO, Cho JS, Kil HK. A comparison of high volume/low concentration and low volume/high concentration ropivacaine in caudal analgesia for pediatric orchiopexy. Anesth Analg. 2009;109:1073–8.
10. Wang Y, Guo Q, An Q, Zhao L, Wu M, Guo Z, Zhang C. Clonidine as an additive to local anesthetics in caudal block for postoperative analgesia in pediatric surgery: a systematic review and meta-analysis. Front Med (Lausanne). 2021;8:723191. https://doi.org/10.3389/fmed.2021.723191.
11. Xing M, Liang X, Li L, Liao L, Liang S, Jiang S, Li J, Zhang C, Zou W. Efficacy of caudal vs intravenous administration of α2 adrenoceptor agonists to prolong analgesia in pediatric caudal block: a systematic review and meta-analysis. Paediatr Anaesth. 2020;30:1322–30.
12. Zhu C, Zhang S, Gu Z, Tong Y, Wei R. Caudal and intravenous dexamethasone as an adjuvant to pediatric caudal block: a systematic review and meta-analysis. Paediatr Anaesth. 2018;28:195–203.
13. Tobias JD. Caudal epidural block: a review of test dosing and recognition of systemic injection in children. Anesth Analg. 2001;93:1156–61.
14. Lewis MPN, Thomas P, Wilson LF, Mulholland RC. The "whoosh" test. Anaesthesia. 1992;47:57–8.
15. Giraud F, Fontana A, Mallet J, Fischer LP, Meunier PJ. Sciatica caused by epidural gas. Four case reports. Joint Bone Spine. 2001;68:434–7.
16. Talwar V, Tyagi R, Mullick P, Gogia AR. Comparison of "whoosh" and modified "swoosh" test for identification of the caudal epidural space in children. Pediatr Anesth. 2006;16:134–9.
17. Tsui B, Leipoldt C, Desai S. Color flow Doppler ultrasonography can distinguish caudal epidural injection from intrathecal injection. Anesth Analg. 2013;116:1376–9.
18. Verghese ST, Mostello LA, Patel RI, Kaplan RF, Patel KM. Testing anal sphincter tone predicts the effectiveness of caudal analgesia in children. Anesth Analg. 2002;94:1161–4.

19. Dave NM, Garasia M. A comparison of the effectiveness of predictors of caudal block in children-swoosh test, anal sphincter tone, and heart rate response. J Anaesthesiol Clin Pharmacol. 2012;28(1):17–20. https://doi.org/10.4103/0970-9185.92428. PMID: 22345939; PMCID: PMC3275964.
20. Berde C, Greco C. Pediatric regional anesthesia. Anesth Analg. 2012;115:1259–62.
21. Bendon AA, Venkataraju A, Shah A, Cooper N, Vashisht R. Information provision for caudal analgesia and the process of consent. Paediatr Anaesth. 2014;24(10):1111–2. https://doi.org/10.1111/pan.12504. PMID: 25196290.

Croupy Cough and O_2 Desaturation in Ex-Premature Toddler

Pooja Gupta

1 Case Presentation

A 20-month-old male presents for bilateral inguinal hernia repair. Medical history is significant for preterm birth at 29 weeks with a NICU stay of 3 weeks during which time he was intubated for 1 week due to respiratory failure. Since discharge, patient has been otherwise healthy except for some reactive airway disease requiring nebulizer treatment when he has an upper respiratory tract infection. He has had a croupy cough whenever he gets a cold, but it resolves with cool mist. He is otherwise not on any daily medications and has no known medication allergies. He lives with three siblings, his parents, and grandparents who smoke regularly. Parents report that he had a runny nose about 3 weeks ago lasting for 3 days but deny any fever, cough, or change in activity level. He has never had anesthesia before and there is no family history of adverse events with anesthesia.

Following mask induction with oxygen and sevoflurane, the patient has some upper airway obstruction that is alleviated with the use of an appropriately sized oral airway. After IV placement, and a bolus of propofol, the resident is able to successfully intubate the patient on her second attempt with the help of a stylet. There is some resistance to advancing the 3.5 cuffed endotracheal tube right at the level below the cords. The patient coughs a few times on the second attempt and another bolus of propofol is administered. The case proceeds uneventfully and the patient is extubated deep after an oral airway is placed. Immediately after extubation, the patient develops noisy breathing which seems to be somewhat alleviated with positioning the head and application of jaw thrust.

P. Gupta (✉)
Children's National Hospital, George Washington University, Washington, DC, USA
e-mail: pgupta4@childrensnational.org

S. T. Verghese (ed.), *Anesthesia STAT! Acute Pediatric Emergencies in PACU*,
https://doi.org/10.1007/978-3-031-24396-7_14

Twenty minutes after the patient is dropped off in the post-anesthesia care unit (PACU), the nurse calls stating that the patient is stridulous with a barking cough like a seal and that his oxygen saturation is 90–94% even with supplemental oxygen by face mask.

2 Discussion

2.1 What Is the Differential Diagnosis for this Child?

Desaturation in an ex-preterm infant after general anesthesia is a common post-operative complication with a wide variety of potential causes. It is imperative to use information about the patient's history, intraoperative course, and postoperative presentation to narrow down the differential diagnosis and treat the underlying cause to prevent progression to respiratory failure. The differential diagnosis for this patient includes soft tissue mechanical airway obstruction, residual paralysis from muscle relaxation, respiratory depression from narcotic administration, bronchospasm, laryngospasm, exacerbation of an underlying viral upper respiratory tract infection (URI), exacerbation of underlying bronchopulmonary disease, or post-extubation croup.

2.2 The Patient Received No Muscle Relaxant and Only 0.5 mcg/kg of Fentanyl Intraoperatively. Upon Evaluation, He Is Awake, Responsive, and Tachypneic with Stridor, Chest Retractions on Inspiration, and a Seal-like Barking Cough. There Is No Wheezing Present on Auscultation of the Lungs. What Is the Most Likely Diagnosis?

As this patient received no muscle relaxant, residual paralysis is not possible. He is awake, responsive, and tachypneic which also reduces the likelihood of this being due to respiratory depression from narcotic administration. The lack of wheezing and audible breath sounds eliminates bronchospasm, exacerbation of underlying bronchopulmonary disease, and laryngospasm as well. While this could be due to an exacerbation of an underlying viral upper respiratory tract infection or bronchopulmonary disease, the child had no symptoms to indicate the presence of an URI prior to this anesthetic other than a runny nose 3 weeks ago.

Given his history of intubation after birth and croupy cough with a cold, he likely already had some element of subglottic narrowing. This coupled with recent airway manipulation from two intubation attempts and some coughing after intubation likely caused subglottic swelling which is resulting in a barking cough. The most likely diagnosis is, therefore, post-extubation croup.

2.3 What Is Post-extubation Croup?

Croup is a symptom complex which includes stridor, hoarse voice, and a seal-like barking cough. When severe, croup can cause respiratory distress with evidence of retractions of suprasternal, intercostal, and subcostal muscles in a child (Fig. 1). Croup can be caused by viral laryngotracheitis, laryngotracheobronchitis, spasmodic croup, and post-extubation croup.

The overall incidence of post-extubation croup is found to be around 0.1–1% [1]. Post-extubation croup is inspiratory stridor developing immediately after extubation and up to 24 h post-extubation [2]. Symptoms can often resemble viral croup and include inspiratory stridor, chest retractions, hoarseness, and barking cough which may progress to respiratory failure [3]. Symptoms vary in terms of onset and severity; however, symptoms requiring treatment often present within the first hour after extubation [1].

Stridor is caused by turbulent gas flow through a narrowed segment of the airway and produces a high-pitched sound. The point during the respiratory cycle at which stridor occurs elucidates which portions of the airway are compromised by narrowing or obstruction.

Inspiratory stridor is seen with narrowing of the laryngeal or supraglottic regions.

Expiratory stridor results from narrowing of the intrathoracic airway.

Biphasic stridor stems from narrowing of both the larynx and subglottic regions [3].

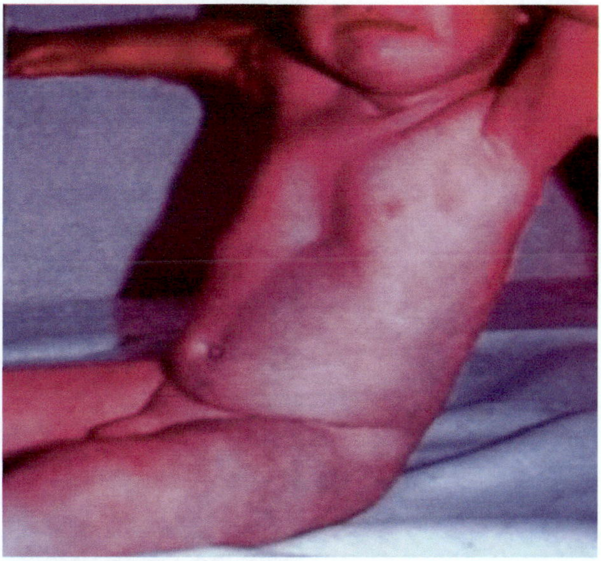

Fig. 1 Typical chest retraction in a child with croup

Compression from the endotracheal tube on the tracheal and subglottic mucosa causes inflammation and edema resulting in luminal narrowing of the airway producing stridor once the endotracheal tube is removed [2]. Decreasing the diameter of the airway lumen causes increased airway resistance as airway resistance is inversely proportional to the fourth power of the radius of the trachea with laminar flow. With turbulent airflow, resistance is increased even further to the fifth power of the radius of the trachea [3]. As the subglottic region in infants is smaller than that of adults, the same degree of edema seen in adults will result in a much more significant increase in resistance for the infant [4].

Glottic and subglottic narrowing from croup can be visualized radiographically and is termed the "steeple sign." The normal cylindrical airway lumen becomes narrowed resembling a church steeple (Fig. 2).

Although edema is one of the more common causes for post-extubation stridor, Tadie et al. found through fiberoptic endoscopic evaluation that granulation tissue, obstructive fibrinous pseudo membrane, and saliva-inducing obstruction can also cause post-extubation stridor [5].

One of the most used systems for grading the severity of croup is the Westley Clinical Score. This system has five clinical categories each given a numerical value with zero representing normal or absent and the highest number representing severe distress.

The clinical categories in **Westley Clinical Score** (Table 1) include level of consciousness, cyanosis, stridor, air entry, and retractions [6].

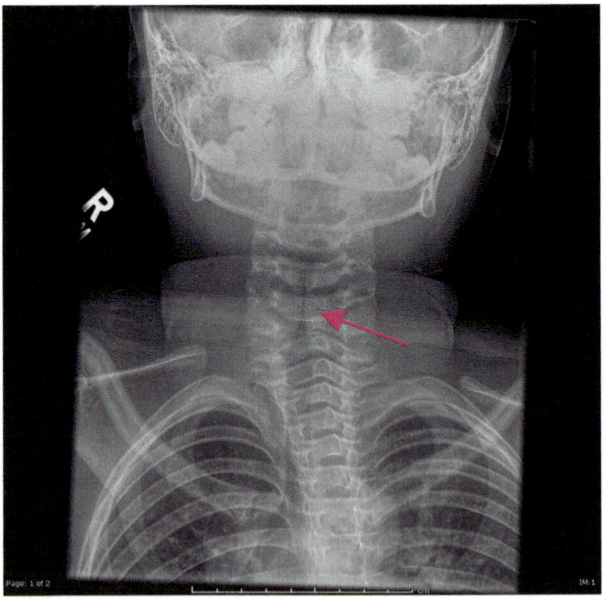

Fig. 2 X-ray of a child's neck with croup (arrow) showing the typical "steeple sign." (Photo courtesy of Dr. Narendra Shet)

Table 1 Westley Clinical Score

	0	1	2	3	4	5
Level of consciousness	Normal, sleeping					Disoriented
Cyanosis	Normal				Cyanosis with agitation	Cyanosis at rest
Stridor	Normal	Stridor with agitation	Stridor at rest	–	–	–
Air entry	Normal	Decreased	Severely decreased	–	–	–
Retractions	None	Mild	Moderate	Severe	–	–

An overall score of less than 2 indicates mild croup, 3–7 indicates moderate croup, and greater than 8 indicates severe croup [3]. This grading system can be a useful tool to quickly measure the overall severity of post-extubation croup and to measure clinical improvements with treatment.

2.4 What Are the Risk Factors for Developing Post-extubation Croup?

There are many risk factors for post-extubation croup, and these can be divided into patient-related, anesthetic, and surgical factors.

Patient-related factors include less than 4 years of age, concomitant upper respiratory tract infection, history of reactive airway disease, history of smoke inhalation, and history of subglottic stenosis [1]. Subglottic stenosis can be seen in patients with Down syndrome, it can also be associated with congenital anomalies such as tracheoesophageal fistula, or it can be acquired if the patient has a history of prolonged intubation in the neonatal period [3] (Fig. 3a–c).

This patient has many risk factors for post-extubation croup. Specifically, he is 20 months old, had a history of preterm birth, was intubated for 1 week, had a history of croupy cough with colds, and had regular second-hand smoke inhalation from his parents and grandparents' smoking. Given this patient's high risk for post-extubation croup, a discussion with the parents about this postoperative sequela would have been helpful during the preoperative interview.

Anesthetic risk factors for the development of post-extubation croup include prolonged mechanical ventilation; repeated or traumatic intubation; use of a tight-fitting endotracheal tube as demonstrated by a high leak pressure (>25 cm H_2O), coughing, or straining on the endotracheal tube; and the administration of copious fluids or transfusions [3, 7, 8].

Surgical risk factors for the development of post-extubation croup include frequent changing of head positioning, head and neck surgery, and patient positioning other than supine [1].

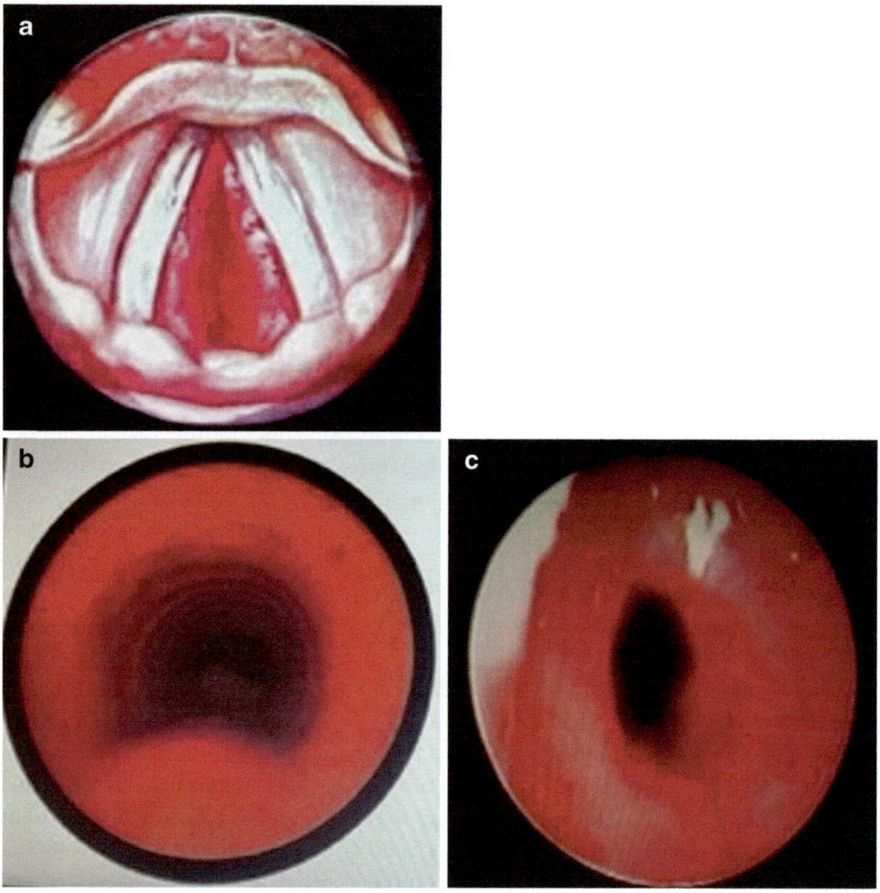

Fig. 3 (**a**) Direct laryngoscopic view of subglottic swelling. (**b**) Normal view. (**c**) Subglottic stenosis. Bronchoscopic view of normal subglottis and subglottic stenosis

2.5 What Are the Key Features of a Pediatric Airway?

Classically, there are five main anatomic features that differentiate a neonatal or pediatric airway from that of an adult. First, neonates and infants have large tongues that can obstruct the airway and may be difficult to navigate during laryngoscopy. The contribution of tongue size to upper airway obstruction, however, is rather minor as MRI studies have shown that the tongue grows in proportion to the bony oral cavity [4]. Second, compared to the adult epiglottis, the infant epiglottis is shorter, narrower, omega shaped, and angled away from the tracheal axis making it difficult to displace during laryngoscopy [4, 9]. Third, the infant larynx is located more cephalad at the level of C3–4 as compared to C4–5 in the adult. This results in an acute angulation of the plane of the tongue to the glottic opening and can make visualization of the airway during laryngoscopy more challenging [9]. Fourth, in the infant the anterior attachment of the vocal cords is located more caudally, thus altering the angulation between the vocal cords and trachea as compared to the adult where the vocal cords are situated more perpendicular to the trachea. This can result in difficulty when attempting to pass an endotracheal tube especially with nasal intubations [4]. Fifth, the cricoid cartilage is functionally the narrowest portion of the upper airway reaching adult sizes by 10–12 years of age [4]. Thus, an endotracheal tube that easily passes through the vocal cords may not pass the subglottic region or cause edema or trauma at the subglottic region [8].

2.6 What Are the Factors Affecting Work of Breathing?

There are several factors impacting the work of breathing. It is important to understand these factors as compromising or impeding any of them can predispose infants and children to respiratory failure.

Infants have a much higher respiratory rate secondary to their increased oxygen consumption. For full-term neonates, their oxygen consumption is 5–7 mL/kg/min as compared to that of an adult which is 2–3 mL/kg/min [4]. To accommodate this increased oxygen consumption, neonates and infants have a much higher baseline respiratory rate.

Work of breathing can also be viewed as resistance to airflow [4]. For laminar flow, airway resistance is inversely proportional to the radius of the airway to the fourth power. For turbulent flow, airway resistance is inversely proportional to the radius of the airway to the fifth power. Whether airflow is laminar or turbulent is determined by the Reynolds number (Reynolds number = (linear velocity × diameter × gas density)/gas viscosity). A low Reynolds number (<1000) correlates with laminar flow and a high Reynolds number (>1500) correlates with turbulent flow [10]. As pediatric airways are much smaller than those of adults, any decrease in airway caliber has a much greater impact on resistance to airflow and thus work of breathing.

The primary muscle of respiration in infants is the diaphragm. However, infants have more type II or fast-twitch low-oxidative or quick to fatigue muscle fibers than type I or slow-twitch high-oxidative or slow to fatigue muscle fibers. The percentage of type I muscle fibers comprising the diaphragm increases with age [4].

Overall, increased oxygen consumption, greater increase in resistance to airflow with any slight decrease in airway caliber, and the easy fatiguability of the diaphragm render infants and young children much more prone to respiratory fatigue and subsequent failure.

2.7 Does Endotracheal Tube Sizing and the Presence or Absence of a Cuff Matter?

Traditional practice in pediatric anesthesia was to use uncuffed endotracheal tubes for children under 8 years of age due to concerns for causing airway trauma or edema leading to post-extubation croup with the use of a cuffed endotracheal tube [11]. Many studies have been performed comparing cuffed endotracheal tubes to uncuffed endotracheal tubes in pediatrics, and overall, there is no difference between the two regarding the incidence of post-extubation croup [2]. In fact, with uncuffed endotracheal tubes, there are an increased number of tube exchanges and movement of the endotracheal tube during mechanical ventilation which can cause airway trauma and edema. The use of cuffed endotracheal tubes in small children not only provides a reliable sealed airway at cuff pressures of <or=20 cm H2O but also reduces the need for endotracheal tube exchanges, without increasing the risk for post-extubation stridor compared with uncuffed tracheal tubes [12, 13]. Cuffed endotracheal tubes carry several additional advantages including less anesthetic gas contamination, reduced aspiration risk, better mechanical ventilation, and the ability to adjust the amount of air in the cuff to account for changes in air leak with varying levels of sedation or alterations in patient positioning [2, 11].

While cuffed endotracheal tubes have some advantages over uncuffed endotracheal tubes, selecting the correctly sized tube for the patient is of utmost importance to prevent airway trauma that may lead to post-extubation croup. A commonly used formula is age/4 + 4 and when using a cuffed endotracheal tube using a tube 0.5 mm smaller than derived from the eq. [2]. When choosing an endotracheal tube size for an infant with suspected subglottic narrowing, as in the presented case, it is prudent to start with a further 0.5 mm smaller tube size than calculated.

Air leak tests are often used to determine whether an endotracheal tube is the correct size for a patient. It is the minimum amount of air pressure as measured by a manometer needed to produce an audible gust of air as auscultated by stethoscope over the larynx [7]. When using a cuffed endotracheal tube, the air leak should be audible with the cuff fully deflated, then the cuff should be slowly inflated until the leak is just occluded at 20 cm H_2O [2]. While the air leak test is routinely used, data does not support that it is predictive of post-extubation stridor in children less than 7 years of age [3, 7].

2.8 What Are Microcuff Tubes and Their Advantages?

Another more recent advancement has been the introduction of Microcuff tubes. These are low-pressure, high-volume polyurethane cuffed endotracheal tubes that allow for the benefits of having a cuffed endotracheal tube in place while allaying some of the concerns regarding cuff pressures and their effect on airway mucosa. The polyurethane material used produces a very thin membraned cuff which allows for an adequate seal at low pressures. Multiple studies have investigated post-extubation stridor or acquired subglottic pathology after prolonged intubation with Microcuff tubes and have shown a low incidence of any sequela [14, 15] (Fig. 4).

An ideal pediatric cuffed tube must have a high-volume low-pressure cuff which can seal at pressures less than 20 cm H_2O. It must have depth markings and its placement should be with the cuff placed just below the cricoid ring with the tip of the tube in the midpart of the trachea. In this optimal position, there is significant margin of safety for head flexion and extension.

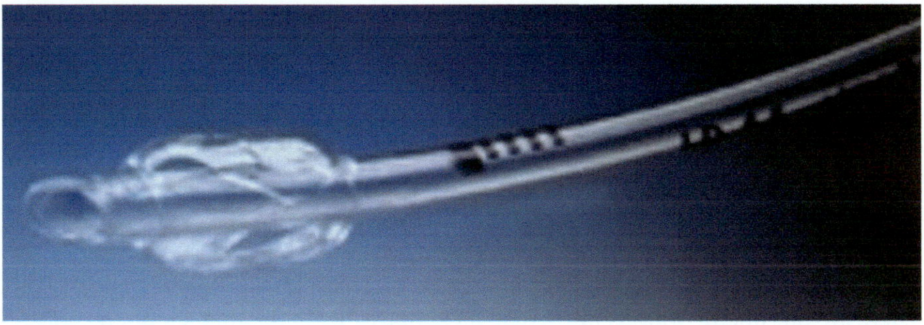

Fig. 4 Microcuff®

2.9 Are There Any Strategies That Can Be Employed to Prevent Post-extubation Croup?

There are several strategies that can be employed in the preoperative and intraoperative settings to help prevent post-extubation croup. Any patient presenting with a recent viral upper respiratory infection should be postponed if the case is not emergent in nature, especially if the case would require prolonged intubation times.

All efforts should be made to avoid multiple or traumatic intubation attempts by optimizing patient positioning, having appropriately sized airway equipment available, ensuring adequate depth of anesthetic prior to laryngoscopy, utilizing muscle relaxant as indicated, and having experienced personnel perform the laryngoscopy [2]. In the case presented, given the patient's history of preterm birth with 1 week intubation and croupy cough with colds, subglottic narrowing should have been suspected. Adequate depth of anesthetic and muscle relaxant administration should be ensured prior to any airway manipulation to prevent coughing or bucking during intubation. Finally, a smaller-sized endotracheal tube should have been selected and introduced with the cuff fully deflated until the cuff was just below the vocal cords. Overall, in this patient, every effort should have been made to ensure first-pass success in intubation to minimize airway manipulation and prevent exacerbation of pre-existing subglottic narrowing.

Dexamethasone IV can be given as prophylaxis to alleviate any airway swelling that may develop due to multiple or traumatic intubation attempts, prolonged intubation, and airway surgery or to any patient at high risk for post-extubation airway obstruction [1].

Facilitating a smooth extubation can also help prevent post-extubation croup as bucking or forceful coughing around an endotracheal tube can lead to swelling or subglottic injury which can subsequently lead to post-extubation croup. To ensure a smooth extubation, one can extubate the patient while breathing spontaneously at a deeper plane of anesthesia or administer IV lidocaine or a sedative like propofol or dexmedetomidine prior to extubation [1].

If the patient has been intubated for a prolonged period, a leak test may also be performed to ensure there is no airway edema around the endotracheal tube [2]. To perform a leak test, the cuff should be fully deflated and the endotracheal tube occluded. With the patient spontaneously ventilating, an audible air leak or gust of air should be auscultated either at the mouth or with a stethoscope held over the larynx.

2.10 Could This Case Have Been Done Without Endotracheal Intubation?

There are anesthetic options other than an endotracheal tube that should be considered in a patient with the possibility of having a preexisting subglottic narrowing in order to avoid airway manipulation and possible exacerbation of subglottic narrowing. However, these regional techniques and alternative airway options may fail, and one should always be ready to convert to general endotracheal anesthesia.

Spinal anesthesia may be useful in at-risk patient populations for surgeries below the umbilicus. An alpha 2 antagonist such as dexmedetomidine or clonidine can be safely utilized to facilitate sedation and supplement pain control without causing respiratory depression. A nasal cannula can be used to monitor spontaneous ventilation and CO_2 in these patients [16].

Regional blocks, such as a caudal, may also be beneficial in this patient population for those undergoing surgery below the umbilicus as it will decrease the need for narcotic administration and can be combined with sedation or total intravenous anesthesia (TIVA). An LMA can be placed if airway support is needed. However, smaller-sized LMAs can be difficult to seat reliably in these infants.

2.11 How Do You Manage Post-extubation Croup?

Management of post-extubation croup varies dependent upon the degree of severity. Racemic epinephrine via nebulizer for 7–10 min will produce vasoconstriction and relieve airway obstruction. For mild cases, humidified cool mist can help decrease mucosal edema [8]. Emergence delirium, crying, and agitation can worsen stridor and post-extubation croup and thus should be treated with sedatives [2].

Dexamethasone, as mentioned earlier, has a role as prophylaxis as it decreases airway edema and the incidence of post-extubation croup. While dexamethasone is not an acute treatment, for patients given prophylactic steroids who still develop post-extubation croup, dexamethasone can be given every 4–6 h for 2 days at 0.5 mg/kg up to 40 mg/day to help ameliorate mucosal edema [2, 8, 17]. In the acute setting, aerosolized budesonide can be used to reduce airway edema through its vasoconstrictive effects [1, 2].

For patients presenting with moderate post-extubation croup, nebulized racemic epinephrine should be administered over 5–10 min, as its vasoconstrictive effects will decrease airway edema [8]. Patients who receive racemic epinephrine should be monitored for 4 h as they may develop a resurgence of symptoms [2].

This resurgence of symptoms, also known as a rebound phenomenon, is due to the short duration of action of racemic epinephrine which leads to a return of edema and airway obstructive symptoms as the medication effects wear off. Patients may require repeated treatment every 1–2 h until their symptoms resolve and should be monitored for at least 2 h after the last administration to ensure complete resolution of airway edema [18].

There have been many studies on differing dosages of racemic epinephrine and their efficacy on treating post-extubation croup as well as their systemic effects. One prospective, randomized double-blind study compared nebulized racemic epinephrine 1:1000 at 0.5, 2.5, and 5 mL and found no difference in clinical improvement in post-extubation croup as assessed using the Westley scoring system and thus recommends using 0.5 mL for treatment to minimize the mild systemic effects they found of tachycardia, pallor, and increased blood pressure [19]. Current guidelines recommend using 0.2–0.5 mL of 2.25% racemic epinephrine diluted into 3–5 mL of normal saline and administered over 5–10 min by nebulizer [2] (Fig. 5).

Helium-oxygen (heliox) therapy is a useful adjunct for upper airway obstruction. It has been used since the 1930s in the management of patients with upper airway obstruction. Helium as a component of inspired gas decreases turbulent flow and airway resistance [10, 20]. Heliox has a lower specific gravity and a low density to viscosity ratio and therefore able to decrease the Reynolds number and promote laminar flow [2, 10]. This can help modify gas flow, improve breathing patterns, and

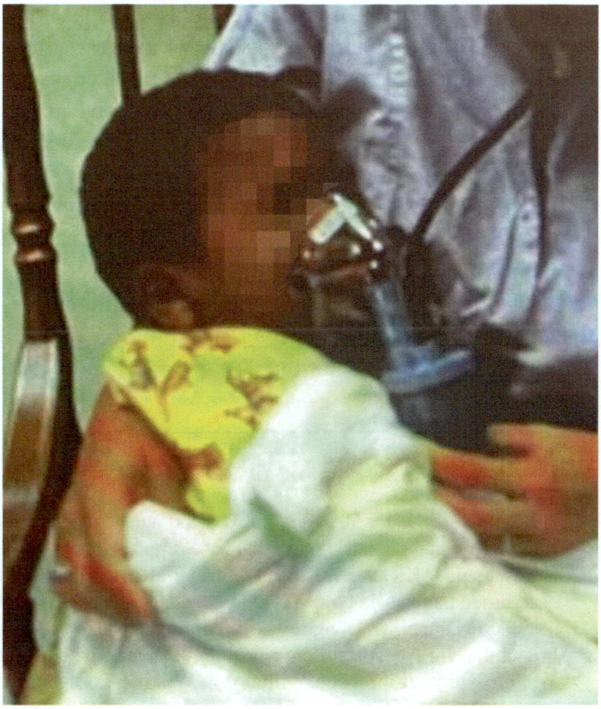

Fig. 5 Racemic epinephrine administration by nebulizer to a child held by a mom in a rocking chair in PACU

decrease work of breathing in a child with stridor especially when racemic epinephrine is not effective. This is however a temporary treatment until other treatments prove effective or the edema resolves on its own. Heliox administration is complex and requires the patient to be admitted to the ICU. Heliox can be administered either through a premixed helium-oxygen tank that contains at least 20% oxygen or with a helium tank and oxygen blender. Either modality requires inline monitoring of inspired oxygen fraction to prevent delivery of a hypoxic mixture [21].

For patients with severe post-extubation croup or impending respiratory failure, reintubation is the recommended management. Patients should be intubated with an endotracheal tube either one half or one full size smaller than was used before [3]. After reintubation it is important to perform a leak test to ensure the endotracheal tube is not too large. The patient should remain intubated for at least 24–48 h for the airway swelling to subside [2].

Post-extubation subglottic upper airway obstruction is not without its own problems because it is associated with threefold greater odds of causing long-term airway morbidity [22]. These patients therefore may represent an at-risk population that should be monitored closely after leaving the ICU. Evaluation by an otolaryngologist may be beneficial to evaluate the degree of airway narrowing and should be recommended prior to discharge.

3 Summary

Ex-premature infants often have occult residual airway problems which become apparent during a general anesthetic as in our patient with post-extubation croup. Careful preoperative assessment and open discussion with the parents and perioperative team (pediatrician, surgeon, perioperative nursing team, and external consultation with ENT surgeon) can help formulate an ideal plan that will allow the patient to undergo a safe anesthetic and optimize their postoperative course.

Facilitating a smooth induction and intubation with minimal airway manipulation, selection of the optimal sized endotracheal tube, early administration of Decadron, and racemic epinephrine by nebulizer in PACU on arrival may mitigate the usual problems if general endotracheal intubation is undertaken. Regional anesthesia with additives to prolong the duration of analgesia may be beneficial by avoiding airway manipulation.

References

1. Kim HJ, Son JD, Kwak K-H. Unexpected and severe postintubation croup after a very short day surgery in a pediatric patient: a case report. Korean J Anesthesiol. 2014;67:287–9.
2. Goldschneider KR, Wu J, Kurth D. Stridor after extubation. In: Clinical pediatric anesthesia: a case-based handbook. New York: Oxford University Press; 2012. pp. 690–698.
3. Yao F-SF, Dinner M, Longhini A. Inflammatory airway disease in childhood: laryngotracheobronchitis. In: Anesthesiology: problem-oriented patient management, 9th ed. Philadelphia: Wolters Kluwer/Lippincott Williams & Wilkins; 2021. pp. 800–810.

4. Coté CJ, Lerman J, Anderson BJ, Fiadjoe JE, Litman RS, Serber JF, Stricker PA, Coté CJ. The pediatric airway. In: A practice of anesthesia for infants and children, 6th ed. Philadelphia: Elsevier; 2019. pp. 297–339.
5. Tadié J-M, Behm E, Lecuyer L, Benhmamed R, Hans S, Brasnu D, Diehl J-L, Fagon J-Y, Guérot E. Post-intubation laryngeal injuries and extubation failure: a fiberoptic endoscopic study. Intensive Care Med. 2010;36:991–8.
6. Westley CR. Nebulized racemic epinephrine by IPPB for the treatment of croup. Am J Dis Child. 1978;132:484.
7. Mhanna MJ, Zamel YB, Tichy CM, Super DM. The "air leak" test around the endotracheal tube, as a predictor of postextubation stridor, is age dependent in children. Crit Care Med. 2002;30:2639–43.
8. Pawar D. Common post-operative complications in children. Indian J Anaesth. 2012;56:496.
9. Estrada C, Carline N, Stayer S, Patel N, Mann D, Hopkins P. Condensed review of pediatric anesthesiology, 2nd ed. 2014.
10. Butterworth JF, Mackey DC, Wasnick JD, Morgan GE, Mikhail MS. Respiratory physiology and anatomy. In: Morgan & Mikhail's clinical anesthesiology, 5th ed. New Delhi: McGraw-Hill; 2014. pp. 487–525.
11. Newth CJL, Rachman B, Patel N, Hammer J. The use of cuffed versus UNCUFFED endotracheal tubes in pediatric intensive care. J Pediatr. 2004;144:333–7.
12. Timmerman K, Thomas JM. Endotracheal tubes in paediatric anaesthesia: the cuffed versus uncuffed debate. S Afr J Anaesth Analg. 2010;16:88–91.
13. Weiss M, Dullenkopf A, Fischer JE, Keller C, Gerber AC. Prospective randomized controlled multi-centre trial of cuffed or uncuffed endotracheal tubes in small children. Br J Anaesth. 2009;103:867–73.
14. Dullenkopf A, Gerber AC, Weiss M. Fit and seal characteristics of a new paediatric tracheal tube with high volume-low pressure polyurethane cuff. Acta Anaesthesiol Scand. 2005;49:232–7.
15. Greaney D, Russell J, Dawkins I, Healy M. A retrospective observational study of acquired subglottic stenosis using low-pressure, high-volume cuffed endotracheal tubes. Pediatr Anesth. 2018;28(12):1136–41.
16. Handlogten K, Warner L, Granberg C, Gargollo P, Thalji L, Haile D. Implementation of a spinal anesthesia and sedation protocol that reliably prolongs infant spinal anesthesia: case series of 102 infants who received spinal anesthesia for urologic surgery. Pediatr Anesth. 2020;30:1355–62.
17. Markovitz BP, Randolph AG. Corticosteroids for the prevention of reintubation and postextubation stridor in pediatric patients: a meta-analysis*. Pediatr Crit Care Med. 2002;3:223–6.
18. Coté CJ, Lerman J, Anderson BJ, Hannallah RS, Brown KA, Verghese ST. Otorhinolaryngologic procedures. In: A practice of anesthesia for infants and children, 6th ed. Philadelphia: Elsevier; 2019. pp. 754–789.
19. da Silva PS, Fonseca MC, Iglesias SB, Junior EL, de Aguiar VE, de Carvalho WB. Nebulized 0.5, 2.5- and 5-ML L-epinephrine for post-extubation stridor in children: a prospective, randomized, double-blind clinical trial. Intensive Care Med. 2011;38:286–93.
20. Grosz AH, Jacobs IN, Cho C, Schears GJ. Use of helium-oxygen mixtures to relieve upper airway obstruction in a pediatric population. Laryngoscope. 2001;111:1512–4.
21. Gupta VK, Cheifetz IM. Heliox administration in the pediatric intensive care unit: an evidence-based review. Pediatr Crit Care Med. 2005;6:204–11.
22. Green J, Ross PA, Newth CJL, Khemani RG. Subglottic post-extubation upper airway obstruction is associated with long-term airway morbidity in children. Pediatr Crit Care Med. 2021;22(10):e502–12. https://doi.org/10.1097/PCC.0000000000002724. PMID: 33833205; PMCID: PMC8490268.

Postop Apnea in An Infant After Spinal Anesthesia for Hernia Repair

Philip dela Merced

Educational Objectives
At the conclusion of this discussion, the learner will be able to:

1. Define the problem of apnea of prematurity and its impact in the perioperative period.
2. Identify risk factors for apnea, including gestational age, post-conceptual age, and anemia.
3. Describe spinal anesthesia in infants and understand its potential complications.
4. Recognize how spinal anesthesia may impact the risk of postoperative apnea, in comparison to general anesthesia.

1 Case Presentation

An 8-week-old male, born at 31 weeks' gestation, is identified to have an incarcerated left inguinal hernia and is thus brought to the operating room for open left inguinal herniorrhaphy. Other pertinent history includes post-delivery intubation for 1 week, as well as history of a small patent foramen ovale not requiring intervention. There is no history of intraventricular hemorrhage, necrotizing enterocolitis, bronchopulmonary dysplasia (BPD), or neurologic abnormality after birth. Following the treatment with caffeine and use of nasal CPAP, he was discharged after 3 weeks, with home monitoring on an apnea monitor, which according to parents had not signified any further apneic events at home.

P. dela Merced (✉)
Department of Anesthesia, Pain, and Perioperative Medicine, Children's National Hospital, Washington, DC, USA
e-mail: pdelamerce@childrensnational.org

S. T. Verghese (ed.), *Anesthesia STAT! Acute Pediatric Emergencies in PACU*,
https://doi.org/10.1007/978-3-031-24396-7_15

On presentation, he weighs 2.9 kg, and his vital signs are stable on room air. After consent is obtained from the parents, the decision is made to provide an awake spinal anesthesia for the surgical procedure. Intravenous line is placed in the saphenous vein on the right leg and D5 LR is administered with the help of an infusion pump. Monitors are placed and the vital signs before the spinal anesthesia and surgery are obtained and recorded on the monitor. After sterile prep and drape, with the infant held in the sitting position by an assistant, spinal space L4–L5 is identified by the anesthesiologist and intrathecal injection of hyperbaric 0.75% bupivacaine dose (1 mg/kg) is performed after easy entry of the spinal needle into the subarachnoid space at the first attempt.

The success of the spinal block is confirmed by the lack of response to sensory stimulus and by the infant's inability to move the legs. Bovie pad is placed with infant maintaining a supine with slight head-up position. The surgical prep starts immediately by the surgeon who is already scrubbed and in a sterile surgical gown, ready to make the surgical incision. The left inguinal herniorrhaphy proceeds without the patient responding to surgical incision or for the remainder of surgical manipulations during the 40-min procedure. No sedation or analgesics are needed intraoperatively, and the patient is transferred to the PACU on a vital sign monitor in stable condition. A complete hand-off is given to the nurse with emphasis to check his blood sugar, keep him warm, and continue monitoring for possible apnea. Although the patient had no intraoperative apneic spells, the possibility of this occurring in the postoperative period is discussed during the hand-off.

After 30 min, PACU nurse calls the anesthesiologist that the patient is having apneic spells lasting about 15–20 s each with bradycardia and drop in oxygen saturation to 94–96% which resolves spontaneously on patient stimulation. The postoperative temperature and blood sugar are both reported to be normal in the infant. The apneic periods continue intermittently for another 20 min, and the anesthesiologist decides to treat it with caffeine. Intravenous caffeine 5 mg/kg is administered in PACU in 2 boluses with a 5-min interval (total 10 mg/kg) with increase in heart rate and blood pressure. He appears more awake, crying, and moving more, and he does not have any more apneic spells during the remainder of his PACU stay. The patient is transferred back to the neonatal intensive care unit with stable vital signs and normal temperature and is monitored overnight without any further apnea problems.

2 Discussion

2.1 What Are the Risk Factors for Postop Apnea in Ex-premature Infants Undergoing Anesthesia?

Infants and neonates are at an increased risk of developing complications when they undergo anesthesia. The risk of perioperative apnea, defined as cessation of breathing for 15–20 s or more, is significantly increased within this patient population [1]. Apnea of prematurity may be defined as less than 20 s often in the presence of desaturation and/or bradycardia [2]. Oxygen desaturation may be defined as saturation ≤80% for ≥4 s, and bradycardia is often defined as heart rate decrease from baseline by <2/3 for ≥4 s [3]. This should be distinguished from periodic breathing, which can be defined as apnea up to 5–10 s, usually during REM sleep, in the absence of either desaturation or bradycardia [3]. While often a normal finding in a healthy neonate, it typically occurs from ages 2–4 weeks, with spontaneous resolution about 6 months of age. If increased in frequency, it can indicate a precursor to other risk factors, including various other illnesses or physiologic stressors, particularly in premature infants.

When considering the risk factors for apnea of prematurity, premature infants are prone to various physiologic insults, including lower birth weight, anemia, electrolyte imbalances, hypoglycemia, hypothermia, and narrow therapeutic windows for oxygen. Additional consideration is to be given to the immaturity of the central nervous system, with a poorly developed respiratory control center contributing to the risk of apnea. The use of intraoperative narcotics may also be a contributor to perioperative apnea when compared to older patient populations. Every effort should be taken to maintain a warm temperature for premature babies in the operating room since a decrease in body temperature can cause apnea in premature infants. Low glycogen stores make them prone to hypoglycemia which can also result in apnea, lethargy, irritability, and seizures [1].

However, age is often seen as the single most important risk factor for apnea, with preterm and ex-premature infants at the highest risk [4].

A retrospective chart review of ex-premature infants undergoing general anesthesia confirmed the results from previous studies regarding the risk predictors for post-anesthesia apnea in them. Low gestational/post-menstrual age, lower weight, and intraoperative narcotic use were considered the cause of one of the apneic events in this study [5].

A study on the incidence of apnea after general anesthesia reported that in ex-premature infants less than 44 weeks of postconceptual age (PCA), there is a higher risk for apnea than in ex-premature infants older than 44 weeks PCA. Based on their findings, they concluded that the maximum long-run risk of apnea after anesthesia in ex-premature infants older than 44 weeks postconceptual age is 5% with 95% confidence [6].

A review of data collected over 12 years described the epidemiological trends among preterm infants with apnea. Although only 7.5% infants were preterm in this study of over 1.38 million births, the diagnosis of apnea was significantly higher. GE reflux and early gestational age were the two predictors of apnea in these preterm babies [7].

Multiple studies have set varying criteria for high-risk ages, but current data cite that those infants less than 60 weeks postgestational age are at risk for anesthesia in the postoperative period [8].

In a landmark study by Coté et al., the investigators analyzed original data from 8 prospective studies from 4 institutions on the risk factors for apnea in 255 infants undergoing inguinal hernia repair under general anesthesia. They excluded infants under spinal or on treatment with caffeine for apnea. The investigators suggested from the combined results of these studies the following:

The probability of apnea in nonanemic infants to be free of apnea in PACU *is* not less than 5% *with 95% statistical confidence until the postconceptual age was* 48 weeks with a gestational age of 35 weeks. This risk *is* not less than 1% *with 95% statistical confidence for the same subset of infants until postconceptual age was* 56 weeks with gestational age 32 weeks *or postconceptual age* was 54 weeks and gestational age 35 weeks [8].

The timing of apnea occurrence is important as well when discussing postoperative apnea. Early apnea is defined as any episode of cessation of breathing within the first 30 min postoperatively, whereas late apnea may occur between 30 min and 12 h postoperatively. Furthermore, data show that early apnea may be a predictor for late apnea [4].

Additional risk factors may include having a history of apneic events or requiring intervention to maintain ventilation, including administration of caffeine/methylxanthine, oxygen support, or positive pressure ventilation [4].

Anemia is another cause for increased incidence of apnea in ex-premature infants undergoing general anesthesia.

Coté et al., in their study, concluded that apnea was *strongly and inversely related to both gestational age and postconceptual age but* anemia to be a significant independent risk factor *in infants less than 43 weeks' post conceptual age* [8].

2.2 What Is Spinal Anesthesia?

Neuraxial blockade is a technique commonly used for many pediatric procedures, either as the primary anesthetic or as an adjunct to postoperative pain control. In spinal anesthesia (SA), awake subarachnoid injection of local anesthetic in infants is used as the primary anesthetic for various general abdominal and urologic procedures, particularly those that are open and infraumbilical [1]. This technique may be chosen to avoid general anesthesia (GA), which will necessitate management of the airway and ventilation of the patient. This may prove useful in the setting of a known or anticipated difficult airway, or patients with a high risk of requiring endotracheal intubation postoperatively. The neonatal population, due to immature lung development and poor respiratory compliance, are often at higher risk of requiring postoperative ventilation following anesthesia [9].

For the procedure, mild sedation may be provided, either preoperatively or intraoperatively, with agents such as dexmedetomidine or ketamine to preserve spontaneous ventilation, though caution should be taken with preterm neonates as they may be more sensitive even to very low doses of sedation. Other means of pacifying young children, after the spinal is performed, would be external environmental factors, such as the use of visual aids and music, and in a neonate or an infant by providing a small amount of high glucose liquid on a pacifier intermittently. Recent studies have shown that intraoperative sedation is not required; electroencephalograms performed on infants undergoing spinal demonstrated increased slow wave activity with decreased beta wave activity, indicating that sleep patterns may occur without the use of pharmacologic sedation [10].

Duration of neuraxial blockade will vary depending on the local anesthetic used for intrathecal injection. Important factors to focus on are the dose of the local anesthetic, baricity, patient position, and the volume of cerebrospinal fluid.

Baricity of the local anesthetic solution used will dictate the spread of local anesthetic in the spinal canal compared to gravity. Hyperbaric solution will therefore spread down in a descending manner with gravity. When using hyperbaric local anesthetic solution, care must be taken to keep patient in a flat supine or slight head-up position which will allow the anesthetic to spread in caudad direction.

Generally accepted practice bases the dose on weight (see Table 1). The use of bupivacaine 0.75% in 8.25% dextrose will typically last 60–90 min, depending on if adjuncts such as dexmedetomidine, clonidine, or epinephrine are used. Because of this, discussion should be held with the surgeon to remain immediately available to make the incision, to reduce the risk of block failure due to prolonged surgical time. If a longer case is anticipated, practitioners may opt to perform a caudal catheter afterward to continue the anesthesia once the spinal bupivacaine is no longer effective. Current practice recommendations do not indicate the use of an intrathecal catheter in these populations, noting the continued unpredictability of spread an increased risk of neurotoxicity and local systemic anesthetic toxicity in infants.

During the performance of a spinal anesthetic in an ex-premature infant, an intravenous line is first established and 10 ml/kg of D5 LR is given first and all the hemodynamic monitor measurements, i.e., heart rate, blood pressure, respiratory rate, and oxygen saturation on room air, are observed and recorded as baseline for comparison.

Contraindication to neuraxial anesthesia would be those with anatomic abnormalities (such as tethered cord, myelomeningocele), coagulopathy, and with concern for increased intracranial pressure. Though a relative contraindication, caution should be held for infants with history of intraventricular hemorrhage in the newborn period and those with implanted devices in connection with the cerebrospinal fluid, such as those with ventricular shunts.

Significant amounts of research have also explored the impact of general anesthesia (GA) on neurocognitive development, with many citing that GA may cause an increase in the incidence of neuroapoptosis and thus worsen neurocognitive outcomes in long term [11]. However, as part of an international, multicenter, long-term trial, multiple studies have shown that exposure to GA with sevoflurane for under 1 h in early infancy did not alter neurodevelopmental outcomes at either 2 or 5 years of age [11, 12]. Further data have shown that, in addition to the purported advantages of avoiding airway manipulation and neurodevelopmental outcomes, SA may reduce the risk of moderate hypotension, which may influence cerebral autoregulation and further confer cerebral protection [13].

Table 1 Suggested dosage protocol for intrathecal bupivacaine 0.75% in 8.25% dextrose

Weight, in kg	Dose (mg/kg)
Less than 5	1
5–10	0.5
10–15	0.4

2.3 What Are the Complications of Spinal Anesthesia (SA)?

Regional anesthetic techniques, including SA, can lead to various complications, including neurologic deficits, local anesthetic systemic toxicity (LAST), infection, cardiovascular collapse, respiratory depression, or postdural puncture headache [14]. These complications are often exceedingly rare, with studies citing the risk as less than 1% between all regional techniques. In comparison to SA performed in adults, the preganglionic sympathetic blockade, and thus significant hypotension or bradycardia, when a high spinal is obtained is often not seen; this is largely due to the immaturity of the sympathetic nervous system as well as anatomic differences in spinal cord area and physiologic differences in cerebrospinal fluid flow, volume, and pressure [1]. It is vital to remember during the procedure that a high spinal may be inadvertently caused by lifting the lower extremities and trunk upward, which may cause any hyperbaric intrathecal local anesthetic to flow by gravity to the cephalad levels. While a very rare complication, this has been shown to cause high spinals and its avoidance is highly recommended.

One additional complication of SA would be failure of the anesthetic to last appropriately long enough till the completion of the procedure and the need for conversion to GA. Failure of SA can be largely due to failure to access the subarachnoid space, obtaining blood instead of CSF on attempted access, or failure of injecting the appropriate amount of local anesthetic into the cerebrospinal fluid [15]. The success rate of SA varies among providers and centers; however, no current data has shown a relation between failure of SA and specific risk factors, including age, weight, or operator experience.

To assist the proceduralist in gaining access to the intrathecal space for a successful SA, mild sedation may be utilized using various agents, such as midazolam or dexmedetomidine. While albeit a small risk, some data have shown that these agents may influence other complications seen, including bradycardia, hypoventilation, or apnea [16]. However, many providers and centers will opt for this supplemental medication to further increase the success rate of SA and reduce the conversion to GA.

2.4 Is There a Difference in Risk of Postoperative Apnea Between General Anesthesia and Regional Anesthesia?

The number of preterm newborns surviving neonatal period has increased because of significant improvements in neonatal intensive care. Because of the renewed interest in spinal anesthesia, many studies have sought to delineate its advantages, if any, over general anesthesia. With regard to postoperative apnea, the overall risk has not been found to be reduced using any regional anesthetic technique in lieu of GA, including the use of SA [4]. However, it can be noted that the risk of early apnea can be reduced through the use of regional techniques, although no evidence has shown that it mitigates late apnea. Further data show that the level of intervention that may be required to treat the apnea is lower with regional techniques, when compared to GA [4].

Clinically, this becomes important when considering the intended anesthetic plan for patients undergoing these procedures, as well as the level of observation required postoperatively. Many providers still consider a reduction of early apnea, as well as obviating the need for oxygen supplementation or invasive airway management, as advantages in comparison to the administration of GA for cases such as herniorrhaphies and other open lower abdominal/urologic procedures. Additional advantages currently being investigated include the use of SA and its ability to improve postoperative analgesia and reduce opiate consumption [17, 18].

In order to effectively reduce the risk of apnea, in the absence of physiologic abnormalities, elective surgeries should be reconsidered and delayed until deemed safer and more feasible, typically once the patient is over 60 weeks postgestational age. Urgent and emergent surgeries should have their risks stratified in accordance with the risks of the intended anesthetic plan.

2.5 If Postoperative Apnea Is Identified, What Is the Expected Course?

The importance of identifying postoperative apnea, even in the absence of clinical intervention, holds significant weight in determining the need for extended observation. Without a significant difference in late apnea between patients receiving regional anesthesia and GA, preterm and ex-premature infants under 60 weeks are still recommended to have 12 h of monitoring postoperatively to ensure no cardiorespiratory compromise, with the highest risk population being those under 45 weeks' postconceptual age. More importantly, the monitoring should occur with providers who are trained in neonatal airway management and can intervene rapidly if necessary.

If postoperative apnea occurs, supportive care is the recommended treatment plan. This may include oxygen supplementation, even requiring endotracheal intubation if apnea is persistent and life threatening. Data suggest that the prophylactic administration of caffeine may reduce the incidence of postoperative apnea; a meta-analysis of three trials compared administration of caffeine during or immediately after induction of anesthesia and found that use of caffeine was associated with reduction of postoperative apnea and bradycardia [19]. Recent data suggest that caffeine is truly effective in treating apnea of prematurity, citing doses of 10 mg/kg in the postoperative period, to a max loading dose of 20 mg/kg. However, further data is needed to show if this truly improves outcomes intraoperatively and is suggested to be limited to patients with the highest risk factors [19]. Other data show that SA may have less clinically significant apnea when compared with GA though this claim should be investigated further [4].

History of intubation and need for prolonged mechanical ventilation, use of CPAP and the use of caffeine for apnea treatment during the neonatal period, and discharging with an apnea monitor on are significant clinical information to be elicited during preoperative interview of the ex-premature infant's parents. Frequent apneas indicated by home monitor alarms should be obtained since this indicates serious underlying cause and prediction of its recurrence in the immediate postoperative period.

2.6 What Are the Risks in This Particular Ex-premature Patient?

2.6.1 What Is His Age?

He was born at 31 weeks (gestational age) and now 8 weeks (natal age) which makes him 39 weeks of postgestational age.

2.6.2 Does His Natal Age Add to His Risk of Post-operative Apnea?

He is now 8 weeks of natal age which places him at increased risk for apnea because of the presence of *physiologic anemia of the newborn* which occurs at this time.

2.6.3 What Is Physiologic Anemia of the Newborn?

Physiologic anemia occurs at 8–12 weeks of age due to a decrease in erythropoietin (EPO) levels in the blood. The newborn on emerging from intrauterine hypoxic atmosphere to an independent life outside which is hyperoxic in comparison will produce less EPO. The switch from fetal hemoglobin to adult hemoglobin also places the infant at risk for this physiologic anemia [20].

2.6.4 How Does Caffeine Prevent Apnea of Prematurity?

Caffeine is the most effective and well-established treatment drug for apnea of prematurity. Its use can decrease the incidence of apnea and intermittent hypoxemia with periodic breathing and allow early wean and extubation success in preterm infants from mechanical ventilation [21].

Caffeine stimulates central nervous and cardiovascular systems and increases minute ventilation, metabolic rate, oxygen consumption, catecholamine secretion, skeletal muscle tone, and contractility of the diaphragm. Its specific effect of stimulation of the respiratory center in the medulla and of increasing peripheral chemoreceptor activity terminates apnea and initiates breathing. Therefore, the beneficial effects of caffeine on newborn respiratory efforts seen from earlier neonatal studies make this a valuable drug to prevent and treat postoperative apnea [21].

The pathophysiology of apnea of prematurity is from immaturity of the brain stem respiratory center as well as the central and peripheral chemoreceptor responses. There is diminished neuromuscular control of the upper airway leading to collapse and obstruction. Infants less than 28 weeks of gestation have apnea of prematurity-related symptoms, which decreases to 20% at 34 weeks and less than 10% beyond 34 weeks' gestation [22].

3 Summary

This is a case of an ex-premature infant now 39 weeks of postconceptual age who undergoes a unilateral hernia repair for incarcerated hernia and experiences postoperative apnea in PACU following an uneventful spinal anesthesia. Risk factors identified include age, weight, and anemia. The history of his discharge to go home from NICU included caffeine, and continuous apnea monitor points to the etiology of persistent central apnea from immature control of the brain stem respiratory centers. Prophylactic caffeine may have helped prevent the postoperative apnea because when administered in PACU it prevented further incidence of apnea. Continuous monitoring and timely intervention helped prevent the problem of persistent apnea and intubation in PACU. The story highlights that postoperative apnea can occur, even if general anesthesia and sedatives are avoided in a 39-week ex-premature infant. Despite a successful spinal with no sedatives, infants less than 44 weeks of postconceptual age, with existing anemia, are prone to postoperative apnea compared to an infant born full term with same natal age of 8 weeks. While this apnea may have occurred with either SA or GA, the lack of airway manipulation in this particular infant prevents the need for further postoperative ventilation and associated airway problems.

References

1. Davis PJ, Cladis F. Smith's anesthesia for infants and children. 9th ed. Philadelphia, PA: Elsevier; 2017.
2. National Institutes of Health Consensus Development Conference on Infantile Apnea and Home Monitoring, Sept 29 to Oct 1, 1986. Pediatrics. 1987;79:292–9.
3. Zhao J, Gonzalez F, Mu D. Apnea of prematurity: from cause to treatment. Eur J Pediatr. 2011;170(9):1097–105. https://doi.org/10.1007/s00431-011-1409-6.
4. Davidson AJ, et al. Apnea after awake regional and general anesthesia in infants: the general anesthesia compared to spinal anesthesia study—comparing apnea and neurodevelopmental outcomes, a randomized controlled trial. Anesthesiology. 2015;123(1):38–54.
5. Fanelli D, Kim D, King TS, Weller GE, Dalal PG. Recovery characteristics in neonates following general anesthesia: a retrospective chart review. Cureus. 2021;13(7):e16126.
6. Malviya S, Swartz J, Lerman J. Are all preterm infants younger than 60 weeks post conceptual age at risk for postanesthetic apnea? Anesthesiology. 1993;78:1076–81.
7. Regenbogen E, Zhang S, Yang J, Shroyer A, Zhu C, DeCristofaro J. Epidemiological trends among preterm infants with apnea. A twelve-year database review. Int J Pediatr Otorhinolaryngol. 2018;107:86–92. https://doi.org/10.1016/j.ijporl.2018.01.036. Epub 2018 Jan 31
8. Cote CJ, Zaslavsky A, Downes JJ, Dean Kurth C, Welborn LG, Warner LO, Malviya SV. Postoperative apnea in former preterm infants after inguinal herniorrhaphy: a combined analysis. Anesthesiology. 1995;82:809–22. https://doi.org/10.1097/00000542-199504000-00002.
9. Mammel D, Kemp J. Prematurity, the diagnosis of bronchopulmonary dysplasia, and maturation of ventilatory control. Pediatr Pulmonol. 2021;56(11):3533–45. https://doi.org/10.1002/ppul.25519. Epub 2021 Jun 1. PMID: 34042316
10. Whitaker EE, Chao JY, Holmes GL, Legatt AD, Yozawitz EG, Purdon PL, Shinnar S, Williams RK. Electroencephalographic assessment of infant spinal anesthesia: A pilot prospective observational study. Paediatr Anaesth. 2021;31(11):1179–86. https://doi.org/10.1111/pan.14294. Epub 2021 Sep 24. PMID: 34510633; PMCID: PjMC8530954
11. Davidson AJ, et al. Neurodevelopmental outcome at 2 years of age after general anaesthesia and awake-regional anaesthesia in infancy (GAS): an international multicentre, randomised controlled trial. Lancet. 2016;387(10015):239–50.
12. McCann ME, de Graaff JC, Dorris L, et al. Neurodevelopmental outcome at 5 years of age after general anaesthesia or awake-regional anesthesia in infancy (GAS): an international, multicentre, randomised, controlled equivalence trial. Lancet. 2019;393:664–77.
13. McCann ME, et al. Differences in blood pressure in infants after general anesthesia compared to awake regional anesthesia (GAS study-a prospective randomized trial). Anesth Analg. 2017;125(3):837–45.

14. Walker BJ, Long JB, Sathyamoorthy M, et al. Complications in pediatric regional anesthesia. Anesthesiology. 2018;129(4):721–32.
15. Frawley G, Bell G, Disma N, et al. Predictors of failure of awake regional anesthesia for neonatal hernia repair. Anesthesiology. 2015;123(1):55–65.
16. Bong CL, et al. A pilot study of dexmedetomidine sedation and caudal anesthesia for inguinal hernia repair in infants. Paediatr Anaesth. 2016;26(6):621–7.
17. Chen FK, Li LT, Kelleher CM, Liu CA. Infant spinal anesthesia reduces postoperative pain scores and pain medication consumption in infants undergoing inguinal herniorrhaphy. J Pediatr Surg. 2020;55(12):2840–3.
18. Whitaker EE, Williams RK. Epidural and spinal anesthesia for newborn surgery. Clin Perinatol. 2019;46(4):731–43.
19. Henderson-Smart DJ, Steer P. Prophylactic caffeine to prevent postoperative apnea following general anesthesia in preterm infants. Cochrane Database Syst Rev. 2001;4:CD000048.
20. Widness JA. Pathophysiology of anemia during the neonatal period, including anemia of prematurity. NeoReviews. 2008;9(11):e520. https://doi.org/10.1542/neo.9-11-e520. PMID: 20463861; PMCID: PMC2867612
21. Abdel-Hady H, Nasef N, Shabaan AE, Nour I. Caffeine therapy in preterm infants. World J Clin Pediatr. 2015;4(4):81–93. https://doi.org/10.5409/wjcp.v4.i4.81. PMID: 26566480; PMCID: PMC4637812
22. Erickson G, Dobson NR, Hunt CE. Immature control of breathing and apnea of prematurity: the known and unknown. J Perinatol. 2021;41(9):2111–23. https://doi.org/10.1038/s41372-021-01010-z. Epub 2021 Mar 12. PMID: 33712716; PMCID: PMC7952819

Persistent Vomiting After Eye Muscle Surgery

Nina Rawtani

Educational Objectives

- Utilize prophylactic methods of postoperative nausea and vomiting in pediatric patients undergoing strabismus surgery.
- Execute anesthetic plan and recognize possible postoperative problems after pediatric strabismus surgery.
- Define risks, treatment options, and complications of postoperative nausea and vomiting.
- Strategize options for treatment of persistent postoperative nausea and vomiting in the pediatric population.

1 Stem Case

A 5-year-old 21 kg young girl is undergoing bilateral strabismus surgery late on a Thursday afternoon. She is otherwise healthy except for a history of motion sickness. After a thorough preoperative assessment, the anesthesia team determines that she has been NPO appropriate since last night with no recent URI symptoms. The patient has no history of prior surgery or anesthesia, but her mother states that she has significant motion sickness and tends to throw up if the car ride is long. The plan for anesthesia includes general anesthesia with an endotracheal tube. Her parents agree with the plan and the patient walks back while chatting about her friends at summer camp. Induction is smooth with a mask induction, followed by placement of a 22 g PIV in the left hand and easy intubation with a 5.0 cuffed ETT after a bolus of propofol. The surgeon proceeds with the procedure.

N. Rawtani (✉)
Division of Anesthesiology, Sedation and Perioperative Medicine, Children's National Hospital—George Washington University, Washington, DC, USA
e-mail: nrawtani@childrensnational.org

S. T. Verghese (ed.), *Anesthesia STAT! Acute Pediatric Emergencies in PACU*,
https://doi.org/10.1007/978-3-031-24396-7_16

1. *Although this patient is healthy, what medical conditions are associated with a child having ocular problems that may require surgical intervention?*

   Patients with ocular impairments may have syndromes known for a difficult airway, such as Pierre Robin syndrome, Treacher Collins syndrome, Apert syndrome, Crouzon disease, mucopolysaccharidosis, and glycogen storage disease [1]. Children with certain muscle diseases may have congenital strabismus and have a high risk of malignant hyperthermia [2]. Of note, strabismus surgery itself is not associated with malignant hyperthermia.
2. *Does the history of motion sickness increase her chance of vomiting after anesthesia and surgery?*

   Motion sickness does increase her chance of vomiting afterward. Several studies have shown that motion sickness is a reliable predictor of increased risk of PONV. In assessing patient risk for PONV, the most reliable independent predictors include female gender, history of PONV, history of motion sickness, nonsmoker, and younger age [3].
3. *In your preop interview and informed consent, do you explain to the parent the high incidence of vomiting that can occur in their child because of motion sickness as well as her surgery?*

   With the increased risk of PONV due to the patient's independent risk factors and the type of procedure, it is important to discuss with the parent the higher-than-average incidence of postoperative nausea and vomiting for our patient. Informed consent within the realm of pediatric anesthesia is complex and unique. Consent is obtained by the parent or legal guardian of the patient but should still include essential elements. Informed consent includes a description of the plan, alternatives, risks, benefits, discussion of uncertainties, assessment of comprehension, and solicitation of a decision [4].
4. *What is your plan for prevention of postoperative nausea and vomiting (PONV) for this patient?*

   Anesthetic management to prevent PONV is a multimodal approach that includes adequate hydration, pharmacologic treatments, avoidance of certain medications, and even anesthetic type. Some institutions have protocolized plans for strabismus surgery. Creating a toolbox or a protocol for PONV prevention during strabismus surgery has been shown to reduce incidence of postoperative nausea and vomiting [5]. Preoperative and intraoperative hydration can decrease PONV by allowing clears up to 2 h before procedure and giving intravenous fluids during the procedure.

   Pharmacological treatments include serotonin (5HT) antagonists, steroids, butyrophenones, and antihistamines. Initially, a combination of 5-HT_3 antagonists and steroids can be highly effective at PONV prevention [1]. A combination of ondansetron and dexamethasone has been shown to decrease PONV in comparison to either agent alone. Gastric emptying after intubation in combination with this multimodal approach can aid in PONV prevention [6].

   Avoiding opioids or using short-acting opioids and nonopioid analgesics can also help in decreasing the risk of PONV. Avoiding nitrous oxide and volatile inhalational agents is shown to decrease the incidence in those at higher risk of

PONV. These patients may benefit from a total intravenous anesthetic (TIVA) approach, especially with a known history of PONV. A TIVA approach has been shown to decrease PONV as well as emergence agitation but can increase the oculocardiac reflex [7]. In a meta-analysis of 4 randomized trials of 558 children who underwent strabismus surgery, the researchers compared the effectiveness of a single pharmacologic prophylaxis to that of TIVA and found that both were equally effective in preventing vomiting in the postoperative period with similar time in the PACU. The children in the TIVA group took significantly less time to resume drinking and eating compared to the non-TIVA group. They concluded that the emetogenic effect of inhalational anesthetic can be compensated adequately by administering a single prophylactic antiemetic medication [8].

5. *She has been NPO since last night and the case is starting at 2:30 PM*

   How much fluid should you plan on giving intraop for a prolonged fast? Is there a need to check blood sugar?

   Intraoperative hydration with a balanced salt solution at 30 mL/kg can greatly decrease the incidence of PONV [9]. Preoperatively, allowing clears up to 2 h before surgery can decrease dehydration as well. With the prolonged fasting time in this patient, maintenance IV fluids with dextrose or a preoperative glucose check may be valuable for patient. However, initial bolus hydration should be an isotonic solution without dextrose.

6. *Why is preventing PONV important? What are the complications of PONV that can lead to patient morbidity in the pediatric population?*

   Nausea is the sensation of feeling sick with the inclination to vomit. Vomiting is the act of retching and forcefully expelling the stomach's contents out of the mouth. It is one of the most common complaints from parents in the recovery area. PONV can lead to dehydration, delayed discharge, prolonged stay in the post-anesthesia care unit (PACU), parental and surgeon's dissatisfaction, and even unplanned admission for patients [10].

   In specific ophthalmic cases, the increased intraocular pressure with retching and vomiting can be deleterious for patient's eye wound closure and cause increased bleeding; it is imperative that every effort is taken to eliminate vomiting.

7. *What is the mechanism for nausea and vomiting in pediatric patients?*

   Several areas in the central nervous system contribute to vomiting including the emetic center, the nucleus of the solitary tract, area postrema, and chemoreceptor trigger zone (CTZ). These areas receive a stimulus from peripheral or central areas that trigger a response [11]. The sensation of nausea or vomiting is an instinctive defense reaction in the body caused by the somato-autonomic nerve reflex integrated in the medulla oblongata [12]. Certain medications or situations are associated with the release of 5-hydroxytryptamine (5-HT) from enterochromaffin cells. These cells are in the intestinal mucosa and the brainstem. The 5-HT then binds to the 5-HT_3 receptors located on adjacent vagal afferent nerves which result in the vomiting reflex.

8. *Why are children undergoing strabismus surgery at an increased risk for PONV?*

   It has been shown that nausea and vomiting after strabismus surgery can occur in 45–85% of cases [9]. Strabismus surgery can cause altered visual perception, which is hypothesized to cause an oculo-emetic reflex, which is similar to the oculocardiac reflex [11]. Studies show that the more extraocular muscles (EOM) involved in the surgery, the greater the incidence as well. Involvement of certain EOM, such as the inferior oblique muscle, can increase the risk as well.

9. *Other than strabismus surgery, what are other risk factors for postoperative nausea and vomiting?*

   Risk factors include history of motion sickness, migraine, previous history of PONV, duration of anesthesia >30 min, female, nonsmoking status, and younger age. Of note, a lower incidence is seen in children <3 years of age.

   Certain types of surgeries other than strabismus surgery can also increase the risk of PONV. Pediatric surgeries with a higher incidence include strabismus repair, adenotonsillectomy, hernia repair, orchiopexy, penile surgery, laparoscopy, brain surgery, and certain ENT procedures. Manipulating certain areas, such as balance, vasomotor activity, salivation, respiration, and bulbar control to the emetic center can also affect risk [11].

   Certain medical conditions, electrolyte abnormalities, and medications like chemotherapy are mediated by the vomiting center and the chemoreceptor trigger zone. These factors can increase baseline nausea and thus PONV. Specifically, opioids given during anesthesia can increase nausea and vomiting, and it is documented in strabismus surgery as well.

   The Eberhart score is an evaluation method to determine propensity for PONV. The scoring range is 1–4 with a point each for surgery ≥30 min, age ≥ 3 years old, strabismus surgery, and history or family history of PONV [10].

10. *You plan to give ondansetron and dexamethasone intraoperatively. What is the mechanism of each medication?*

    Ondansetron is a selective serotonin 5-HT_3 antagonist that binds to the 5-HT_3 receptors on the vagal afferent neurons in the gastrointestinal tract and the brainstem [13]. It's structure which is similar to serotonin allows it to bind to the receptors [14]. It has a relatively good safety profile and is approved by the FDA for use in children older than 1 month. This medication shows superior efficacy in reducing postoperative nausea and vomiting in children [15]. The dosage range is 0.05–0.15 mg/kg with a maximum dose of 4 mg. Thus, ondansetron is considered a first-line antiemetic in children undergoing strabismus surgery and should be administered before the end of surgery.

    Ondansetron in combination with dexamethasone is significantly more effective than ondansetron or dexamethasone alone. Dexamethasone is a corticosteroid that has an antiemetic as well as an anti-inflammatory effect. The antiemetic action is thought to act at the vomiting center [10]. Intravenous dosing in children is 0.15–0.5 mg/kg with a maximum dose of 8–10 mg.

11. *What are some of the side effects of ondansetron?*

    Ondansetron is generally well tolerated in pediatric patients. Theoretically, ondansetron can also antagonize the effects of the Bezold-Jarisch reflex (reflex bradycardia), which is in part due to stimulation of the 5-HT_3 receptors in the vagal nerve endings. It is utilized in higher doses in patients undergoing chemotherapy and has been seen to have minimal side effects such as headache (2–8%), constipation (1–3.5%), and diarrhea (2%) [15].

    Of note, the clearance of ondansetron decreases with age [14]. This is likely due to age-related decrease in hepatic function. Furthermore, the plasma clearance is decreased in patients with hepatic impairment. Ondansetron undergoes first-pass metabolism by the liver using the enzymes CYP1A1/2, CYP3A, and CYP2D6. Any change in enzyme activity can alter the metabolism of the medication as well.

12. *How does ondansetron affect the QTc interval? What are our concerns with QTc prolongation?*

    High dose of the drug can prolong the QTc interval and thus not recommended in those with congenital long QT syndrome. The QTc interval prolongation by ondansetron is similar to the effect seen after administration of droperidol. QT interval prolongation can predispose patients to fatal arrhythmias such as torsade de pointes. The incidence of congenital QT prolongation in the general population is estimated to be 1:2500. Pediatric patients with this syndrome may not have been diagnosed at the time of surgery, and possibility of potential adverse events must be considered when administering this medication [16].

    Adverse events can occur due to long QT syndrome and medication interaction. It has been noted during emergence from anesthesia specifically in patients with long QT syndrome who have been given neuromuscular blockade reversal (anticholinesterase anticholinergic drugs) in combination with ondansetron at an incidence of 5.9% [17]. Compared with sugammadex, reversal of nondepolarizing blocking agent with neostigmine is associated with QT prolongation under general anesthesia [18]. In clinical practice, it is customary not to administer neostigmine and ondansetron simultaneously. In addition, sevoflurane is known to prolong the QTc interval. It's combination with ondansetron can increase this undesirable effect in children [19]. Thus, ECG monitoring is essential when the antiemetic is administered.

13. *What is your plan for intraoperative and postoperative analgesia?*

    A multimodal method can include acetaminophen, intravenous NSAIDs, topical local anesthetic, and minimal opioid usage [7]. Nonsteroidal anti-inflammatory drugs (NSAIDs) and acetaminophen are effective medications in providing analgesia in pediatric strabismus surgery. Pain scores were comparable in patients who had NSAIDS versus intravenous opioids. However, opioids can increase PONV; thus, minimizing opioids is a reasonable approach.

    Of note, ondansetron may decrease the efficacy of acetaminophen. A randomized controlled trial on children undergoing tonsillectomy concluded that intravenous administration of 0.1 mg/kg ondansetron reduces the analgesic action of intravenous acetaminophen [20].

14. *The surgeon begins the procedure, and the heart rate decreases rapidly to 30 beats per minute. What do you do?*

    The likely cause is the oculocardiac reflex. The oculocardiac reflex (OCR) also known as Aschner reflex or trigeminovagal reflex (TVR) is a vagal bradycardia triggered by trigeminal stimulation. It involves the ophthalmic branch of the trigeminal and vagus nerves. The reflex can be triggered when traction is applied to the extraocular muscles or pressure on the globe. This causes afferent signals to travel via the trigeminal nerve and produce an efferent signal through the vagal nerve. The vagal response is highly variable and can range from bradycardia to junctional rhythm to asystole. OCR is defined as a heart rate reduction of more than 20% following globe pressure or traction of the extraocular muscles in comparison to baseline heart rate [21]. Sometimes arrest of spontaneous respiration accompanies the bradycardia. The effect if left untreated can lead to hypoperfusion and possibly asystole and cardiac arrest. ECG monitoring during muscle manipulation is therefore of paramount importance.

    OCR is more common with the medial rectus muscle due to the need for increased traction to access it. Light anesthesia and hypercarbia can also cause OCR. The use of opioids and dexamethasone may increase the incidence of OCR.

    The initial and most effective treatment includes stopping the stimulus by asking the surgeon to release the traction. In addition, anticholinergic medication, atropine or glycopyrrolate, can be given to increase the heart rate. Another dose can be given if the bradycardia persists. Intravenous fluids can be given to aid in increasing the intravascular volume and blood pressure in the patient. Deepening the anesthetic and adequate ventilation can also aid in decreasing the risk of OCR. Dexmedetomidine has also been found to decrease OCR. Alternate treatments include applying topical lidocaine to interrupt the signaling from the OCR or intravenous ketamine [9].

15. *What are other intraoperative complications of strabismus surgery?*

    Oculorespiratory reflex is a change in respiratory effort during surgery due to muscle traction and is often seen in children. Globe perforation, retinal detachment, slipped muscle, and lost muscle can also been reported during strabismus surgery [7].

16. *The patient is slightly to the side tilted breathing spontaneously with good tidal volumes and no response to oral suctioning stimulation. What are the advantages and disadvantages of a deep extubation in children undergoing ocular surgery?*

    A deep extubation refers to the removal of the endotracheal tube while the patient is under deep anesthesia without airway reflexes and spontaneously ventilating. Deep extubation can prevent the increase in intraocular pressure which can occur with awake extubation with the patient coughing and bucking against the endotracheal tube [22]. The increase in intraocular pressure can further cause surgical complications, such as bleeding, visual problems, or suture unraveling. If deep extubation is planned, dexmedetomidine can be used at a dose of 0.5 mcg/kg to reduce oculocardiac reflex and PONV [23].

    Disadvantages of a deep extubation include airway complications, such as airway obstruction, cough, desaturation, laryngospasm, aspiration, and breath holding. A deep extubation should be avoided if the patient has a difficult airway and full stomach or if the practitioner is uncomfortable with the technique. Placing the spontaneously breathing patient in the lateral position and removing the endotracheal tube at a deeper level of anesthesia after suctioning the mouth are helpful to prevent laryngospasm and airway obstruction.

17. *What are other alternatives to general anesthesia for strabismus surgery? What are the advantages and disadvantages, particularly in children?*

    Regional anesthesia with ophthalmologic regional block can be used as a primary anesthetic technique in adults but may be difficult for children. The patient would be awake and may be uncomfortable during muscle traction intraoperatively. This method can reduce OCR, PONV, and emergence delirium but is not an ideal approach for children. Similarly, topical anesthesia may be advantageous for adults but unsuitable for children [7].

18. *You proceed to remove the endotracheal tube and assess that she is breathing normally. You place the patient on her side and move her to the stretcher and proceed to PACU. The patient is stable in the recovery area with stable vital signs and appears comfortable in her lateral position. After your hand-off, you explain to the PACU nurse that the reason for avoiding narcotics in the PACU was deliberate because you would like to be informed if she starts vomiting. About 20 min later, you receive a call from the PACU nurse stating that the young girl is awake and has started vomiting. You decide to assess the patient, and when you arrive, the patient has a low blood pressure on the monitor and has vomited twice already. What is your next course of action?*

    Treatment of the low blood pressure should include intravenous fluids and medications that may aid in increasing the blood pressure. The low blood pressure could also be contributing to the nausea that the patient is having.

    Guidelines state that if no prophylaxis or dexamethasone alone was used as initial antiemetic therapy, then a serotonin antagonist should be administered [11, 24]. In this patient's case, both a serotonin antagonist and a second agent have been used. The next step is to use a drug from a different class. If triple therapy with 5-HT_3 antagonist and two other agents were used within 6 h of surgery, then do not repeat initial therapy. Use a drug from a different class or administer a small bolus of propofol as needed. If it has been greater than 6 h, then repeat regimen of the 5-HT_3 antagonist can be used.

    Several other medications can also aid in reducing nausea for the patient. Antiemetic classes include serotonin antagonists, corticosteroids, butyrophenone, neurokinin antagonists, anticholinergics, and dopamine antagonists. Other medications may include dexmedetomidine and propofol while in PACU.

19. *What alterative pharmacological options can be used for PONV?*

    Serotonin 5-HT_3 antagonists and corticosteroids include ondansetron and dexamethasone, which have already been given as first-line agents to this patient. Other 5-HT_3 antagonists include granisetron and ramosetron. Oral granisetron administered prior to anesthesia was found to be effective in the first 24 h after strabismus surgery [11]. Intravenous granisetron at a dose of 40 mcg/kg is the lowest effective dose for PONV. Intravenous ramosetron is comparable to granisetron as well. Palonosetron is another medication used in the same class.

Droperidol is a butyrophenone that has been shown to reduce nausea in conjunction with ondansetron. However, its risks of extrapyramidal symptoms and drowsiness as well as its black box warning due to QT prolongation have led to decreased usage in the United States. The warning recommends a 12-lead EKG to be done before the use of droperidol and to continue monitoring 3 h post-administration. A low dose of droperidol is suggested as a second-line antiemetic in Great Britain and Ireland [7].

NK-1 receptor antagonists include aprepitant (Emend). This medication has a long half-life and may even be more effective in comparison to ondansetron [25]. This agent is used to treat patients who are at higher risk of adverse outcomes due to PONV from chemotherapy or those who cannot use the first-line medications.

Metoclopramide is a commonly used antiemetic for treatment of PONV when prophylaxis has failed. Metoclopramide is a dopamine antagonist that is a gastrokinetic medication. High doses can be associated with extrapyramidal side effects, but lower doses can be used for nausea and vomiting.

Scopolamine is an anticholinergic that can be used as a patch typically placed before the anesthetic. It is more effective as a routine antiemetic prophylaxis because of its slow onset of action. In addition, side effects include drowsiness, visual disturbances, and dry mouth, and it should not be detached or moved while placed on the patient. Thus, scopolamine is typically used for higher-risk patients. It is a single-dose patch at 1.5 mg delivered over 72 h. Younger children may have to use a lower dose than the standard adult dosing, and it does not have FDA approval for pediatric patients [10]. Advantages include long-term effectiveness and cost-effectiveness.

Gabapentin is a γ-aminobutyric acid analog that is typically used to treat neuropathic pain but may decrease PONV through a decrease in tachykinin neurotransmission [10]. It may also decrease opioid consumption and emergence delirium in children. It has been shown to aid in refractory vomiting postcraniotomy.

Dexmedetomidine is an α-2 agonist acting as a sedative and analgesic [25]. It can aid in minimizing opioid use, thus decreasing incidence of PONV. Clonidine is also an α-2 agonist with promising results in children undergoing strabismus surgery. Propofol is a sedative that is used in small doses mainly for adults for nausea and vomiting in PACU [11]. Dimenhydrinate is another antiemetic used that can produce sedation in patients. Midazolam, a benzodiazepine, is a sedative that has been used in conjunction with other medications for PONV [26]. Ketamine is a nonselective antagonist of the *N*-methyl-D-aspartate (NMDA) receptor, which can be useful as a morphine-sparing analgesic and thus may help in small doses to reduce nausea in combination with other therapies [10].

20. *The PACU nurse is wondering if she should discharge the patient home since she is awake and alert. She is still nauseous and has not had anything to drink. What is your plan?*

A trial of fluids by mouth may be appropriate. However, studies have shown that withholding oral fluid intake in the PACU until the patient is ready can also decrease the incidence of PONV [9].

21. *What other nonpharmacological options are there for PONV?*

    Alternative therapies in aiding nausea may be considered [11]. One such method is acupuncture at the PC6 acupoint or acupressure of the P6 point [10]. This pressure point is located on the inner or palm side of the wrist about 2–4 cm from the wrist crease between the tendons of the palmaris longus and flexor carpi radialis muscles. Wristbands with acupressure concentration on the P6 point have been worn to prevent nausea in the perioperative period. Several studies have shown the effectiveness of reducing nausea and vomiting. When compared to standard anti-emetic medications, PC6 acupoint stimulation shows no difference.

    Isopropyl alcohol is another alternative method shown to reduce PONV, although transient with recurrence within 20–60 min. The technique includes inhaling an isopropyl alcohol wipe and repeating up to three times [11].

    Honey has been used as an adjunct therapy to other medications and effective in reducing use of pain medications through enhanced analgesia effect [10].

22. *The patient feels better but after about an hour she begins gagging and vomiting. What is your next course of action?*

    At this point, it is appropriate to consider overnight admission for the patient to receive intravenous fluids and observation. Persistent PONV can lead to dehydration, electrolyte abnormalities, and even surgical complications. After discussion with parents, the ophthalmologist on call, and the hospitalist, the patient is admitted to the floor with continuous monitoring and hydration via intravenous fluids. After an uneventful night on the floor, she woke up without nausea, ready to eat her breakfast and eventually discharged to go home.

References

1. Labovsky K. Anesthesia for ophthalmic procedures. In: Ellinas H, Matthes K, Alrayashi W, Bilge A, editors. Clinical pediatric anesthesiology. New York, NY: McGraw Hill; 2021.
2. Bourdeu K, Bayes J, Eappen S. Anesthesia for ophthalmic surgery. In: Longnecker DE, Mackey SC, Newman MF, Sandberg WS, Zapol WM, editors. Anesthesiology. 3rd ed. New York, NY: McGraw-Hill Education; 2017.
3. Apfel CC, Heidrich FM, Jukar-Rao S, et al. Evidence-based analysis of risk factors for postoperative nausea and vomiting. Br J Anaesth. 2012;109(5):742–53. https://doi.org/10.1093/bja/aes276.
4. Gentry KR, Lepere K, Opel DJ. Informed consent in pediatric anesthesiology. Paediatr Anaesth. 2017;27(12):1253–60. https://doi.org/10.1111/pan.13270.
5. Ali U, Tsang M, Igbeyi B, et al. A 4-year quality improvement initiative reducing postoperative nausea and vomiting in children undergoing strabismus surgery at a quaternary paediatric hospital. Paediatr Anaesth. 2019;29(7):690–7. https://doi.org/10.1111/pan.13664.
6. Smith PV, Walton DS. Prevention of vomiting after general anesthesia for pediatric ophthalmic surgery. AANA J. 2001;69(1):39–43.
7. Chua AW, Chua MJ, Leung H, Kam PC. Anaesthetic considerations for strabismus surgery in children and adults. Anaesth Intensive Care. 2020;48(4):277–88. https://doi.org/10.1177/0310057X20937710.

8. Schaefer MS, Kranke P, Weibel S, Kreysing R, Ochel J, Kienbaum P. Total intravenous anesthesia vs single pharmacological prophylaxis to prevent postoperative vomiting in children: a systematic review and meta-analysis. Paediatr Anaesth. 2017;27(12):1202–9. https://doi.org/10.1111/pan.13268.
9. Lobaugh L, Nguyen V. Strabismus. In: Freeman BS, Berger JS, editors. Anesthesiology core review: part two advanced exam. New York, NY: McGraw-Hill Education; 2016.
10. Kovac AL. Postoperative nausea and vomiting in pediatric patients. Paediatr Drugs. 2021;23(1):11–37. https://doi.org/10.1007/s40272-020-00424-0.
11. Kovac AL. Management of postoperative nausea and vomiting in children. Paediatr Drugs. 2007;9(1):47–69. https://doi.org/10.2165/00148581-200709010-00005.
12. Endo T, Minami M, Hirafuji M, et al. Neurochemistry and neuropharmacology of emesis - the role of serotonin. Toxicology. 2000;153(1–3):189–201. https://doi.org/10.1016/s0300-483x(00)00314-0.
13. Tyers MB, Freeman AJ. Mechanism of the anti-emetic activity of 5-HT3 receptor antagonists. Oncology. 1992;49(4):263–8. https://doi.org/10.1159/000227054.
14. Huddart R, Altman RB, Klein TE. PharmGKB summary: ondansetron and tropisetron pathways, pharmacokinetics and pharmacodynamics. Pharmacogenet Genomics. 2019;29(4):91–7. https://doi.org/10.1097/FPC.0000000000000369.
15. Culy CR, Bhana N, Plosker GL. Ondansetron: a review of its use as an antiemetic in children. Paediatr Drugs. 2001;3(6):441–79. https://doi.org/10.2165/00128072-200103060-00007.
16. McKechnie K, Froese A. Ventricular tachycardia after ondansetron administration in a child with undiagnosed long QT syndrome. Can J Anaesth. 2010;57(5):453–7. https://doi.org/10.1007/s12630-010-9288-2.
17. Nathan AT, Berkowitz DH, Montenegro LM, Nicolson SC, Vetter VL, Jobes DR. Implications of anesthesia in children with long QT syndrome. Anesth Analg. 2011;112(5):1163–8. https://doi.org/10.1213/ANE.0b013e3182121d57.
18. Yamashita Y, Takasusuki T, Kimura Y, Komatsuzaki M, Yamaguchi S. Effects of neostigmine and sugammadex for reversal of neuromuscular blockade on QT dispersion under propofol anesthesia: a randomized controlled trial. Cardiol Ther. 2018;7(2):163–72. https://doi.org/10.1007/s40119-018-0119-9.
19. Lee JH, Park YH, Kim JT, Kim CS, Kim HS. The effect of sevoflurane and ondansetron on QT interval and transmural dispersion of repolarization in children. Paediatr Anaesth. 2014;24(4):421–5. https://doi.org/10.1111/pan.12339.
20. Nikooseresht M, Nasrolahi M, Hajian P, Moradi A. The effects of ondansetron on the analgesic action of intravenous acetaminophen after tonsillectomy in children: a triple-blind randomized controlled trial. Oxid Med Cell Longev. 2021;2021:6611740. https://doi.org/10.1155/2021/6611740.
21. Arnold RW. The oculocardiac reflex: a review. Clin Ophthalmol. 2021;15:2693–725. https://doi.org/10.2147/OPTH.S317447.
22. Veyckemans F. Tracheal extubation in children: planning, technique, and complications. Paediatr Anaesth. 2020;30(3):331–8. https://doi.org/10.1111/pan.13774.
23. Li S, Liu T, Xia J, Jia J, Li W. Effect of dexmedetomidine on prevention of postoperative nausea and vomiting in pediatric strabismus surgery: A randomized controlled study. BMC Ophthalmol. 2020;20(1):86–3. https://doi.org/10.1186/s12886-020-01359-3.
24. Gan TJ, Belani KG, Bergese S, et al. Fourth consensus guidelines for the management of postoperative nausea and vomiting. Anesth Analg. 2020;131(2):411–48. https://doi.org/10.1213/ANE.0000000000004833.
25. Cao X, White PF, Ma H. An update on the management of postoperative nausea and vomiting. J Anesthesiol. 2017;31(4):617–26. https://doi.org/10.1007/s00540-017-2363-x.
26. Riad W, Marouf H. Combination therapy in the prevention of PONV after strabismus surgery in children: Granisetron, ondansetron, midazolam with dexamethasone. Middle East J Anaesthesiol. 2009;20(3):431–6.

Blindness After Bone Marrow Harvest in a Healthy Patient

Gregory Lessans

1 Stem Case

An 8-year-old previously healthy male presents to the OR for bone marrow harvest and subsequent donation to his sibling. His weight is 24 kg, and he looks small for his age. He has no history of prior anesthetics, he takes no medications and has no known drug allergies. General anesthesia is induced using an inhalational technique of 8% sevoflurane in 100% oxygen. A peripheral IV is placed and he is intubated with intravenous lidocaine, propofol, and rocuronium. A caudal block is attempted for postoperative pain relief but soon abandoned after two unsuccessful attempts resulting in a "bloody tap". The patient is turned prone for optimal positioning for marrow harvesting. The procedure proceeds and finishes uneventfully, and when the patient is repositioned supine at the end of the case, a drop in SPO2 to the 70s is noted, while he was coughing and bucking on the tube as he emerged from anesthesia. Positive pressure ventilation became difficult, and bronchospasm is suspected. An IV bolus of propofol is used successfully and the patient is extubated to face mask and transferred to the PACU.

Twenty minutes following sign-out, the PACU anesthesiologist is called to the bedside because the patient is exhibiting severe agitation. After the patient is reoriented and calmed down, the source of the agitation is verbalized by him stating that he cannot see at all. Parents are near him and look alarmed because he is frantically touching objects and them saying repeatedly "I can't see anything! Help me please, I think I am blind!"

G. Lessans (✉)
Department of Anesthesiology, Pain and Perioperative Medicine, Children's National Hospital, Washington, DC, USA

S. T. Verghese (ed.), *Anesthesia STAT! Acute Pediatric Emergencies in PACU*,
https://doi.org/10.1007/978-3-031-24396-7_17

1.1 How Common Is Post-operative Visual Loss (POVL)?

Postoperative visual loss (POVL) is a rare but devastating complication. In a literature review of perioperative visual loss after non-ocular surgeries, the author concluded that the incidence was 0.002% of all surgeries and as high as 0.2% of cardiac and spine surgeries [1, 2], widely considered to be the "higher-risk" procedures for POVL [3, 1]. While any segment of the visual pathway can be implicated in POVL, the most common site for permanent injury is the optic nerves, mainly from ischemia.

While POVL is rare, other eye injuries do occur under general anesthesia with more prevalence. In addition to vision loss, these injuries include direct trauma to the eye, keratopathy, or chemical injuries suffered while under general anesthesia.

1.2 Are There Specific Risk Factors That Make POVL More Likely?

While it remains a rare complication, POVL has been shown to be associated with a variety of risk factors.

Positioning complications have been shown to increase the chance of POVL, with prone positioning leading to a higher risk of POVL [4]. Ocular perfusion pressure (OPP) is equal to the difference between mean arterial pressure (MAP) and intraocular pressure (IOP). Multiple studies have shown that in the prone position, IOP can rise dramatically leading to a lower ocular perfusion pressure, putting the patient's vision at risk. Additionally, any positioning that results in any pressure on the face or eyes has been shown to increase the chance of POVL. Use of orthopedic and/or neurosurgical operating room tables that may lead to pressure on the eyes is particularly concerning, and patients should be positioned with extreme caution and care.

Traditionally, POVL was thought to be a complication specific to the very old and very sick, but newer research has shown that younger patients were among the highest-risk patients for POVL. **Patient-specific** factors include male gender and age < 18 years leading to a higher likelihood of POVL [2]. Additionally, pathologic states during which oxygen delivery may be compromised, including hypotension and anemia, or the need for vasoconstrictive agents also increases the risk of visual complications.

Procedure-specific risks: Studies have repeatedly shown that spinal and cardiac procedures have been most implicated in POVL [2, 5], especially in ischemic optic neuropathy and retinal vascular occlusion (see below). Some of the reasons for this include their long operative length and increased chance of hypotension and blood loss and transfusion, all states that can lead to hypoperfusion of the ocular structures.

1.3 Which Risk Factors Exist in Our Patient Who Presents for Bone Marrow Harvest?

Allogenic bone marrow transplantation is used to treat diseases ranging from genetic disorders to leukemias. Harvesting bone marrow can be painful; therefore, it is often performed under general endotracheal anesthesia with narcotic supplementation and sometimes with caudal anesthesia if feasible for postoperative pain relief. The donors are usually healthy, and after intubation they are **turned prone** for the harvesting procedure. Harvesting can be a time-intensive **process**, with the average procedural length approaching 90 min or more (Buisson et al.).

1.4 What Is the Differential Diagnosis for Postoperative Visual Loss?

The differential diagnosis for POVL is limited and will be directed by patient comorbidities and procedure-specific risks. The differential includes:

- Corneal abrasion (unilateral or bilateral)
- Ischemic optic neuropathy (ION) (anterior or posterior (AION or PION))
- Retinal vascular occlusion
- Cortical blindness.

2 Corneal Abrasions Describe the Presentation, Natural Course and Treatment of Corneal Abrasions

Corneal abrasion is a complication well known to most anesthesiologists, as they are the most common perioperative ocular complication. Incidence has been shown to be as high as 0.013% to 0.17% of surgeries not involving the eye [2]. Symptoms generally present in the 1–3 h following surgery and are described as a "foreign object sensation" in the eye [4].

There are several reasons general anesthesia can predispose a patient to a corneal abrasion. These include physical contact with the globe during induction, maintenance, or emergence from anesthesia, especially inadvertently by a poorly fitting ventilation mask or from a patient scratching their eye upon awakening. Additionally, tear production that keeps the surface of the eye lubricated may be inhibited or depressed which can lead to a drier eye more susceptible to abrasion.

For this reason, prompt and correct taping of the eyelids as soon as the patient loses consciousness is important to lower the risk of corneal abrasions. Some anesthesiologists use ointment or eye drops to keep the eye moist, though no added benefit has been demonstrated for this practice [6].

Signs and symptoms of corneal abrasion include burning, itching, and a "sharp sensation" in the eye. Pain is generally worse with blinking and patients will often refuse to open their eyes to prevent the pain from returning. When the eyes are open, patients can exhibit photophobia and blurred vision. Physical exam findings can include excessive tear production, miosis, redness, and irritation.

It should be noted that, in general, complete visual loss is rare and unexpected from a corneal abrasion. This said, pediatric patients often have limited ability to discern and describe their symptoms, especially when distressed, in pain, or while recovering from anesthesia. It is not uncommon to hear complaints of complete blindness when the true cause is pain and irritation from a new corneal abrasion.

Given their relative frequency, there are often department-specific guidelines for treating corneal abrasions that specifically request ophthalmologist available for in-patient consultation, to come to the bedside for a full fundoscopic exam. In large academic centers, for instance, it is not uncommon to have an ophthalmologist evaluate for more serious issues before prescribing eye drops for pain and/or antibiotics. In outpatient surgery or smaller centers, often it is up to the anesthesiologist to diagnose (and follow up on) corneal abrasions. Generally, most treatment protocols will call for a quick examination of the eye, for foreign bodies and saline irrigation to wash out any objects that may be present, followed by prescribing antibiotic drops or ointment and discharge home with follow-up with the ophthalmologist within 1–3 days. In some situations, the anesthesiologist can perform a fluorescein dye exam which allows for quick and easy identification of abrasions of the cornea; however, anesthesiologist's comfort with this exam varies based on practice setting, training, experience, etc.

Newer protocols that allow for streamlined treatment of uncomplicated corneal abrasions by anesthesiologists have been shown to be effective and potentially decrease the time to treatment and cost of care. Requesting a consultation with the inhouse ophthalmologist should be done as soon as possible and prior to discharging the patient home since this can become a medicolegal problem if correct diagnosis and treatment are not undertaken for the patient.

3 Ischemic Optic Neuropathy: Symptoms, Pathophysiology, and Prevention

Ischemic optic neuropathy (ION) is characterized by acute damage to the optic nerve by an acute compromise in its blood supply. Unlike corneal abrasion, it is generally painless and leads to complete loss of visual fields in the affected eye. Most commonly in spinal fusions and cardiac surgery, the rate of this complication in these surgeries has continued to drop in the past two decades, likely from the use of less-invasive surgical techniques.

Symptoms are most described immediately after emergence from anesthesia, though delayed presentation of 1–2 days has been reported.

Two subtypes of ION exist: AION and PION. In AION there is swelling of the head of the optic nerve when viewed radiographically, whereas in the case of PION there is no such swelling. Incidence of AION is far more common than PION.

Risk factors for both AION and PION include any state in which blood supply may be compromised. As discussed above, these include hypotension, anemia, and positioning in which pressure may be inadvertently placed on the globe, preventing free blood flow. Multiple studies have shown that both cardiac surgery and spinal fusions are the surgeries during which ION occurs most frequently.

When ION is suspected, an immediate ophthalmologic consult is warranted. A fundoscopic exam as well as a test of all visual fields is of paramount importance. Usually imaging such as MRI can be considered to rule out other intracranial pathologies. Further diagnosis is usually directed by ophthalmologists and may include an arterial biopsy as well as an injection of fluorescent dye to evaluate for compromised blood flow.

Given the pathophysiology of the disease, the mainstay of treatment revolves around decreasing the swelling around the optic nerve. Long-term steroids are usually prescribed and have varying success depending on patient condition and disease severity.

From an anesthesiologist's perspective, it is most important to recognize patients who may be at risk for this complication and to manage their blood pressure promptly and aggressively to prevent low perfusion states. As with all patients, proper positioning must be ensured to prevent any state in which flow in the retinal artery or its vascular bed may be decreased. Protection of the eyes by application of a complete covering and avoidance of pressure on the globe during positioning and throughout surgery is vital in children maintained in the prone position.

4 Retinal Vascular Occlusion: Etiology and Natural Course

Retinal vascular occlusion (RVO) is an aptly named condition during which blood flow into, or out of, the retina is compromised. As in ischemic optic neuropathy, retinal vascular occlusion is most common in cardiac and spinal surgery and thought to occur from either embolic phenomena or vascular compression states. As with other ocular injuries, poor positioning can lead to decreased blood flow and cause retinal vascular occlusion.

A large US study of over five million cardiac procedures from 1998 to 2013 showed that the risk retinal arterial occlusion during cardiac surgery was significantly higher for patients with carotid stenosis, a history of CVA, hypercoagulability, giant cell arteritis, and diabetes [7].

Another traditional risk factor for RVO is a retrobulbar block performed by ophthalmologists during surgical procedures. Instillation of local anesthetic in and around the retina can lead to increased venous pressure preventing adequate blood flow to the retina.

With RVO, painless visual loss is demonstrated immediately following or soon after surgery. Similar to ION, an ophthalmologic consultation and fundoscopic exam are warranted immediately while excluding other organic causes of visual loss. After diagnosis, treatment focuses on decreasing swelling in the optic vasculature by intravitreal injection of corticosteroids or antivascular endothelial growth factor medications.

5 Cortical Blindness: Etiology and Course

The pathophysiology of cortical blindness does not depend on vascular compromise to the structures of the eye. Instead, symptoms result from ischemia of the optic cortex of the brain. Cortical blindness results in a loss of visual fields with a *normal* ophthalmologic examination of the eye as well as normal pupillary responses [8]. Since the perfusion of the visual cortex is fed via "watershed" blood supply, it is particularly vulnerable to injury caused by low perfusion states. This is illustrated in Fig. 1, where blood supply to the **central retinal artery** is shown to be the most distal from its supplying vessels (the carotid, middle cerebral, and anterior cerebral arteries). Thus, cortical blindness is likely to co-present with other neurologic symptoms including nausea or sensory deficits, unlike the other diagnoses described above.

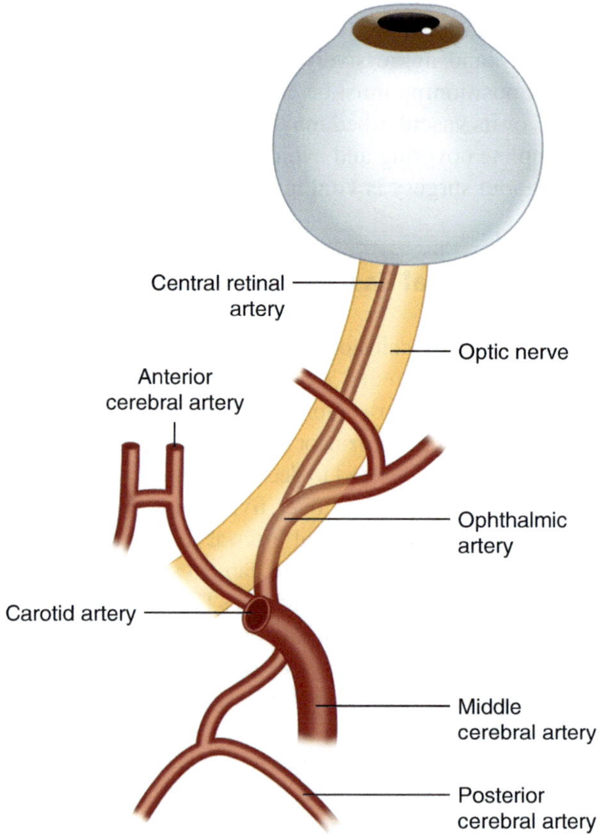

Fig. 1 Blood supply to the optic nerve and eye

Cortical blindness is also of particular concern to the pediatric anesthesiologist, as studies have shown consistently that patients under 18 years of age have a higher prevalence of cortical blindness than their adult counterparts [9].

Like other etiologies of POVL, cortical blindness is most likely from poor perfusion states. These include vascular accidents during surgery, prolonged states of poor perfusion including anemia and hypotension or blood loss, as well as prone positioning.

In general, symptom presentation can tend to be later than in ION or RVO. CT or MRI findings can demonstrate infarct injuries in the occipital lobe of the affected side, while fundoscopic exam traditionally remains normal.

6 Could This Be Related to the Failed Caudal Attempts in Our Patient?

Vision loss after neuraxial anesthesia is an exceedingly rare complication. After literature review, only ten such cases have been described, all of whom were adult patients presenting lumbar epidural injections [10]. No pediatric case reports of blindness following either epidural or caudal anesthetics were found. The most likely explanation for these patients is retinal hemorrhage following a rapid rise in cerebrospinal fluid pressure during medication administration. Although the attempted caudal on our patient was unsuccessful, any contribution to the patient's ocular symptoms from caudal attempt would be extremely unlikely.

6.1 What Is the Goal in Assessing This Patient?

When a pediatric patient complains of postoperative visual loss, a great deal of stress and anxiety can be expected—from both the patient and their family. An astute anesthesiologist will approach the complication with a sense of calm and quickly work through their differential. As in any acute neurologic changes, the clinician must quickly determine whether an acute, evolving neurologic insult (i.e., stroke) is evolving in real time. A rapid and thorough neurologic exam should be completed, and if any non-ophthalmologic deficits are revealed, stat cranial imaging should be undertaken.

Assuming visual loss remains the only finding, the anesthesiologist should have a low threshold for an ophthalmologic consult for a full fundoscopic exam.

As in most neurologic complications, a rapid diagnosis is key for establishing a treatment plan that gives the patient the best chance of a full recovery.

In conclusion, while rare, POVL is an alarming and devastating postoperative complication. By identifying the patient and procedure-specific risk factors, anesthesiologists are empowered to prevent these events. A working knowledge of the most common conditions responsible for POVL allows for an expedient and robust management strategy should this complication occur.

References

1. Warner ME, Warner MA, Garrity JA, MacKenzie RA, Warner DO. The frequency of perioperative vision loss. Anesth Analg. 2001;93(6):1417–21. table of contents
2. Shen Y, Drum M, Roth S. The prevalence of perioperative visual loss in the United States: a 10-year study from 1996 to 2005 of spinal, orthopedic, cardiac, and general surgery. Anesth Analg. 2009;109(5):1534–45.
3. Newman NJ. Perioperative visual loss after nonocular surgeries. Am J Ophthalmol. 2008;145(4):604–10. https://doi.org/10.1016/j.ajo.2007.09.016. PMID: 18358851; PMCID: PMC2989384
4. Grixti A, Sadri M, Watts MT. Corneal protection during general anesthesia for nonocular surgery. Ocul Surf. 2013;11(2):109–18.
5. Michelle Stephenson CE. Diagnosing and managing ischemic optic neuropathy [Internet]. Reviewofophthalmologycom 2010 [cited 2021 Dec 20]. https://www.reviewofophthalmology.com/article/diagnosing-and-managing-ischemic-optic-neuropathy
6. Orlin SE, Kurata FK, Krupin T, Schneider M, Glendrange RR. Ocular lubricants and corneal injury during anesthesia. Anesth Analg. 1989;69(3):384–5.
7. Calway T, Rubin DS, Moss HE, Joslin CE, Beckmann K, Roth S. Perioperative retinal artery occlusion. Ophthalmology. 2017;124(2):189–96.
8. Moslemi MK, Soleimani M, Faiz HR, Rahimzadeh P. Cortical blindness after complicated general anesthesia in urological surgery. Am J Case Rep. 2013;14:376–9.
9. Goni V, Tripathy SK, Goyal T, Tamuk T, Panda BB, Bk S. Cortical blindness following spinal surgery: very rare cause of perioperative vision loss. Asian Spine J. 2012;6(4):287–90.
10. Young WF. Transient blindness after lumbar epidural steroid injection: a case report and literature review. Spine. 2002;27(21):E476–7.

Further Reading

Buisson C, Attia J, Barrier G. Anesthésie et don de moelle osseuse chez l'enfant [Anesthesia and bone marrow harvesting in children]. Ann Fr Anesth Reanim. 1989;8(2):90–2. French. https://doi.org/10.1016/s0750-7658(89)80158-3.

Huo R, Burden SK, Hoyt CS, Good WV. Chronic cortical visual impairment in children: aetiology, prognosis, and associated neurological deficits. Br J Ophthalmol. 1999;83(6):670–5.

Harvard.edu. [cited 2021 Dec 20]. https://anesthesia.bidmc.harvard.edu/Policies/Clinical/Clinical/Guidelines/Guideline%20for%20perioperative%20corneal%20abrasion.pdf

Kaur K, Khanduri N, Sachdeva S, Singh R, Bhardwaj M, Bala M. A study to evaluate ocular changes in patients undergoing spine surgery in the prone position. J Anaesthesiol Clin Pharmacol. 2021;37(4):580–5. https://doi.org/10.4103/joacp.JOACP_428_19. Epub 2022 Jan 6. PMID: 35340948; PMCID: PMC8944359Lichter JR, Marr LB, Schilling DE, Hudson ME, Boretsky RH, Barad RF, et al. A department-of-anesthesiology-based management protocol for perioperative corneal abrasions. Clin Ophthalmol. 2015;9:1689–95. https://www.ncbi.nlm.nih.gov/labs/pmc/articles/PMC4574851/

Hayreh SS. Anterior ischemic optic neuropathy. Ophthalmology. 1987;94(11):1488–502. https://my.clevelandclinic.org/health/diseases/15770-anterior-ischemic-optic-neuropathy

Merckmanuals.com. [cited 2021 Dec 20]. https://www.merckmanuals.com/home/eye-disorders/optic-nerve-disorders/ischemic-optic-neuropathy

Roth S, Moss HE. Update on perioperative ischemic optic neuropathy associated with non-ophthalmic surgery. Front Neurol. 2018;9:557.

Tachycardia and Hypertension in a Teen After Goiter Surgery

Claude Abdallah

Goals

1. Understand the physiological and biological changes associated with hyperthyroidism and thyrotoxicosis.
2. Discuss the management of anesthesia in a patient with hyperthyroidism.
3. Evaluate the postoperative complications of thyroidectomy.
4. Discuss the perioperative diagnosis and management of a thyroid storm.

1 Stem Case

The patient is an 18-year-old female, with a history of anxiety and depression, scheduled for total thyroidectomy secondary to Graves' disease with the presence of suspicious thyroid nodules on biopsy. Numerous attempts to manage her disease with antithyroid medications in the past were unsuccessful because she was non-compliant to clinical or laboratory follow-up visits. Finally, it was clear that surgical removal was the only option to control her disease. After discussion with the patient and her parents by the endocrinology and the surgical teams, she was scheduled for a total thyroidectomy the following week.

Patient was assessed preoperatively by a preop clinical care (POCC) team, and appropriate recommendations for fasting and premedication need were suggested.

Patient was evaluated again in the preop area by the anesthesiologist: she was described as a thin, nervous-looking young woman with features of hyperthyroidism mainly with exophthalmos. As the conversation progressed, she became more tearful, agitated, and anxious and is expressing ambivalent feelings about undergoing surgery.

C. Abdallah (✉)
Division of Anesthesiology, Children's National Hospital, Washington, DC, USA
e-mail: cabdalla@childrensnational.org

S. T. Verghese (ed.), *Anesthesia STAT! Acute Pediatric Emergencies in PACU*,
https://doi.org/10.1007/978-3-031-24396-7_18

During the preop interview, she stated that she was taking her scheduled medications for the last week, and although she denied any diarrhea or sweating, she appeared to have bilateral hand tremors and baseline tachycardia. Her heart rate was 100 bpm and BP 145/75 mm Hg with normal temperature and normal oxygen saturation on room air. She was given the oral premedication after the consent was signed by herself and her parents.

Anxiety improved after administration of 20 mg po midazolam, and since her pregnancy test (HCG) was negative, she was wheeled to the operating room for the planned surgery.

1. *What are the clinical signs, symptoms, and manifestations of hyperthyroidism? How would you evaluate a patient with hyperthyroidism preoperatively?*
2. *What is the etiology, criteria for diagnosis, and treatment options for this disease?*
3. *How would you optimize, prepare, and manage this patient intraoperatively?*
4. *What are some of the common problems that can occur after thyroid surgery in patients with inadequate medical control?*
5. *What are some of the highlights to remember while positioning and intubating these patients? Is there a need for specialized endotracheal tubes?*

After an uneventful surgery for removing her large goiter (Fig. 1), trachea was extubated deep and the integrity of the vocal cords ascertained, with patient appearing comfortable with stable vital signs.

She was sedated, breathing spontaneously, and continuing to receive intravenous fluid during her transfer to the recovery room with supplemental oxygen via a mask.

Approximately an hour postoperatively, the PACU nurse called the anesthesiologist to report that the patient had become restless. She was reported to be agitated, tachycardic with a HR of 145 bpm, hypertensive with 160–170/100 mm Hg with a respiratory rate of 45/min. Despite escalation of pain control with intravenous morphine, she was showing signs of an acute postoperative thyroid hyperactivity.

Once at the bedside, the diagnosis of a "thyroid storm" in the postoperative period was made and treatment started immediately. Intermittent intravenous propranolol was administered to treat elevated blood pressure and heart rate. Small doses of dexmedetomidine were also given and patient was instructed to be kept Nil Per Os and to continue receiving intravenous fluids. She responded to the drugs administered and became sedated with lower heart rate, BP, and respiratory rate. An hour later, patient woke up and complained of having dysphagia and dyspnea, and the PACU anesthesiologist was called urgently to assess. Upon arriving at the bedside, it was evident that there was an expanding hematoma under the incision site which needed urgent surgical evacuation. The need to establish an airway support in the form of endotracheal intubation if the hematoma evacuation is delayed was also clear to the attending anesthesiologist. The surgeon arrived promptly and evacuated the hematoma rapidly at the bedside and the patient was taken back without delay to the OR for surgical re-exploration.

Fig. 1 Surgical exposure of the goiter (Photo Courtesy of Dr. P. Mudd)

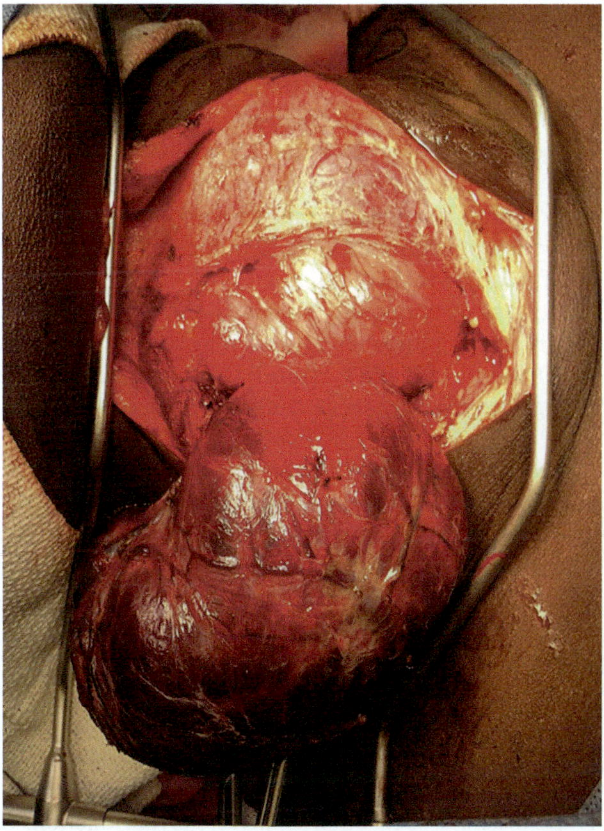

1. *What are the possible complications after a surgical procedure involving the thyroid gland?*
2. *How would you manage these complications?*
3. *What are the precipitating factors for occurrence of a "thyroid storm"?*
4. *Is a thyroid storm post-total thyroidectomy possible?*
5. *How do you manage a postoperative thyroid storm?*

2 Discussion

The hypothalamus releases thyrotropin-releasing hormone (TRH), which traverses the pituitary stalk and stimulates release of thyroid-stimulating hormone (TSH) from the anterior pituitary. TSH is released into the circulation and controls production and release of T_4 and T_3. Some T_3 is secreted by the thyroid, but most is produced by deiodination of T_4 in peripheral tissues. Both T_4 and T_3 are bound to carrier proteins (principally thyroid-binding globulin, TBG) in the circulation.

2.1 Different Steps Involved in Thyroid Hormone Synthesis

1. Uptake of iodide. Iodide from the bloodstream is concentrated in thyroid cells by an active transport mechanism.
2. Iodination of thyroglobulin. Thyroglobulin, a large glycoprotein rich in tyrosine, is enzymatically iodinated and stored in the thyroid follicles.
3. Coupling reactions: the mono-iodotyrosine and diiodotyrosine moieties within the thyroglobulin molecule are coupled to one another to form triiodothyronine (T_3) and thyroxine (T_4).
4. Release of hormones. T_3 and T_4 are enzymatically cleaved from thyroglobulin within the follicular cell and released into the bloodstream. T_3 and T_4 inhibit release of TSH and to a much smaller degree the release of TRH, thus establishing a negative feedback control mechanism.

The thyroid secretes thyroxine (T_4) and triiodothyronine (T_3), which influence basal metabolic rate and cardiac and neurological functions. Diseases of the thyroid may manifest by quantitative or qualitative alterations in hormone secretion, enlargement of the gland, or both. Under- or overproduction of thyroid hormones is usually reflected in decrease or increase of serum T_4 and T_3 levels. When TBG is elevated or low, the free thyroxin index (FTI) corrects serum T_4 for alterations in binding protein and thus provides an index of thyroid status [1, 2].

2.2 Different Types of Thyrotoxicosis

1. Disorders associated with thyroid hyperfunction: due to excess production of TSH (rare) or an abnormal thyroid stimulator such as Graves' disease/trophoblastic tumor or intrinsic thyroid autonomy such as a hyperfunctioning adenoma/toxic multinodular goiter.
2. Disorders not associated with thyroid hyperfunction: due to disorders of hormone storage such as subacute thyroiditis/chronic thyroiditis with transient thyrotoxicosis or an extrathyroidal source of hormone such as thyrotoxicosis factitial/ectopic thyroid tissue (struma ovarii, functioning follicular carcinoma).

Hyperthyroidism in children is most commonly congenital or a result of Graves' disease. Congenital hyperthyroidism is caused by the transfer of maternal thyroid-stimulating immunoglobulins in utero. These infants may be premature, and tachycardia, respiratory distress, and congestive heart failure may be present along with physical appearance of goiter. Conversely, Graves' disease occurs more frequently among adolescents than children and four to five times more frequently among females.

Many symptoms and signs are associated with hyperthyroidism. They are the same for all hyperthyroidism with some exceptions, such as infiltrative ophthalmopathy and dermopathy, which are confined to Graves' disease. The clinical presentation may be dramatic or subtle.

The more common signs of hyperthyroidism (1) goiter; (2) tachycardia; (3) widened pulse pressure; (4) warm, fine, moist skin and fingernails may separate from the nail bed; (5) tremor (97%); (6) eye signs (71%); and (7) atrial fibrillation (10%). In hyperthyroidism, the metabolic rate of the body is increased, causing significant changes in the cardiovascular system, proportional to the severity of the thyroid dysfunction.

The most frequent symptoms of hyperthyroidism (1) nervousness and increased activity (99%), (2) increased sweating, (3) hypersensitivity to heat, (4) palpitations, (5) fatigue, (6) increased appetite, (7) weight loss, (8) tachycardia, (9) insomnia, (10) weakness, and (11) frequent bowel movements. Eye signs noted in patients with thyrotoxicosis include stare, lid lag, lid retraction, and mild degrees of conjunctival injection or edema-producing symptoms including orbital pain, lacrimation, irritation, and photophobia.

Infiltrative ophthalmopathy is a more serious development and is specific for Graves' disease. It is characterized by increased retro-orbital tissue, producing exophthalmos, and by lymphocytic infiltration of the extraocular muscles, producing a spectrum of ocular muscle weakness frequently leading to blurred and double vision. The pathogenesis of infiltrative ophthalmopathy is poorly understood. It may occur before the onset of hyperthyroidism or as late as 15–20 years afterward and frequently worsens or improves independent of the clinical course of hyperthyroidism.

Infiltrative dermopathy, also known as pretibial myxedema (a confusing term, since myxedema suggests hypothyroidism), is characterized by nonpitting infiltration of mucinous ground substance, usually in the pretibial area. The lesion is very pruritic and erythematous in its early stages and subsequently becomes brawny. Like ophthalmopathy, infiltrative dermopathy may appear years before or after hyperthyroidism.

The diagnosis of hyperthyroidism depends on a careful clinical history and physical examination, a high index of suspicion, and routine thyroid hormone determinations. A serum T_4 assay and a T_3 resin uptake test are a highly accurate combination of initial tests for assessing thyroid status. Mild to moderate hyperthyroidism may be difficult to diagnose clinically during pregnancy since many normal parturients experience tachycardia, heat intolerance, and emotional instability. In hyperthyroidism, there is increased T_4, increased RT_3U, and increased T_3, while in pregnancy there is increased T_4, decreased RT_3U, and normal T_3. Age-adjusted normal values are needed because thyroid hormone levels are higher in children [1, 2].

Preoperatively, elective surgery should be deferred until the patient has been rendered euthyroid and the hyperdynamic cardiovascular system has been controlled with a beta antagonist, as evidenced by an acceptable resting heart rate. The child should have received ablation treatment to ensure a euthyroid state confirmed by preoperative thyroid function tests. All drugs being administered to manage the hyperthyroid state should be continued through the perioperative period. One week before surgery, administration of Lugol's iodine solution may be initiated to decrease vascularity and hyperplasia of the overreactive gland.

When surgery cannot be delayed in a symptomatic hyperthyroid patient, the continuous infusion of a beta blocker may be useful for the control of cardiovascular responses evoked by sympathetic nervous system stimulation [3]. Poor control of hyperthyroidism and surgery are associated with an increased risk of the development of thyroid storm.

Anxiety relief is often provided by the oral administration of a benzodiazepine. The use of an anticholinergic drug is not recommended, since such a drug could interfere with the body's normal heat-regulating mechanism and contribute to an increase in heart rate. Evaluation of the upper airway for evidence of obstruction is an important part of the preoperative preparation. A large goiter requires a computed axial tomography scan to determine if tracheal compression or deviation exists. Propranolol may be used preoperatively to control tachycardia [4–6].

Induction of anesthesia is usually achieved with intravenous induction drugs.

Patients do best with premedication with midazolam in the preoperative area followed by a smooth induction with preoxygenation and intravenous line placement followed by intravenous drugs like propofol with frequent checks on hemodynamic stability.

Ketamine is not an appropriate selection because it can stimulate the sympathetic nervous system. Indeed, tachycardia and hypertension have been described after administration of ketamine to euthyroid patients being treated with thyroid hormone replacement. Propofol clearance and distribution volume increase in patients with hyperthyroidism [7, 8].

Assuming the absence of airway obstruction from an enlarged goiter, the administration of succinylcholine or of a nondepolarizing muscle relaxant that will not affect the cardiovascular system may be useful to facilitate intubation of the trachea.

Constant monitoring of body temperature is particularly useful; methods to lower body temperature, including a cooling mattress and cold crystalloid solutions for intravenous infusion, are recommended. The patient with exophthalmos is susceptible to corneal ulceration and drying, and therefore it is important to protect the eyes during the perioperative period. Placement of artificial tears and eye lubricant is advised. Covering both eyes with soft cotton gauge and placing OPSITE over the protuberant eyes completely may be sufficient although goggles have been placed in patients with very protuberant eyes. It is optimal to continue to monitor the eyes to prevent any pressure over it from surgeon's hands or retractors since the surgical site is close to the face.

During positioning of these patients, slight head-up position is often requested by surgeons to allow increased venous drainage of the surgical site [9].

General anesthesia is usually maintained with a combination of inhalational agent and intravenous anesthetics since neuromuscular agents are often avoided. Total intravenous anesthesia (TIVA) can also be achieved with propofol, because of rapid-onset and quick recovery potential. In addition, short-acting narcotics like remifentanil can be given as an infusion for continuous analgesia. Intravenous dexmedetomidine can be helpful to counter sudden increase in heart rate during surgical manipulation of the thyroid. Most commonly, a combination of inhalational anesthetic and intravenous anesthetic is chosen to achieve hemodynamic stability during thyroid surgery.

Intraoperatively, there may be transient episodes of tachycardia and hypertension attributed to increased levels of thyroxine being released during surgical manipulation and can be treated with small doses of propranolol and intravenous dexmedetomidine.

A second intravenous line is usually necessary to be placed to enable the anesthesiologist to draw lab specimens intraoperatively.

The anesthesiologist should be familiar with the proper use and functioning of the neural integrity monitor (NIM) electromyogram (EMG) tracheal tube. The use of the specialized neural integrity monitor electromyogram (NIM EMG) endotracheal tubes to accurately monitor amplitude and latency changes requires optimal placement at the vocal cords to allow neuromonitoring (Fig. 2). Proper understanding of its structure and function is essential for the anesthesiologist. It is frequently being utilized, for the head and neck procedures, when laryngeal nerves could be injured during the process of surgical dissection. Initially, this unique tracheal tube must be positioned so that its color-coded contact band is appropriately placed between the vocal cords.

The aim is to identify the recurrent laryngeal nerve (RLN) and to avoid intraoperative inadvertent RLN palsy which is possible during total thyroidectomy.

Intraoperatively after identification, the RLN is stimulated electrically, and the electric field is converted into an acoustic signal from which the evoked potentials

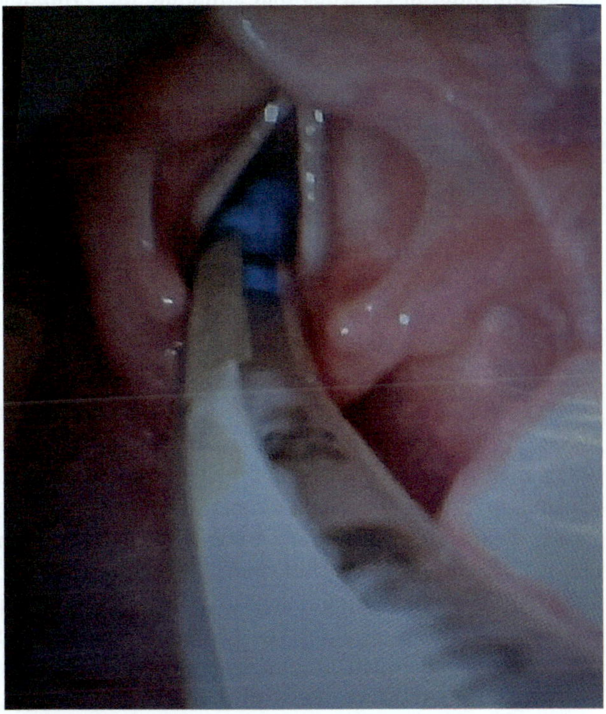

Fig. 2 Use of the specialized neural integrity monitor electromyogram (NIM EMG) endotracheal tubes with optimal placement at the vocal cords (Photo Courtesy of Dr. P. Mudd)

are obtained. A retrospective study of 113 children who underwent thyroid surgery between 2001 and 2019 showed that use of IONM was associated with decreased rate of RLN injury during pediatric thyroid surgery [10, 11].

If the plan is to avoid neuromuscular blockade, the induction can be accomplished by a combination of inhalation agent sevoflurane and intravenous hypnotics and narcotics. When the depth of anesthesia is sufficient for performing a direct laryngoscopy, it is useful to spray the larynx and the vocal cords with 2% lidocaine spray prior to intubation.

If the goiter is large, the difficulty with tracheal intubation is mainly from reduced mobility of the underlying structures. The use of video laryngoscope such as GlideScope has improved visualization of vocal cords and tracheal intubation in patients with potential for difficult airway.

If the special NIM EMG tube is not being used, then neuromuscular paralysis may be used. To facilitate tracheal intubation, a depolarizing agent may be required. Preparalytic, as well as postparalytic, assessment of train-of-four monitoring should be conducted with documentation of the return of neuromuscular function. If requested by the surgeon, the selection of a muscle relaxant should include consideration of the potential impact of this drug on the sympathetic nervous system. Pancuronium is not an appropriate selection, in view of the ability of this drug to increase heart rate and thereby mimic sympathetic nervous system stimulation.

Goals during maintenance of anesthesia for a hyperthyroid patient are to avoid the administration of drugs that stimulate the sympathetic nervous system and to provide sufficient anesthetic depression to prevent an exaggerated response to surgical stimulation. The possibility of organ toxicity owing to altered or accelerated drug metabolism in the presence of hyperthyroidism must also be considered when selecting drugs for maintenance of anesthesia. The use of volatile agents is acceptable. Increased cardiac output and temperature may result in an increased minimum alveolar concentration (MAC) for the volatile agents. High-dose narcotics would be required to provide adequate inhibition of the sympathetic nervous system. Muscle relaxation, as described above, should be avoided, but if requested, the choice of a nondepolarizing agents with minimal cardiac effects is preferable. A prolonged response to nondepolarizing agents may occur in patients with preexisting muscle weakness. Hypercarbia will result in stimulation of the sympathetic nervous system and should therefore be avoided. In the presence of tachycardia, the use of beta blockers during the perioperative period is essential. Treatment of hypotension, if needed, is best achieved with the use of a direct-acting agent such as phenylephrine rather than agents such as ephedrine, which act in part by an indirect mechanism. Constant monitoring of body temperature is essential.

Regional anesthesia with its associated blockade of the sympathetic nervous system is a potentially useful selection for the hyperthyroid patient, assuming there is no evidence of high-output congestive heart failure. Epinephrine is to be avoided in the local anesthetic solution, as systemic absorption of this catecholamine could produce an exaggerated circulatory response.

Every effort must be taken to decrease or possibly eliminate the potential for postoperative vomiting in patients with thyroid surgery. Incidence of vomiting is high in patients after thyroid surgery, and this can increase postoperative bleeding and hematoma formation which can lead to airway obstruction. Vagal stimulation from the surgical manipulation of neck structures during surgery, female gender, age, and history of motion sickness all contribute to increase incidence of postoperative vomiting. Prophylactic treatment with serotonin receptor antagonists (ondansetron, granisetron), anticholinergics (scopolamine), antihistamines (diphenhydramine, promethazine), and corticosteroids (dexamethasone) are recommended to achieve the antiemesis status in the immediate postoperative period [12].

A smooth emergence is desirable after thyroid surgery and can be achieved by a planned deep extubation with spontaneous ventilation or awake extubation without coughing by using lidocaine and titrated doses of dexmedetomidine. It is important to keep in mind that the airway may have developed mucosal edema and some element of tracheomalacia after surgery.

Deep extubation may be requested by some surgeons to prevent coughing on emergence and to document bilateral vocal cord movement and may be accomplished with the use of intravenous lidocaine and dexmedetomidine [13].

Some physicians tend to replace the endotracheal tube with an appropriately sized laryngeal mask airway (LMA) and placement of a fiberoptic bronchoscope to evaluate vocal cord movement. Ultrasound technology can also be used to evaluate vocal cord movement [14].

2.3 Complications of Thyroid Surgery/Resection

Prevention of complications depends on careful preoperative evaluation and operative technique and is enhanced using specific techniques such as intraoperative neuromonitoring. A systematic strategy for detection of complications after thyroidectomy involving a multidisciplinary approach is favorable to a good patient outcome. The two most common early complications of thyroid surgery are hypocalcemia from permanent hypoparathyroidism (20–30%) and recurrent laryngeal nerve injury (5–11%). Bilateral recurrent nerve paralysis resulting in adduction of the vocal cords is a rare life-threatening complication. Postsurgical hypocalcemia is managed by the administration of calcium plus vitamin D for at least 10 days. Recurrent laryngeal nerve paralysis recovers in most cases, and no invasive therapy should be performed for at least 6 months, except for emergency presentations; laryngeal surgery techniques may offer significant improvement if phonation or respiratory sequelae persist beyond 6 months, with inconsistent results [15, 16].

Thyroid storm is a rare life-threatening condition from acute exacerbation of hyperthyroidism and requires diagnosis and immediate treatment. It is caused by the sudden excessive release of thyroid gland hormones into the circulation. It can develop in patients who have long-standing inadequately treated hyperthyroidism and can be induced by surgical manipulation. Thyroid storm, which is rare in children, results from untreated or inadequately treated thyrotoxicosis and may be precipitated by infection, vigorous palpation of the thyroid, trauma, bowel infarction, congestive heart failure, surgery (thyroid and nonthyroid), pulmonary thromboembolism, diabetic acidosis, severe fright, toxemia of pregnancy or labor, lithium or amiodarone treatment, discontinuance of antithyroid medication, or excessive thyroid hormone ingestion and Iodine-131 therapy or radiation thyroiditis.

It may mimic malignant hyperthermia but often lack muscle rigidity, severe acidosis, and myoglobinuria.

Common manifestations include fever (>40 °C), diaphoresis, and disorders of the cardiovascular system (high blood pressure, tachycardia, atrial fibrillation, heart failure), gastrointestinal system (nausea, vomiting), hepatic system (unexplained jaundice), and central nervous system (agitation, delirium, psychosis, seizures). A point scale, Burch-Wartofsky Point Scale [17], is available during the evaluation of the adult patient, to score the possibility of diagnosis of a thyroid storm (Table 1).

Treatment of a thyroid storm must be immediate and should be conducted in an acute/intensive care setting [18]. Blood measurements including thyroid function levels should be drawn. Treatment should consist of an infusion of cooled crystalloid solutions and continuous infusion of a beta blocker (esmolol), to maintain the

Table 1 Burch-Wartofsky point scale [12]

Cardiovascular dysfunction
Tachycardia (bpm)
99–109 → 5 points
110–119 → 10 points
120–129 → 15 points
130–139 → 20 points
≥140 → 25 points
Atrial fibrillation → 10 points
Heart failure
Mild (pedal edema) → 5 points
Moderate (bibasilar rales) → 10 points
Severe (pulmonary edema) → 15 points
Gastrointestinal-hepatic dysfunction
Moderate (nausea/vomiting, abdominal pain, diarrhea) → 10 points
Severe (unexplained jaundice) → 20 points
Central nervous system effects
Absent → 0
Mild (agitation) → 10
Moderate (delirium, psychosis, extreme lethargy) → 20
Severe (seizure, coma) → 30
Temperature (degrees F)
99–99.9 → 5 points
100–100.9 → 10 points
101–101.9 → 15 points
102–102.9 → 20 points
103–103.9 → 25 points
≥104 → 30 points
Precipitant history
Positive → 0 points
Negative → 10 points

Total: <25 → Storm unlikely
Total: 25–45 → Impending storm
Total: >45 → Thyroid storm

Table 2 Management of a thyroid storm

Supportive
• Airway maintenance and oxygen supplementation
• Hemodynamic stability: IV fluids and BP control
Beta blockers (decreases sympathetic hyperactivity) and/or if needed Ca++ channel blockers
• Temperature control: Cooling blanket and acetaminophen. Avoid salicylates: Increase free T4 and free T3 levels
Treat precipitating causes
Pharmaceutical treatment
1. 4 and T3 synthesis inhibition: Methimazole/propylthiouracil (faster action and preferred in pregnancy)
2. T4 and T3 release inhibition: Potassium iodide
3. T4 to T3 conversion inhibition: Steroids, propranolol partially blocks peripheral conversion of T4 to T3

heart rate at an acceptable level. When hypotension is persistent, the administration of cortisol should be considered. Dexamethasone may inhibit the conversion of T_4–T_3, an effect that is additive to propylthiouracil. Aspirin may displace T_4 from its carrier protein and is not recommended for lowering body temperature. It is also important to treat any suspected infection. Ultimately, antithyroid drugs such as propylthiouracil and sodium iodide should be added. Definitive therapy after control of the crisis consists of ablation of the thyroid gland with ^{131} I or surgery [19] (Table 2).

Cooling the patient and fluid resuscitation combined with treatment with beta adrenergic blockers propranolol to counter the effects of circulating thyroid hormone levels is important while labs are being drawn. Titrating small doses of intravenous dexmedetomidine to see its effect in blunting the hemodynamic effects of the thyroid storm can also be tried.

3 Summary

Caregivers should be vigilant about the possibility of occurrence of a thyroid storm in the postoperative period even after total thyroidectomy. This patient was found to be noncompliant to medication intake and showed clinical signs of thyroid storm even after complete removal of the thyroid gland. In the adolescent and young adult, the fractional rate of turnover of T4 in the periphery is normally about 10%/d (half-life, 6.7 d). The half-life of thyroxine is inversely related to the initial serum thyroxine levels. Large quantities of thyroglobulin are released into the blood during surgical manipulation of the thyroid [20]. Metabolic and hemodynamic manifestations of thyrotoxicosis may be masked intraoperatively by anesthetics and sedation and exaggerated in the postoperative period. The diagnosis of a thyrotoxic crisis is made entirely on the clinical findings. Most importantly, there is no difference in thyroid hormone levels between patients with "uncomplicated" thyrotoxicosis and those undergoing a thyroid storm. Any delay in therapy, such as awaiting additional laboratory results, must be strictly avoided, because the mortality rate may rise to 75%. Treatment of a thyroid storm must be immediate and should occur in an intensive care setting. Monitoring in an acute care setting with tight control of blood pressure is often needed to manage a developing thyroid storm. Surgical outcomes after thyroid surgery at a single center in 464 patients with a median age of 15 years reported that six patients required return to the OR for hematoma evacuation including five patients after surgery for Graves' disease [21]. The possibility of acute postoperative thyroid storm leading to acute airway loss from an expanding neck hematoma should be considered in patients with poor medical compliance [22].

References

1. Scott GM, Steward DJ. Diseases of the endocrine system. In: Berry FA, Steward DJ, editors. Pediatrics for the anesthesiologist. New York: Churchill Livingstone; 1993. p. 200–30.
2. Reed Larson PR, Davies T, Hay ID. The thyroid gland. In: Wilson JD, Foster DW, Kronenberg HM, Larsen PR, editors. Williams textbook of endocrinology. 9th ed. Philadelphia, PA: W.B. Saunders Company; 1998. p. 389–515.
3. Zonszein J, Santangelo R, Mackin J, Lee T, Coffey R, Canary J. Propranalol therapy in thyrotoxicosis: a review of 84 patients undergoing surgery. Am J Med. 1979;66:411–6.
4. Farling PA. Thyroid disease. Br J Anaesth. 2000;85(1):15–28.
5. Langley RW, Burch HB. Perioperative management of the thyrotoxic patient. Endocrinol Metab Clin N Am. 2003;32(2):519–34.
6. Streetman DD, Khanderia U. Diagnosis and treatment of graves' disease. Ann Pharmacother. 2003;37:1100–9.
7. Tsubokawa T, Yamamoto K, Kobayashi T. Propofol clearance and distribution volume increase in patients with hyperthyroidism. Anesth Analg. 1998;87:195–9.
8. Kaplan JA, Cooperman LH. Alarming reactions to ketamine in patients taking thyroid medication-treatment with propranolol. Anesthesiology. 1971;35:229–30.
9. Saracoglu A, Altun D, Yavru A, et al. Effects of head position on cerebral oxygenation and blood flow velocity during thyroidectomy. Turk J Anesthesiol Reanim. 2016;44(5):241–6.
10. Ritter A, Hod R, Jauven Y, Shpitzer T, Mizrachi A, Raveh E, Bachar G. Role of intraoperative recurrent laryngeal nerve monitoring for pediatric thyroid surgery: comparative analysis. Head Neck. 2021;43(3):849–57.
11. Atlas G, Lee M. The neural integrity monitor electromyogram tracheal tube: anesthetic considerations. J Anaesthesiol Clin Pharmacol. 2013;29(3):403–4.
12. Won YJ, Yoo JY, Chae YJ, et al. The incidence of post-operative nausea and vomiting after thyroidectomy using three anesthetic techniques. J Int Med Res. 2011;39:1834–42.
13. Hu S, Li Y, Wang S, Xu S, Ju X, Ma L. Effects of intravenous infusion of lidocaine and dexmedetomidine on inhibiting cough during the tracheal extubation period after thyroid surgery. BMC Anesthesiol. 2019;19(1):66.
14. Kandil E, Deniwar A, Noureldine SI, et al. Assessment of vocal cord function using transcutaneous laryngeal ultrasonography and flexible laryngoscopy. JAMA Otolaryngol Head Neck Surg. 2016;142(1):74–8.
15. Christou N, Mathonnet M. Complications after total thyroidectomy. Visc Surg. 2013;150(4):249–56.
16. Akkari M, Makeieff M, Jeandel C, Raingeard I, Cartier C, Garrel R, Guerrier B, Blanchet C, Mondain M. Thyroid surgery in children and adolescents: a series of 65 cases. Eur Ann Otorhinolaryngol Head Neck Dis. 2014;131(5):293–7.
17. Burch HB, Wartofsky L. Life-threatening thyrotoxicosis. Thyroid storm. Endocrinol Metab Clin N Am. 1993;22(2):263–77.
18. Carrol R, Matfin G. Endocrine and metabolic emergencies: thyroid storm. Ther Adv Endocrinolog Metab. 2010;3:139–45.

19. Migneco A, Ojetti V, Testa A, De Lorenzo A, Gentiloni SN. Management of thyrotoxic crisis. Eur Rev Med Pharmacol Sci. 2005;9(1):69–74.
20. Izumi M, Larsen PR. Correlation of sequential changes in serum thyroglobulin, triiodothyronine, and thyroxine in patients with graves' disease and subacute thyroiditis. Metabolism. 1978;27:449–60.
21. Baumgarten HD, Bauer AJ, Isaza A, Mostoufi-Moab S, Kazahaya K, Adzick NS. Surgical management of pediatric thyroid disease: complication rates after thyroidectomy at the Children's Hospital of Philadelphia high-volume Pediatric Thyroid Center. J Pediatr Surg. 2019;54(10):1969–75.
22. Abdallah C, Verghese S. Airway emergency post thyroidectomy: the role of thyroid hormone pharmacokinetics and compliance with treatment. Saudi J Anaesth. 2012;6(3):305.

Prolonged Apnea After Treatment of Laryngospasm in a Child After Botox Injection

Marjorie P. Brennan

Learning Objective
At the end of this educational session, the participants will be able to:

1. Discuss the differential diagnosis of postoperative prolonged apnea.
2. Describe the pathophysiology and the effect of pseudocholinesterase deficiency in patients.
3. Discuss the management of anesthesia in the patient with spastic cerebral palsy.
4. Pros and cons about oral premed and other methods to allay anxiety.
5. Discuss the use of Botox phenol and Dysport in children with CP and the adverse reactions that can occur after its use.

1 Stem Case

A 7-year-old girl with spastic quadriplegia, cerebral palsy, and infantile seizures requires Botox injections. She had developed group b strep at 17 days of life, with multiple cerebral vascular accidents. She has developed some drooling recently and was scheduled for an ENT consult for a selective Botox injection near her salivary gland. She prefers a soft diet now and has had episodes of gagging after solid food. She presents for Botox injection for management of her multiple limb spasticity. She has undergone many Botox injections in the past, but her parents noticed that she was getting more anxious and afraid of these procedures and strongly requested oral premedication with midazolam, which was given in the past. Therefore, she was given 20 mg of oral midazolam before the procedure. Her weight is 34.2 kg, with an ASA Classification of class 2-mild systemic disease.

M. P. Brennan (✉)
Children's National Hospital, Washington, DC, USA
e-mail: mbrennan@childrensnational.org

S. T. Verghese (ed.), *Anesthesia STAT! Acute Pediatric Emergencies in PACU*,
https://doi.org/10.1007/978-3-031-24396-7_19

She was taken to the procedure room with her parents and induced by mask after the placement of monitors. Anesthesia for Botox injections included an inhalation induction with nitrous oxide and sevoflurane. After placement of a peripheral intravenous catheter, propofol 70 mg was administered, and a laryngeal mask airway (LMA) was placed without difficulty. Anesthesia was maintained with sevoflurane and spontaneous ventilation. After Botox injections were completed, the LMA was removed deep. Some secretions were noted in the mouth, and the oropharynx was suctioned. The patient was transported to the postoperative care unit (PACU) in the lateral position breathing oxygen via a Jackson-Rees circuit.

Initial vital signs in the recovery were stable with a pulse oximetry of 98%, HR 94/min with blood pressure 95/56. During handoff to the PACU nurse, the patient developed hiccups and started coughing, and the pulse oximeter reading decreased to 95% and then 90%. Oxygen was being delivered via a facemask placed close to the patient's face. The patient was coughing and retching and developing clinical signs of upper airway obstruction and beginning to look dusky. A Yankauer suction was used to suction out copious secretions in the mouth, which looked pink like the oral premedication that was given to her.

After her mouth was suctioned, the anesthesiologist attempted to assist her breathing, but it was impossible to move air into her trachea and lungs because of suspected glottic closure. Since the laryngospasm could not be overcome with positive pressure, intravenous succinylcholine was administered with a rapidly improved ability to ventilate. Her ventilation was controlled during the period of apnea from the succinylcholine, and her oxygen saturation improved to 98%.

Ten minutes after succinylcholine administration, the patient showed no signs of respiratory effort but had developed an increased heart rate of 125/min and blood pressure of 120/70. Fifteen minutes after succinylcholine, blood pressure had increased to 140/85, and HR had increased to 140/min. An ulnar nerve stimulator was placed, and the train-of-four yielded no twitch.

Apnea after anesthesia has several etiologies, including lingering effects of anesthetic agents such as propofol, opiates, or benzodiazepines. Systemic spread of Botox in a child with cerebral palsy can rarely result in weakness, respiratory distress, or apnea.

Pediatric laryngospasm is a life-threatening event and can be defined as total glottic closure due to reflex constriction of the laryngeal muscles. Laryngospasm can be complete or partial and occurs in a state of decreased inhibition of glottic reflexes with increased stimulation. Common causes of increased stimulation are extubation, secretions or blood irritating the vocal cords, an artificial airway, or a suction catheter. This glottic closure can lead to hypoxemia, negative-pressure pulmonary edema, pulmonary aspiration, and cardiac arrest.

Treatment may initially begin with physical methods such as jaw thrust, immediate application of positive-pressure ventilation, and administration of 100% oxygen.

Pharmacologic interventions have long included succinylcholine because of its rapid onset and short duration of action. Succinylcholine is administered at a dose of 1–2 mg/kg and given with atropine (0.02 mg/kg) to prevent bradycardia. This results in a duration of effect of 5–10 min following a standard dose. Therefore, a period of apnea is expected after administration. When intravenous access is absent, succinylcholine can be administered intramuscularly at a dose of 4 mg/kg. The agent that is commonly used to break laryngospasm currently is intravenous propofol. Propofol has been reported to relieve laryngospasm in most cases effectively. Its use can avoid the need for paralysis and the potential side effects of succinylcholine.

Questions

1. *How did she develop hiccups and laryngospasm after an uneventful anesthetic?*
2. *Could she have developed apnea from the multiple Botox injection?*
3. *Could she have developed an unusual reaction to the Botox or phenol injection?*
4. *What is the cause of apnea immediately after treatment of laryngospasm in PACU with succinylcholine?*
5. *Could the use of propofol avoided this apnea?*

This patient most probably has a rare condition of pseudocholinesterase deficiency that affects 1 per 2000–5000 people. The incidence of heterozygotes for the abnormal enzyme is approximately 1 per 500.

2 Cause of Laryngospasm

It was clear that as she emerged slowly from her anesthetic after reaching PACU that she had vomited and had developed laryngospasm from the copious secretions in her mouth, which included her oral premedication of midazolam 20 mg (volume 10 cc). Children with cerebral palsy commonly have feeding disorders and dysphagia that place them at risk for aspiration with oral intake, with potential pulmonary consequences.

Removal of the LMA deep was well tolerated at the end of the procedure in the OR. She exhibited good respiratory effort initially because she had no respiratory depression from any drugs given during the case. Intravenous Tylenol managed her pain, and she had not received any narcotics intraoperatively. The patient arrived in the PACU in the lateral position, but on emergence she spontaneously turned supine, but she was not sufficiently conscious to cough to expel the secretions in her mouth. She was therefore at risk for pulmonary aspiration and laryngospasm. Children with CP are usually positioned in a lateral or recovery position as they emerge from anesthesia to keep their airway clear and open and thus improve respiratory efforts. It also ensures that any vomit or secretions will drain by gravity to the side of the bed and not be aspirated into the airway. Laryngospasm in PACU is usually treated with propofol. In this scenario, succinylcholine was the only drug readily available to treat the laryngospasm in the anesthesiologist's hand.

Pseudocholinesterase deficiency is an important consideration in patients who develop prolonged apnea after succinylcholine is administered. These patients cannot effectively metabolize the muscle relaxants succinylcholine, mivacurium, and ester type of local anesthetics. Using a muscle relaxant such as succinylcholine to relax the apposed vocal cords during laryngospasm, which is normally short acting, can lead to prolonged paralysis of several hours following its administration. Given the use of succinylcholine and the patient's otherwise unremarkable history, pseudocholinesterase deficiency was the possible diagnosis.

After breaking the laryngospasm and improvement in oxygen saturation with manual ventilation by mask, an endotracheal tube was placed, and ventilation was controlled with 100% oxygen. The patient's temperature was 37.1. Point-of-care testing revealed normal potassium, mild respiratory acidosis (pH, 7.26; carbon dioxide, 52 mmHg; oxygen partial pressure, 328 mmHg; bicarbonate concentration, 19.4 mmol/L; base excess, −4.2 mmol/L).

Fifty-five minutes after arrival in the PACU, endotracheal tube suction slightly increased her blood pressure and heart rate, but spontaneous respiration and movement were not observed.

The patient's body temperature was 37.3 C, and her serum potassium level was within the normal range.

Three hours and 30 min after the arrival in the PACU, the patient showed slight diaphragm and eyelid movement and mild coughing. Four and a half hours after the PACU arrival, the patient regained consciousness with sustained head lift and adequate spontaneous ventilation. The patient was extubated and admitted for overnight observation to PICU and was discharged the next day in stable condition. A blood sample was submitted to measure serum pseudocholinesterase level. This specialized testing was sent to a reference laboratory and revealed a dibucaine number of 22. Family members were also counseled to receive testing. The parents are grateful that this genetic defect in enzyme function was diagnosed and wanted to know how their daughter will be identified as having this deficiency without an identifying marker.

Their question prior to discharge was an important one.

2.1 What Is the Ideal Safe Way for Their Daughter to Undergo Future Anesthesia for Botox Injection?

The anesthesiologist and the PMR physician went over the medical problems that she was developing of drooling and dysphagia and aversion to solid food as she manifested signs of diminished gag reflex and inability to have strong cough to clear her own salivary secretions. In this setting, perhaps oral premedication may not be ideal for her to have as a premedication drug for calming her.

The choice of other avenues of preoperative relaxation was suggested including listening to her favorite music or distractions with children's movies and games that the hospital child life specialists frequently use, which may be better tolerated by her to allay her anxiety prior to the next Botox procedure. TIVA with propofol supplemented with intravenous Tylenol for pain relief could be beneficial if she can breathe well spontaneously with a nasal cannula in place. The most important information they needed to hear was that their daughter's inability to swallow well may put her at risk for general anesthesia by mask or LMA in the future, and so intravenous drugs which will not depress her ventilation could be tried with a nasal cannula for oxygen delivery and a CO_2 monitor side port for evaluating adequacy of her ventilation. If the PMR physician could tolerate her position in the bed slightly tilted to the side position, then it would be advantageous and safer to undergo the next procedure with TIVA.

3 Discussion

Cerebral palsy is the most common motor disorder of childhood, with a reported prevalence ranging from 1 to nearly 4 per 1000 live births or per 1000 children.

Botulinum neurotoxin-A (BoNT-A) injections are used to children suffering from muscle conditions such as spasticity to increase mobility. It is a neurotoxin produced by the bacterium *Clostridium botulinum* and inhibits neuromuscular transmission to nicotine acetylcholine receptors by blocking the presynaptic fusion of acetylcholine-containing vesicles and, thus, muscle activation. By exerting chemodenervation effects at the presynaptic nerve terminal [1], it is effective in pathologies that present with atypical improper muscle contractions. The release of acetylcholine at cholinergic nerve endings is blocked after the neurotoxin is injected into muscle to progress to a temporary denervation and atrophy. Its therapeutic effectiveness was first demonstrated for the management of strabismus and now encompasses treatment of multiple muscular abnormalities. Botox has been effective in treating pathologies of the head and neck and gastrointestinal, urogenital, musculoskeletal, neurological, gynecologic, rheumatologic, and cosmetic disorders (Table 1). Treatment of spasticity with botulinum toxin in children with cerebral

Table 1 Indications for botulinum A toxin injection for children with cerebral palsy (CP).

Localization	Unilateral CP	Bilateral ambulant CP	Bilateral non-ambulant CP
Upper limb	Improved function and aesthetics/appearance	N/A	Pain management Easier caring and positioning Functional and/or cosmetic improvement of hand position
Lower limb	Improved gait	Improved gait	Pain management Easier caring and positioning Improvement of weight bearing Prevention of hip dislocation
Spine	N/A	N/A	Postural management Care Pain management

CP, cerebral palsy; N/A, not applicable.

From: Best Clinical Practice in Botulinum Toxin Treatment for Children with Cerebral Palsy. *Toxins*. May 2015 [3]

Table 2 Comparison of botulinum neurotoxin preparations

	Botox Onabotulinumtoxin A	Dysport Abobotulinumtoxin A	Xeomin Incobotulinumtoxin A
Dosing		1:2 or 1:25 dosing ratio Botox to Dysport (ratio may be up to 1:4 or 1:5 in some studies)	1:1 dosing ratio between Botox and Xeomin
Dilution	2.5-4 U/0.1 mL	10–30 U/0.1 mL	2.5–4 U/0.1 mL
FDA approval granted	2002	2009	2010
Other characteristics		Larger area of action with greater diffusion of spread	Refrigeration not required
Bacterial source	*Clostridium botulinum*	*Clostridium botulinum*	*Clostridium botulinum*

palsy was first described in 1993 to successfully treat upper and lower hypertonia in children [2]. Goals of treatment are increasing range of motion, prevention of contractures, and improved ambulation [3].

Dysport® is an injectable form of a botulinum neurotoxin type A. Dysport is more diluted and spreads quickly compared to Botox (Table 2). Dysport has been demonstrated to be well-tolerated by patient with CP, with a favorable benefit-risk ratio in the treatment of lower limb spasticity. Phenol is a chemical injection that works similarly to botulinum toxin. Botulinum toxin injections are often more effective in smaller muscles, and phenol might be more effective in larger muscles. Phenol is a safe and cost-effective method to reduce spasticity and to improve functions in patients with CP. However, the effect with phenol was short lived when compared to BTX-A injection, and phenol was painful after injection, which may lead to poor follow-up [4]. Xeomin (incobotulinumtoxin A) is a newer injectable neurotoxin FDA approved to treat patients aged 2 years and older who have upper limb spasticity, not including spasticity caused by cerebral palsy.

Injections of BoNT-A are generally safe for the child with cerebral palsy. However, serious adverse events such dysphagia, excessive hypotonia, dyspnea, and aspiration pneumonia have been described in non-ambulant children [5]. A study conducted to assess the risk of adverse drug reactions (ADRs) with botulinum neurotoxin type A (BoNT-A) in children with cerebral palsy (CP) using the World Health Organization global individual case safety report (ICSR) database, VigiBase, showed a higher risk of ADRs with BoNT-A in children than in adults. The most frequent ADR was dysphagia followed by muscular weakness and was lethal in 12% of the cases [6]. The study concluded that in children with CP, the most adverse reactions occurred from a systemic spread of BoNT-A.

4 Management

Pseudocholinesterase (PChE) is a plasma protein enzyme synthesized by the liver that has an enzymatic activity of ester hydrolysis, which is important in the metabolism of several commonly used medications including succinylcholine and mivacurium, as well as aminoester local anesthetics, including cocaine and procaine. **Mivacurium is no longer available in the United States**. Pseudocholinesterase deficiency also known as butyryl cholinesterase deficiency is rare and can be acquired and/or be inherited. Patients may therefore present as heterozygotes with only one gene coding for the abnormal enzyme or as a homozygote with both genes coding for the defective pseudocholinesterase enzyme. Heterozygotes will present a less than 2-h increase in the duration of the neuromuscular blockade after standard succinylcholine dosing. Homozygotes, however, can present with neuromuscular blockade for a clinically significant greater duration (2–3 and up to 8 h). The incidence of patients that present as homozygotes for abnormal pseudocholinesterase enzyme is approximately 1 per 2000–5000 people. The incidence of heterozygotes for the abnormal enzyme is approximately 1 per 500.

Acquired pseudocholinesterase deficiency can also occur in several disease states or with the use of certain drugs. Malnutrition, pregnancy, and the postpartum period, burns, liver disease, kidney disease, hemodialysis, MI, CHF, malignancy, chronic infections, and drugs such as steroids and cytotoxic agents can decrease the production of the pseudocholinesterase enzyme [7].

Laboratory analysis for pseudocholinesterase deficiency can be performed by taking a sample of the patient's plasma and performing a qualitative test of pseudocholinesterase enzyme activity. Dibucaine is an amino amide local anesthetic that will inhibit the activity of the normal variant of the pseudocholinesterase enzyme by 80%. The dibucaine number is the percent of pseudocholinesterase (PChE) enzyme activity that is inhibited by dibucaine. Heterozygotes will have PChE enzyme activity inhibited by approximately 40–60%. Homozygotes will have their enzyme activity inhibited by approximately 20% [8, 9].

Together, the dibucaine number and the PChE enzyme activity results can help to identify individuals at risk for prolonged paralysis following the administration of succinylcholine (Table 3).

Individuals diagnosed with pseudocholinesterase deficiency should inform their doctor and anesthesia provider of their condition before any surgery. The patient's medical record should be updated to reflect the diagnosis of pseudocholinesterase deficiency. Future anesthetics should avoid administration of succinylcholine and

Table 3 Pseudocholinesterase activity and dibucaine number

Pseudocholinesterase deficiency			
	Succinylcholine response	Dibucaine number	Incidence
Homozygous	Normal	70–80	
Heterozygous	Lengthened 50–100%	50–60	1 in 480
Homozygous	Lengthened 4–8 h	20–30	1 in 3200

mivacurium to avoid prolonged neuromuscular blockade and possibly respiratory failure. Family members of patients with pseudocholinesterase deficiency are encouraged to undergo laboratory testing due to a strong genetic component associated with inheriting an abnormal variant of the pseudocholinesterase gene. Patients diagnosed with pseudocholinesterase deficiency should wear a medical alert bracelet or necklace and carry a wallet card. This will allow the healthcare professionals to become aware of the risk if patient needs an emergency surgery.

An ideal anesthetic in a child with cerebral palsy and pseudocholinesterase deficiency will address her situational anxiety without compromising safety. Frequent episodes of care such as medical procedures and hospitalization can be emotionally traumatizing for pediatric patients. The provider should provide age-appropriate and developmentally appropriate information to the patient to combat heightened anxiety levels. No oral premedication should be administered to this patient at high risk for aspiration. Parental presence, music, child life specialists, and virtual reality technologies can help the child cope better with induction.

Consider using an S-Caine patch to start and an intravenous line (iv) while the patient is awake rather than induction with a mask, as in a patient with a full stomach. Inhalation induction in the lateral position with the placement of an iv and LMA while maintaining spontaneous ventilation can also be successful. It is important to be cautious during the removal of the LMA to avoid hiccups and vomiting. Maintain the lateral position en route to the PACU, and if laryngospasm occurs, use propofol. During handoff, specify the need for the lateral position with a pillow at the back of the patient to maintain that position.

5 Summary

The anesthesiologist will often encounter patients with cerebral palsy for various surgical procedures, including Botox injection. Children with CP may be at increased risk for aspiration during general anesthesia by mask if they have developed dysphagia complications from Botox injections. An appropriate anesthetic plan and sedation-analgesic strategy are critical for safe management. Though a rare condition, pseudocholinesterase deficiency may lead to prolonged paralysis and fatal complications. Supportive care should be provided when the diagnosis is suspected, and a PChE level and dibucaine number should be obtained. Good communication with the patient and family is essential, including offering genetic testing to the patient and to all the members of the family.

References

1. Multani I, Manji J, Hastings-Ison T, Khot A, Graham K. Botulinum toxin in the management of children with cerebral palsy. Paediatr Drugs. 2019;21(4):261–81. https://doi.org/10.1007/s40272-019-00344-8. PMID: 31257556; PMCID: PMC6682585
2. Bjornson K, Hays R, Graubert C, Price R, Won F, McLaughlin JF, Cohen M. Botulinum toxin for spasticity in children with cerebral palsy: a comprehensive evaluation. Pediatrics. 2007;120(1):49–58. https://doi.org/10.1542/peds.2007-0016. PMID: 17606561; PMCID: PMC1920182
3. Strobl W, Theologis T, Brunner R, Kocer S, Viehweger E, Pascual-Pascual I, Placzek R. Best clinical practice in botulinum toxin treatment for children with cerebral palsy. Toxins. 2015;7:1629–48. https://doi.org/10.3390/toxins7051629.
4. Gonnade N, Lokhande V, Ajij M, Gaur A, Shukla K. Phenol versus botulinum toxin a injection in ambulatory cerebral palsy spastic diplegia: a comparative study. J Pediatr Neurosci. 2017;12(4):338–43. https://doi.org/10.4103/jpn.JPN_123_17. PMID: 29675072; PMCID: PMC5890553
5. Naidu K, Smith K, Sheedy M, Adair B, Yu X, Graham HK. Systemic adverse events following botulinum toxin a therapy in children with cerebral palsy. Dev Med Child Neurol. 2010;52(2):139–44. https://doi.org/10.1111/j.1469-8749.2009.03583.x. PMID: 20412252
6. Montastruc J, Marque P, Moulis F, Bourg V, Lambert V, Durrieu G, Montastruc JL, Montastruc F. Adverse drug reactions of botulinum neurotoxin type A in children with cerebral palsy: a pharmaco-epidemiological study in VigiBase. Dev Med Child Neurol. 2017;59(3):329–34. https://doi.org/10.1111/dmcn.13286. Epub 2016 Sep 28. PMID: 27682175
7. Trujillo R, West WP. Pseudocholinesterase deficiency. 2022 Jul 12. In: StatPearls [Internet]. Treasure Island, FL: StatPearls Publishing; 2022. PMID: 31082076
8. Cornelius BW, Jacobs TM. Pseudocholinesterase deficiency considerations: a case study. Anesth Prog. 2020;67(3):177–84. https://doi.org/10.2344/anpr-67-03-16. PMID: 32992329; PMCID: PMC7530809
9. Zhang C, Cao H, Wan ZG, Wang J. Prolonged neuromuscular block associated with cholinesterase deficiency. Medicine (Baltimore). 2018;97(52):e13714.

Seizures in a Child After Caudal Block for Circumcision

Andrew T. Waberski

Objectives

1. Describe the clinical presentation of seizures in the perioperative setting.
2. Understand immediate management of seizure activity in the post-anesthesia care unit (PACU).
3. Evaluate the pathophysiologic causes of seizures in the PACU.
4. Describe the management strategy of patients with local anesthetic systemic toxicity (LAST).

1 Case History

A 10-month-old 9 kg boy presents to the PACU after a circumcision revision. Prior to handoff, standard monitors are placed and 2 L/min blow by mask oxygenation is instituted. His initial vital signs include heart rate of 110 bpm, blood pressure of 89/40 mmHg, SpO_2 of 99%, respiratory rate of 23 bpm, and axillary temperature of 36.1C. A 24 gauge antecubital IV catheter is infusing lactated Ringer's solution.

The handoff report describes an uncomplicated general anesthetic with straightforward single-shot caudal analgesia. Easy mask induction with sevoflurane, a 24 gauge IV was placed in the foot, and 11 mL of 2% ropivacaine was administered via a caudal block injection. Anesthesia was maintained with a laryngeal mask airway and sevoflurane. The patient's medical history is significant for a low-birthweight and benign hemangioma requiring propranolol. The patient was extubated awake in the operating room and was comfortable to move to the bed with no issues during transport. The anesthesiologist remarks that the patient seems more lethargic and sleepier after emergence and extubation than he had anticipated. Following handoff, you are alerted to a new progressively noisy breathing pattern. While repositioning

A. T. Waberski (✉)
George Washington University School of Medicine, Washington, DC, USA
e-mail: awabersk@childrensnational.org

S. T. Verghese (ed.), *Anesthesia STAT! Acute Pediatric Emergencies in PACU*,
https://doi.org/10.1007/978-3-031-24396-7_20

the airway, you notice the patient's head is difficult to manipulate due to a sustained head tilt, and the patient's saturation has dropped to 90%. On further examination of breathing patterns, you witness repetitive bilateral upper limb jerking movements and diffused leg spasms.

2 What Are Typical Symptoms and Signs of Seizures?

Classic signs of seizures are changes in level of consciousness and uncontrolled jerking or spastic movements. Notably, there are many pediatric myoclonic and nonepileptic events that have similar signs to seizures. These seizure-like events occur in the absence of an aura or postictal state and have specific clinical clues for differentiation by age and provoking features [1]. As the pattern of seizure is specific to its cerebral origin and global effect, the clinical signs of a seizure may have variable expression between patients and may be numerous per patient. The seizure is characterized by its origin, quality, and progression. Seizures can begin as focal cortical amplifications or generalized involving the whole cortex. The seizure itself can produce varying degrees of rhythmic movements, sustained stiffness, or loss of tone or awareness. Additional descriptors detail the seizure progression, to involve other areas of the cortex, and whether the patient's level of consciousness is impaired. The presentation of a seizure influences the diagnostic modalities including EEG, CT scan, or MRI [2].

The level of consciousness following anesthesia or sedation may mask clinical and subclinical seizure activity. Physical examination and assessment of vital signs are immediate diagnostic tools that will alert providers to patterns of movement consistent with seizures. Patients emerging from anesthesia and sedation may present with somnolence, disorientation, confusion, and uncontrolled movements of various presentations. This is especially true during stage 2 of an anesthetic wakeup; patient's present with disconjugate gaze, altered mental status, erratic and obstructive breathing patterns, and uninhibited movements.

3 What Initial Steps Should You Perform to Manage Patients Experiencing Convulsive Movements?

Initial steps to manage convulsive movements and seizures include standard anesthetic practice measures to ensure safety and stability. Strong convulsive movements can have unforeseen and unanticipated harmful effects to a patient. Protect the head and limbs from noxious injury against the stretcher and stretcher rails. Prevent the patient from accidentally dislodging medical devices including monitors, IVs, and oral airways.

Acute changes in neurologic function necessitate immediate vital sign assessment and stabilization. This can be achieved with continuous monitoring of oxygen saturation and respiratory rate in addition to visual inspection and auscultation of respiratory dynamics.

For airway management, provide manipulation that maintains airway patency and ensures adequacy of ventilation and oxygenation. Relief of upper airway obstruction can best be performed by head tilt, chin lift, and, if necessary, an oral airway to relieve tongue obstruction. Consider supplementing oxygenation with nasal cannula, non-rebreathers, or supportive mask ventilation. In cases of severe airway obstruction and hypoxia that are not relieved by basic airway maneuvers, measures to place advanced airway techniques (endotracheal tube placement) should be taken.

Blood pressure and heart rate management include standard PACU practices. For unstable blood pressures in the setting of rhythm disturbances, CPR protocols should be followed. Management may include chest compressions, cardioversion, defibrillation, fluid resuscitation, and inotrope administration in serial fashion until return of spontaneous circulation. In the setting of stable blood pressures, any arrythmias management should be continued with cardiology consultation.

The patient's airway is repositioned to a head tilt position and obstructed patterns of breathing are stabilized. Supplemental oxygen is provided with 6 L/min of mask blow-by. Following repositioning of the airway and supplemental oxygen administration, the patient's oxygen saturation rises to 98% with a respiratory rate of 20. Blood pressure is 95/45 mmHg and temperature is measured at 36.2 °C. The patient continues to have repetitive jerking and spastic limb movements and remains unresponsive for this period now of 2 min.

Assessment of the patient vital signs shows no fever, normal blood pressure and perfusion state, and normal oxygenation. Delineation based on operative case and perioperative state can delineate reasons for seizure occurrence.

4 What Significant Patient Medical History Findings Predispose the Patient to Unprovoked Seizures?

New onset clinical seizures can be either provoked or unprovoked. Unprovoked seizures are typically exacerbations of chronic epileptic disease. While the etiology of seizures is difficult to discern in the acute setting, patients with a history of epilepsy may present with postoperative seizures. Seizures in patients with epilepsy may be attributed to perioperative risk factors.

History of epilepsy predisposes patients to postoperative seizures. Epilepsy treatment with antiseizure medications should be routinely continued through the perioperative state, unless indicated by the surgical procedure. In the preoperative period, a thorough review of antiepileptic prescription medication, recent doses, and upcoming scheduled doses can ensure that the patient's predisposing seizure history is optimized. Review of patient specific seizure characteristics with the patient and family can help clinicians discern seizure activity based on medical history. Adherence to scheduled antiepileptic medications throughout the perioperative period will also decrease the risk of seizure activity. Missed doses within the preoperative period predispose patients with epilepsy to unprovoked postoperative seizures.

5 What Intraoperative Events Predispose Pediatric Patients to Seizures in the Postoperative Period?

Hypoxia predisposes patients to depressed neurologic function and can illicit electrical disturbances in the form of dizziness, altered mentation, seizures, or coma. The pathologic state in which the supply of oxygen is diminished beyond the demand of the brain places risk of prolonged injury to cerebral cells. Patients with prolonged hypoxia due to intraoperative cardiopulmonary failure may present with clinical or subclinical seizures. The occurrence of seizure activity is most appreciated within a week of the neurologic insult. Additionally, hypotension and low perfusion states also can cause severe depression of neurologic function and predispose the patient to seizures [3]. As the anesthetic was uncomplicated and there were no reports of hypoxia or hypotension, it is unlikely that this provoked seizures. Furthermore, it is imperative to continue to support cerebral function by maximizing supply and minimizing metabolic demand during a seizure. As such the goals of care are to support the cardiopulmonary system and suppressing seizure activity.

In pediatrics, fevers can provoke seizures, most commonly between the ages of 6 months and 5 years old. These febrile seizures typically present with recurrence and are strongly associated with a rise in temperature and diagnosed when other mechanisms of seizures have been ruled out. In this scenario this is unlikely because the patient is afebrile and has no medical history of triggered seizures with fevers [1].

6 What Laboratory Measurements Will Help Determine the Cause of Seizures?

Electrolyte abnormalities may present initially as seizures. Most commonly sodium, calcium, and magnesium disturbances across the neuronal membranes can cause overactivation and suppression of electrical activity. Seizures present more readily in patients with severe hyponatremia, hypocalcemia, and hypomagnesemia. Clinical causes of these electrolyte disturbances include cardiac, endocrine, and renal disorders in addition to medication side effects. This patient received balanced electrolytes in lactated Ringer's solution and presented with no medical history that would elevate suspicion for electrolyte abnormalities [4].

Hypoglycemia is a major predisposing factor to acute neurologic changes. The degree of hypoglycemia can vary in symptom presentation from dizziness and light headedness to seizures and coma [5].

7 What Predisposing Perioperative Factors Could Lead to Hypoglycemia in the Postoperative Period?

Preoperative fasting guidelines for pediatric patients limit the oral intake to minimize the chance of severe respiratory complications from aspiration. Prolonged fasting times have often been debated and revolve around patient comfort, aspiration risk, and risk of severe sequelae following aspiration. Current NPO guidelines for pediatric anesthesia recommend stopping all food at 8 h, formula at 6 h, milk at 4 h, and clear liquids at 2 h prior to the procedure. These guidelines have been debated for decades with concern for the low risk of severe pulmonary complications, discomfort for patients, and maintaining oral scheduled medications [6]. Furthermore, fasting can be lengthened unintentionally as scheduled case may be delayed throughout the course of the operating room day. Prolonged fasting times place patients at risk for undiagnosed intraoperative hypoglycemia. An earlier report in an infant who had seizures perioperatively due to unplanned prolonged fasting of 13 h showed a blood sugar value of 25 mg/dL and was successfully treated with 20 mL of intravenous dextrose 25% [7].

Hypoglycemia can also be caused by preoperative medications administered for disease states. Insulin is a commonly administered medication in the perioperative setting. Any patient taking insulin or diabetic medication should have glucose levels strictly monitored to prevent and treat severe fluctuations. Beta-blocking agents may interfere with glucose transport, but this is seen most commonly in patients requiring insulin treatment. Propranolol has been found to cause hypoglycemia in infants, but most commonly at higher doses. This population is predisposed to hypoglycemia from low glycogen stores [8].

A blood sample is taken for rapid point-of-care testing, electrolytes are within normal range, and the glucose level is normal, at 89 mg/dL.

8 What Intraoperative Medications Predispose Patients to Seizures in the Postoperative Period?

Several anesthetic medications predispose patients to seizures. For patient with a history of unprovoked seizures, anesthetics may induce seizures by lowering the threshold. Drugs including local anesthetics, ketamine, etomidate, methohexital, sevoflurane, isoflurane, enflurane, and opioids have all been implicated in provoking seizures. However, EEG evidence of seizure activity in nonepileptic patients is indeterminate for patients receiving opioids, ketamine, and propofol [9]. Much of the reported seizure activity with induction of anesthesia can be attributed to myoclonic movements, and clinical diagnosis of seizures without EEG testing is not specific.

Local anesthetic systemic toxicity (LAST) exists with absorption in highly vascular areas or inadvertent intravenous injection during regional anesthesia technique. Technique for local anesthetic administration should include intermittent negative blood aspiration and visualization with ultrasound of local anesthetic spread to minimize change of direct intravenous injection. Local anesthetic toxicity can present with neurologic dizziness, confusion, changes in level of consciousness, convulsions, or seizures. Local anesthetics both activate NMDA receptors and GABA receptors resulting in an array of dose-dependent severity of clinical presentation. High dose toxicity can present as with cardiac arrythmias, hyper and hypotension, or cardiac arrest [10]. Maximal dosing for toxicity should be calculated and checked prior to administration; patients most at risk for toxicity are newborns and infants, as well as patients with hepatic and renal impairment. Absorption rates should be considered when placing local anesthetics with caution at highly vascular regions. In decreasing absorption order, those are the intercostal, caudal, brachial plexus, femoral, and subcutaneous areas. Maximal dosing for toxicity should be calculated for direct intravenous local anesthetics for analgesia from intravenous anesthetics. Additionally, the cumulative effect of multiple local anesthetics in different regions can also be toxic. Infants are predisposed to toxicity, likely from low plasma protein levels resulting in an increased free fraction of long-acting local anesthetics [11]. As most pediatric regional anesthetic techniques are performed under general anesthesia, the clinical signs of local anesthetic toxicity may be rare.

Review of medications at bedside reveals that the patient received 11 mL of 2% ropivacaine for caudal anesthesia, sevoflurane, and 100 mL of intravenous lactated Ringer's fluid. Localanesthetic systemic toxicity (LAST) is suspected, and the lipid emulsion is emergently requisitioned. The patient is monitored for signs of cardiopulmonary instability.

9 What Risks Are Associated with Developing LAST?

The risk of LAST is dependent on the LA injected, technique used to produce the block, and patient predispositions. Highly lipohilic local anesthetics increase the susceptibility to toxicity, and this is true for bupivacaine. However, newer local anesthetics, ropivacaine and levobupivacaine, were developed to produce the same analgesic potency with fewer cardiotoxic effects, attributed to a lower degree of lipophilicity. Although studies have shown that the clinical safety profile of ropivacaine is superior to levobupivacaine, but it still has potential to produce systemic toxicity at high doses. At present, ropivacaine has the greatest margin of safety of all long-acting local anesthetics [12]. It is imperative for patient safety that anesthesiologists and recovery room nurses understand the pharmacokinetic mechanisms with which local anesthetics produce local anesthetic systemic toxicity.

The vascular supply to the site and the total amount of local anesthetic (LA) determine the peak plasma concentration and systemic absorption and potential for toxicity. It is the free unbound LA presented to an organ that determines the clinical and toxic effects. Organs with higher percentage of perfusion, namely, the brain, heart, and liver, receive a higher proportion of unbound LA relative to poorly perfused organs. The poorly protein bound amino ester (procaine and chloroprocaine) have higher peak plasma concentrations as compared to aminoamide LAs (lidocaine, bupivacaine, ropivacaine) which are highly protein bound to alpha-L-acid glycoprotein. With regard to metabolism, the amino ester LAs undergo rapid hydrolysis by plasma cholinesterase, while amino amide LAs undergo a lengthier enzymatic metabolism by the hepatic cytochrome P450 enzymes increasing the exposure and potential for toxicity.

10 What Cerebral Nervous and Cardiovascular Signs Are Characteristic in LAST?

All local anesthetics can produce LAST. The ideal dose of LA that should be utilized is the lowest dose that achieves the desired degree of analgesia. In adult studies 40% of LAST cases had an atypical presentation [13]. Seizures are the most common severe CNS presentation of LAST (68–77%) [14, 15]. Awake adult patients have described perioral numbness, agitation, confusion, audio, and visual disturbances. As the quantity of LA in plasma increases, the cortical inhibitory pathways are regulated by blocked sodium channels which compromise regulatory inhibitory depolarization. Clinically, this can manifest in an awake patient as sensory and visual changes, muscle contractions, and seizures. Further rise in LA in plasma disrupts the excitatory neuronal pathways resulting in loss of consciousness, coma, and respiratory arrest. Adult studies have shown that one third of the reported cases of LAST began with neurological signs followed by manifestations of cardiac abnormalities like rhythm disturbances and one fifth presented with cardiac arrhythmias [15].

LA blockage of sodium channels impairs normal cardiac conduction by affecting the bundle of His producing rhythm disturbances. Decrease in the propagation of action potential from LA induces ECG changes that include prolongation of PR, QRS, and ST intervals and result in tachyarrhythmias and bradyarrhythmias. QT interval prolongation by potassium channel blockade can exacerbate the rhythm disturbances. In addition, the blockade of sodium, calcium, and potassium exchange transporters reduces intracellular calcium for adequate cardiac contractility [15].

11 What Are the Phases of LAST?

Patients who develop LAST present with a biphasic clinical picture, initial neurologic excitement followed by inhibition. Cardiovascular effects can begin with dysrhythmias, myocardial depression, decreased contractility, and systemic vascular resistance [15]. The ratio of local anesthetic dose required to cause cardiovascular collapse (CC) to the drug dose required to cause seizures (CN) is known as the CC/CN ratio, and a low CC/CCN ratio translates to a more potent cardiotoxic drug, and those with a higher CC/CN ratio, namely, ropivacaine and levobupivacaine, have a greater safety margin. Local anesthetics also have intrinsic vasoactive properties that may prolong their duration and slow systemic absorption [16]. A review of published reports of LAST over 30 years concluded that only 60% of cases followed the classic clinical pattern of progressive worsening of neurologic symptoms of seizures and coma followed by hemodynamic instability and cardiovascular collapse. Forty percent of the cases exhibited only cardiovascular collapse without evidence of CNS symptoms [17].

12 How Do You Reduce the Risk of LAST?

Preventing LAST can best be done by maintaining periprocedural safety routines when using local anesthetics. Several systems and individual best practice techniques in regional and local anesthetic can ensure patient safety. These best practices start with calculation and checking the total local anesthetic dose and total drug daily dose based on kilogram weight of the patient. Additionally, administering a regional and neuraxial anesthetic block comes with avoidance of vascular puncture by way of ultrasound avoided vascular injury and frequent aspiration during placement of local anesthetic. Epinephrine doses have been used to prolong the duration of the block and indicate early vascular puncture; doses range from 1:200,000 to 1:400,000. Characteristic t-wave morphologies present early in vascular injection and resolve quickly but can help alert the practitioner to LAST.

Ultrasound-guided neuraxial and regional anesthesia are gaining popularity because of the ease of obtaining adequate visual field, avoiding vascular and neuronal injury, and high success rates with local anesthetic placement. In infants and small children, the visualization of the caudal space, ability to measure the distance of the epidural space from the skin in the viewed image, and seeing the widening or distension of the epidural space caused by the drug injected are helpful predictors of successful caudal puncture and administration of the local anesthetic drug [18].

Repeated exposure to local anesthetics during the procedure can further exacerbate the toxic dose. Avoidance of redosing neuraxial and regional anesthetics for prolongation of blockade reduces the risk of toxicity. Repeated failed attempts at neuraxial techniques increase the risk of complications including nerve injury, hematoma, and vascular injection. In circumstances when the caudal block is difficult or requires repeated attempts, an effort should be made to abandon the block for alternative analgesic modalities, including the dorsal penile nerve block.

13 What Is the Treatment for Patients with Suspected LAST?

In suspected local anesthetic toxicity, total dose and amount of different local anesthetics should be confirmed. Local anesthetic boluses and infusions should be discontinued immediately. Treatment begins based on symptomatology. Mild symptoms of dizziness, light headedness, twitching, and tinnitus can resolve without intervention. These symptoms must be watched closely for progression of toxicity in the post-anesthesia care unit. Treatment of severe local anesthesia toxicity follows the Pediatric Advanced Life Support (PALS) standards for cardiopulmonary resuscitation. This includes respiratory support, control of arrythmias, volume resuscitation, medication administration, and chest compressions when indicated. In the case of ventricular arrythmias, amiodarone is recommended over lidocaine. Additionally, vasopressin, calcium channel blockers, and beta blockers should be avoided during resuscitation.

Severe central nervous system local anesthetic toxicity presents as tonic-clinic seizures, unresponsiveness, and coma. Treatment of seizures revolves around suppression of excitatory neuronal pathways with benzodiazepines and intravenous anesthetics. Midazolam and lorazepam can be used to treat the active seizure in local anesthetic toxicity [10].

14 What Is Lipid Emulsion Therapy for the Treatment of LAST?

Treatment of severe local anesthetics toxicity includes lipid emulsion therapy. The proposed mechanism is inactivation by lipid sink and lipid shuttle of local anesthetics. The lipid sink mechanism of action is reabsorption of lipophilic form of local anesthetic from vascular-rich organs into the plasma followed by lipid shuttle and redistribution of local anesthetics to the muscles and liver. Additional protective mechanisms of lipid emulsion therapy are proposed to include improved systemic vascular resistance, enhanced contractility, and increased preload by volume expansion. It is also postulated that lipid emulsion therapy mitigates ischemia-induced cardiovascular biochemical and cellular changes.

Lipid emulsion formulations are offered as 20% lipid emulsions with mixed long-chain and medium-chain fatty acids. Propofol is a 10% lipid emulsion and is not a suitable substitute for lipid emulsion therapy; in addition, the cardiovascular depressant effects of propofol should warrant exclusion from its administration in the setting of LAST [19].

The initial intravenous lipid emulsion (ILE) therapy is 1.5 mL of 20% lipid solution administered over 2 min for patients less than 70 kgs. This is then followed by a continuous infusion of 0.25 mL/kg/min. Repeated boluses and continuation of infusion may be necessary if continuous cardiopulmonary resuscitation efforts were required [10, 11]. The recommend maximum dose is 12 mL/kg.

Although rare, side effects of ILE include allergic reaction (severe egg allergy), hyperlipidemia, and hypercoagulability. These side effects should not withstand early and definitive treatment for the patient with local anesthetic toxicity but should be recognized and not withstanding of appropriate treatment of LAST. Toxicity of ILE presents with hypertriglyceridemia, liver dysfunction, acute pancreatitis, and acute kidney injury and is more common in high-dose lipid emulsion therapy or impaired lipid metabolism and storage.

In the treatment of cardiovascular collapse from LAST, *local anesthetics for ventricular arrythmias are strictly prohibited. Amiodarone is the preferred antiarrhythmic medication. In addition, low doses of epinephrine are preferred as higher doses impair lipid therapy. Epinephrine doses exceeding 10mcg/kg have detrimental effects to increasing lactate and worsen metabolic acidosis. Vasopressin, calcium channel blockers, and betablockers should also be avoided.*

Intravenous lipid emulsions have been used to treat other life-threatening lipophilic drug toxicities in children with beneficial outcomes. These drugs include amitriptyline, diltiazem, bupropion, dosulepin, lamotrigine, quetiapine, and verapamil [20, 21]. A recent practical guide for the management of systemic toxicity by local anesthetics published by the Japanese society of anesthesiologist is a helpful tool to follow for all anesthesiologists who perform nerve blocks [22].

Following the administration of 2 mg of midazolam and 1.5 mL of 20% lipid solution administered over 2 min, the patient's convulsive activity is suppressed. The patient's vital signs are within normal limits and the patient is waking up but drowsy and uncomfortable. The patient is admitted to ICU for monitoring overnight and continued neurologic evaluation.

15 Summary

Local anesthetic systemic toxicity is a potentially lethal condition. The prevention, clinical presentation, and management of LAST should be appreciated by the clinician and recovery team. Ultrasound-guided regional and neuraxial technique, correct drug calculations, and avoidance of vascular injection are best ways to mitigate LAST. Additionally, recovery room personnel and providing clinicians should have a sound understanding of the local anesthetic drug characteristics, markers of toxicity, and therapies for LAST. Timely administration of ILE for immediate treatment of LAST improves morbidity and mortality. ILE therapy requires dose calculation and administration by trained professionals. Resuscitation from LAST with advanced life support skills should include maintaining adequacy of ventilation and oxygenation, maintaining cardiovascular stability, correction of abnormal laboratory values, and treatment of seizures. LAST requires post-resuscitation continuous monitoring in an intensive care setting and stabilization. With the advent of ILE therapy, successful resuscitation from LAST has become possible. Maintaining a high level of clinical suspicion and ability to treat LAST promptly can be lifesaving.

References

1. Fine A, Wirrell EC. Seizures in children. Pediatr Rev. 2020;41(7):321–47. https://doi.org/10.1542/pir.2019-0134.
2. Fisher RS, et al. Operational classification of seizure types by the International League Against Epilepsy: Position Paper of the ILAE Commission for Classification and Terminology. Epilepsia. 2017;58(4):522–30.
3. Zhou KQ, McDouall A, Drury PP, Lear CA, Cho KHT, Bennet L, Gunn AJ, Davidson JO. Treating seizures after hypoxic-ischemic encephalopathy-current controversies and future directions. Int J Mol Sci. 2021;22(13):7121. https://doi.org/10.3390/ijms22137121. PMID: 34281174; PMCID: PMC8268683
4. Nardone R, Brigo F, Trinka E. Acute symptomatic seizures caused by electrolyte disturbances. J Clin Neurol. 2016;12(1):21–33. https://doi.org/10.3988/jcn.2016.12.1.21. PMID: 26754778; PMCID: PMC4712283
5. Imad H, Zelano J, Kumlien E. Hypoglycemia, and risk of seizures: a retrospective cross-sectional study. Seizure. 2015;25:147–9. https://doi.org/10.1016/j.seizure.2014.10.005. Epub 2014 Oct 17. Erratum in: Seizure. 2017; 45:132. Johan, Zelano [corrected to Zelano, Johan]; Eva, Kumlien [corrected to Kumlien, Eva]. PMID: 25455725
6. Fawcett WJ, Thomas M. Pre-operative fasting in adults and children: clinical practice and guidelines. Anaesthesia. 2019;74(1):83–8. https://doi.org/10.1111/anae.14500. Epub 2018 Nov 30. PMID: 30500064

7. Maze A, Samuels SI. Hypoglycemia-induced seizures in an infant during anesthesia. Anesthesiology. 1980;52:77. https://doi.org/10.1097/00000542-198001000-00017.
8. Holland KE, Frieden IJ, Frommelt PC, Mancini AJ, Wyatt D, Drolet BA. Hypoglycemia in children taking propranolol for the treatment of infantile hemangioma. Arch Dermatol. 2010;146(7):775–8. https://doi.org/10.1001/archdermatol.2010.158.
9. Voss LJ, Sleigh JW, Barnard JP, Kirsch HE. The howling cortex: seizures and general anesthetic drugs. Anesth Analg. 2008;107(5):1689–703. https://doi.org/10.1213/ane.0b013e3181852595. PMID: 18931234
10. Dontukurthy S, Tobias JD. Update on local anesthetic toxicity, prevention and treatment during regional anesthesia in infants and children. J Pediatr Pharmacol Ther. 2021;26(5):445–54. https://doi.org/10.5863/1551-6776-26.5.445. Epub 2021 Jun 28. PMID: 34239395; PMCID: PMC8244955
11. Lönnqvist PA. Toxicity of local anesthetic drugs: a pediatric perspective. Paediatr Anaesth. 2012;22(1):39–43. https://doi.org/10.1111/j.1460-9592.2011.03631.x. Epub 2011 Jun 14. PMID: 21672079
12. Zink W, Graf BM. The toxicity of local anesthetics: the place of ropivacaine and levobupivacaine. Curr Opin Anaesthesiol. 2008;21(5):645–50. https://doi.org/10.1097/ACO.0b013e32830c214c. PMID: 18784493
13. Neal JM, Bernards CM, Butterworth JF 4th, Di Gregorio G, Drasner K, Hejtmanek MR, Mulroy MF, Rosenquist RW, Weinberg GL. ASRA practice advisory on local anesthetic systemic toxicity. Reg Anesth Pain Med. 2010;35(2):152–61. https://doi.org/10.1097/AAP.0b013e3181d22fcd. PMID: 20216033
14. El-Boghdadly K, Chin KJ. Local anesthetic systemic toxicity: continuing professional development. Can J Anaesth. 2016;63(3):330–49. https://doi.org/10.1007/s12630-015-0564-z. Epub 2016 Jan 29. PMID: 26830640
15. Gitman M, Barrington MJ. Local anesthetic systemic toxicity: a review of recent case reports and registries. Reg Anesth Pain Med. 2018;43(2):124–30. https://doi.org/10.1097/AAP.0000000000000721. PMID: 29303925
16. El-Boghdadly K, Pawa A, Chin KJ. Local anesthetic systemic toxicity: current perspectives. Local Reg Anesth. 2018;11:35–44. https://doi.org/10.2147/LRA.S154512. PMID: 30122981; PMCID: PMC6087022
17. Di Gregorio G, Neal JM, Rosenquist RW, Weinberg GL. Clinical presentation of local anesthetic systemic toxicity: a review of published cases, 1979 to 2009. Reg Anesth Pain Med. 2010;35(2):181–7. https://doi.org/10.1097/aap.0b013e3181d2310b. PMID: 20301824
18. Kil HK. Caudal and epidural blocks in infants and small children: historical perspective and ultrasound-guided approaches. Korean J Anesthesiol. 2018;71(6):430–9. https://doi.org/10.4097/kja.d.18.00109. Epub 2018 Aug 8. PMID: 30086609; PMCID: PMC6283718
19. Ok SH, Hong JM, Lee SH, Sohn JT. Lipid emulsion for treating local anesthetic systemic toxicity. Int J Med Sci. 2018;15(7):713–22. https://doi.org/10.7150/ijms.22643. PMID: 29910676; PMCID: PMC6001420
20. Presley JD, Chyka PA. Intravenous lipid emulsion to reverse acute drug toxicity in pediatric patients. Ann Pharmacother. 2013;47(5):735–43. https://doi.org/10.1345/aph.1R666. Epub 2013 Apr 23. PMID: 23613099
21. Havan M, Kendirli T, Özcan S, Doğan MT, Yiğit AO, Uçar T. A successful treatment with intravenous lipid emulsion therapy in a child with verapamil poisoning. Turk J Emerg Med. 2021;21(4):217–20. https://doi.org/10.4103/2452-2473.329626. PMID: 34849436; PMCID: PMC8593422
22. Safety Committee of Japanese Society of Anesthesiologists. Practical guide for the management of systemic toxicity caused by local anesthetics. J Anesth. 2019;33(1):1–8. https://doi.org/10.1007/s00540-018-2542-4. Epub 2018 Nov 11. PMID: 30417244

Hyperthermia in a Child After Dental Rehabilitation: Is This M.H

Domiciano Jerry Santos

A 5-year-old Hispanic, 15-kilogram (kg) female came to the ambulatory center with the history of acute situational anxiety for dental rehabilitation surgery. Parents speak only Spanish and through a video Spanish interpreter her medical history was gathered. Her past medical history included reactive airway disease, frequent upper respiratory infections (URIs), and many ear infections from age 2. Her surgical history includes two sets of bilateral myringotomy tubes placed at age 2 and 4, when she also underwent adenoidectomy. Four weeks ago, she had a runny nose (rhinorrhea) which resolved but she did not have fever nor an associated cough. The patient's younger brother is currently sick at home with a cough and fever. From the parents' report, she has had no issues with anesthesia or surgery in the past. Both parents reported that there was no anesthesia-related death in their respective families. Dad did volunteer that his uncle who had emergent surgery did not make it out of the operating room due to complications during surgery. However, he did not have any details regarding that death. The patient has no known drug allergies (NKDA). She does not currently take daily medications. Her only preoperative test was a COVID-19 negative PCR.

She was appropriately nervous, but the amount of midazolam to reduce anxiety that was given PO was much less than the dose intended for her, because she threw up the oral premed a few minutes after the administration. She had a difficult inhalation induction with a combination of nitrous oxide at 70% and 6% sevoflurane. After placing an intravenous (IV) catheter, oxymetazoline spray was sprayed intranasally into both nostrils for vasoconstriction. The anesthetic was deepened with a bolus of propofol. The nasal intubation was traumatic with the blood pooling in the back of the oral pharynx. A cuffed endotracheal nasal (RAE) tube was placed via the right nostril with confirmed auscultation of bilateral breath sounds and the cuff

D. J. Santos (✉)
Children's National Medical Center, Washington, DC, USA
e-mail: dsantos@childrensnational.org

S. T. Verghese (ed.), *Anesthesia STAT! Acute Pediatric Emergencies in PACU*,
https://doi.org/10.1007/978-3-031-24396-7_21

inflated immediately. Unfortunately, crackles were heard in the right lung field. A suction catheter was inserted, and scant amount of blood and pink-colored oral pre-med was removed. After some positive pressure breaths, the nasal RAE tube was suctioned again with the removal of a small amount blood. The crackles resolved and a quick lavage of the lungs with normal saline was done. The lavage fluid was suctioned out and appeared clear without any blood. Though the lungs were clear on auscultation, the compliance of the lungs was reduced. Discussion about cancelling the procedure between the dentist and the anesthesiologist ended when the dentist pointed out that the parents were not compliant about the child's dental care. And it was with much difficulty that the parents had finally agreed to come for this scheduled surgery. The case finally started based on the need for treating the child's dental caries without postponement.

Since the beginning of the anesthetic, she had been tachycardic and hypotensive. Since she had been NPO for a long time, this was treated with a fluid bolus of lactated Ringer's solution. After 150 cc of lactated Ringer's solution, the hypotension resolved but her heart rate remained high, ranging 115–120 beats per minute. The anesthetic maintenance plan was for one minimum alveolar concentration (MAC) of sevoflurane and less than 1 mcg/kg of fentanyl because of the planned dental extractions. Ondansetron was given prophylactically to prevent postoperative nausea and vomiting (PONV). Local injection of lidocaine with epinephrine was given prior to extractions, and she responded with tachycardia and hypertension. Since she had mild oozing from the extracted teeth, the postop order to give intravenous ketorolac was discontinued.

The dental procedure was completed eventually. There were some episodes of sudden tachycardia and desaturation which resolved with manual ventilation. Prior to extubation, auscultation revealed mild wheezing bilaterally. She was then given multiple doses of albuterol within the breathing circuit. The wheezing improved. The plan was for an awake extubation. Upon emergence, the patient coughed repeatedly, and the endotracheal tube had white secretions which became more apparent when she coughed. Suctioning the nasal RAE tube produced thick white secretions. After these coughing spells, the patient would remain apneic. After four episodes of coughing followed by apnea, the patient finally opened her eyes and attempted to self-extubate and remove the nasal RAE tube. The nasal RAE tube was eventually removed by the provider and patient was turned on her side to lie in the lateral (recovery) position.

Unfortunately, the patient began coughing again and it was clear that she was not exchanging air effectively. She was quickly returned to the supine position. A jaw thrust was attempted with positive pressure ventilation (PPV). But her chest rise was minimal, and no end-tidal CO_2 was recorded. PPV was attempted until the saturation began to decrease below 94% and then IV propofol was administered to break the laryngospasm. However, during the movement from recovery position to supine, the IV had become dislodged. Immediately, 3 mg/kg of succinylcholine (45 mg) was given intramuscularly into the left deltoid muscle. The laryngospasm was relieved eventually, and her oxygen saturation improved with PPV. A second IV was successfully replaced. After several minutes, the patient returned to breathing spontaneously with an occasional cough; she was placed again in the recovery position to allow for drainage of secretions. When vital signs were stable and she was breathing well without coughing or pauses, the patient was transported to the post-anesthesia recovery room under some blankets.

During the hand-off to the recovery room nurse, the heart rate was 122 bpm, and the blood pressure was 110/89 and the temperature was 37.9 °C. The anesthesia team attributed the elevated temperature to the warm blankets and that it was perhaps this higher temperature which caused the increased heart rate and BP. Instructions were given to allow her to emerge lying on her side and to monitor her vitals closely.

The anesthesia team was called back to bedside of the patient after 15 min because she now had a heart rate of 130 bpm and blood pressure was still elevated at 120/92, and her temperature was 40.1 °C. She still coughed on occasion with some crackles in the right lower lobe. She had no blankets on her and a cool compress was placed on her forehead by the PACU nurse. She was drowsy but not fully awake.

The nurse asks the question for clarification, if IM atropine was also given along with succinylcholine IM injection and it was affirmed that only succinylcholine was given and that the effect of tachycardia was perhaps due to the warm blankets.

1 What Is the Differential Diagnosis and Workup for Fever for this Postoperative Patient?

Postoperative fever is not uncommon following surgery. The most obvious cause in the postoperative period is an infectious process from a surgical site infection, respiratory pathology, or urinary tract infection. Another very common reason for gradual rise of temperature during full dental rehabilitation surgery in children could be covering the patient with impermeable drapes and warm blankets. Effective means of cooling efforts to decrease the rise in temperature and to preserve normothermia include ambient forced-air cooling using tent-like draping [1]. Other causes of fever can be related to the inflammatory process of surgery, the physiologic stress of surgery, phlebitis, postoperative anemia, drug reaction, or very rarely malignant hyperthermia [2]. The onset and rate of rise of the fever can provide a wealth of information about the cause of the fever.

Fevers within the first few hours of surgery are more commonly secondary to inflammatory changes. The amount of damage to tissue during surgery is directly correlated to the amount of circulating inflammatory markers like Interleukin-6 (IL-6). The higher amount of inflammatory makers has direct effect on the severity of the fever in the first few hours after surgery [3]. Fortunately for patients, fevers related to inflammatory charges are usually short lived with minimal sequalae. For patients with fever who are hemodynamically stable, the cause is most likely due to inflammatory changes. Treatment is usually temperature control with antipyretics. Other more insidious causes of immediate postoperative fever are malignant hyperthermia, pulmonary embolism, necrotizing soft tissue infections, and adrenal insufficiency. These are fortunately rare in occurrence.

Malignant hyperthermia is a lethal medical condition associated with exposure to inhalational anesthetic agents and succinylcholine (a depolarizing muscle relaxant). After exposure to one of these triggering agents, a hypermetabolic response is triggered. This leads to fever, increase in heart rate, increase in end-expired carbon dioxide (CO_2) despite increases in minute ventilation, and muscle rigidity. The fever can rise dramatically 1–2 °C every 3–5 min. Treatment requires prompt diagnosis and treatment with dantrolene [4].

Pulmonary embolism can lead to immediate postoperative fever. This is usually low-grade fever. The cause of the embolism could be septic thrombophlebitis. Patients with pulmonary embolism typically complain of shortness of breath and chest pain. They are tachypneic, tachycardiac, hypotensive, and hypoxic and have low-expired CO_2. Diagnosis is usually based on computed tomography (CT), and treatment is mainly supportive (vasopressors and ventilatory support) and anticoagulation [5].

Necrotizing soft tissue infections usually present with very high immediate postoperative fever and pathognomonic physical findings such as "dishwater drainage," edema, induration, and extreme pain. Prompt surgical treatment is needed with drainage, antibiotics, and supportive therapies.

Lastly, adrenal insufficiency can present as an immediate postoperative fever. The associated signs and symptoms are not specific. A careful review of the patient's medical is warranted. Adrenal insufficiency can be primary leading to direct damage to the adrenal gland. It can also be secondary adrenal insufficiency, which is more common from hypothalamic pituitary disease-causing hypopituitarism. Secondary adrenal insufficiency can be caused by exogenous or endogenous steroids causing suppression. Treatment is supportive therapy along with steroids and treatment of any electrolyte disturbances [3].

Timing of the onset of the fever is key. Other more common causes of fever are wound infection, atelectasis, pneumonia, urinary infection, phlebitis in the immediately postoperative period, and occasionally sepsis if the wound was already infected prior to surgery. These causes are most likely seen after the first postoperative day and not in the recovery unit. To determine the cause of immediate hyperthermia in PACU, anesthesiologists need a focused diagnostic workup, including labs and radiologic studies.

For our patient, her fever occurred immediately after surgery. This does narrow the differential diagnosis. More focused investigation is warranted to decide the next course of action.

2 Could This Immediate Postoperative Fever Be Due to Inflammatory Changes?

The cause of her fever could be from inflammatory changes. Dental surgery can cause some trauma to the gums; however, the trauma in dental surgery is minor typically and does not cause as much tissue damage like an open bowel surgery. A high fever might be more expected in an open bowel surgery because of the amount of tissue damage and higher inflammatory response. Tissue damage is minimal to the gums during dental surgery, and a large inflammatory response would not be likely seen. If she was hemodynamically stable and this was just inflammatory response, the expectation would be a low-grade fever which would be self-limiting. If the fever continued, a short course of antipyretics could be helpful to decrease the fever. Our patient's fever was high in PACU and continued to rise which is not very typical for fever related to inflammatory changes. A clinical study to detect the risk of bacteremia from nasotracheal intubation in children undergoing dental treatment under general anesthesia reported the most common bacteria in positive cultures to be *Streptococcus* viridans [6]. Another study compared the use of antibiotics and placebo in children (mean age: 3.5) undergoing dental extractions under general anesthesia and reported the incidence of bacteremia to be significantly high in the placebo group. Bacteremia occurred from a variety of bacterial species mainly Gram-positive cocci and for a longer duration after dental extractions. Amoxicillin was shown to have a significant impact on the incidence, nature, and duration of bacteremia after nasal intubation; dental restorative, and cleaning procedures; and dental extractions [7].

3 Could This Fever Be Related to Malignant Hyperthermia?

Malignant hyperthermia (MH) is an autosomal dominant disorder of skeletal muscles with incomplete penetrance and variable expression. The disorder is dependent on exposure to a triggering agent. Halogenated anesthetics and succinylcholine, a depolarizing muscle relaxant, are the known triggering agents for MH. The usual clinical presentation is tachycardia, increased CO_2 production, hyperthermia, and rigidity.

Tachycardia can be due to many other factors in the postoperative setting. Tachycardia is a nonspecific sign and can be related to pain from surgery, secondary to hypotension/hypovolemia, fever from infection, medications, emergence from anesthesia, or anxiety.

The increased CO_2 production is because of the hypermetabolic process that occurs in MH. MH causes a dysregulation of the calcium channel in the skeletal muscles leading to contraction and rigidity. Eventually, this leads to depletion of ATP stores and metabolic acidosis. Under general anesthesia this is typically discovered by rising end-tidal CO_2 concentration despite adequate or increasing minute ventilation. In the postoperative period, patients may have a rise in minute ventilation to compensate for the metabolic acidosis which may not be noticeable.

Hyperthermia can be the first or one of the last signs of MH. In a study by Larch et al., 63.5% of presentations of MH had hyperthermia as one of the first three signs of the disorder [8]. Like tachycardia, it can be attributed to many other factors. During a MH crisis, the increase in temperature can be quite dramatic, typically increasing 1–2 °C every 3–5 min [4]. Severe hyperthermia above 41 °C can lead to multiorgan system failure, DIC, and death.

Other clinical signs include muscle rigidity, contractures, myoglobinuria from myocyte death, and rhabdomyolysis. Muscle rigidity is a very specific sign of MH, presenting in 50–80% of patients [9]. Late clinical signs include hypoxia, altered mental status, pulmonary edema, cardiac arrythmias, electrolyte abnormalities like hyperkalemia, heart failure, and disseminated intravascular disseminated (DIC) [9].

For our patient, she presented with the nonspecific signs of tachycardia and fever. She was exposed to two triggering agents during the case, an inhalational anesthetic (sevoflurane) and IM succinylcholine (a depolarizing neuromuscular blockade). In the recovery room, since she was not intubated, it would be hard to accurately quantify her CO_2 production. However, we can use her respiratory effort as a reflection of her minute ventilation and use a nasal cannula with a CO_2 side port to assess her breath-by-breath CO_2 on the monitor. If her respiratory rate was elevated, it could be evidence that she is compensating for the increased CO_2 production. The dramatic rise in temperature over a short period of time is key in deciding if this is a MH crisis. Because MH has high morbidity and mortality if untreated, diagnosis and treatment should be promptly initiated for MH patient.

4 Did This Child Have Risk Factors for Malignant Hyperthermia?

The incidence of MH is reported between 1:10,000 and 1:250,000 in all ethnic groups. It is seen in males more often and young people with the median age of 18.3. MH can present after the first exposure to a triggering agent but on average usually presents during the third exposure to a triggering agent [4].

5 Pathophysiology of MH

Malignant hyperthermia shows an autosomal dominant pattern with incomplete penetrance and variable expression. The prevalence of a genetic mutation which makes someone susceptible to MH is 1:2000 to 1:3000 [10]. The most common and studied mutation is on chromosome 19 which is also the genetic coding site for the ryanodine receptor type 1 (RYR1). A defect in the excitation-contraction coupling of calcium in the sarcolemma in the muscle causes uncontrolled rise in myoplasmic calcium when a patient with this mutation is exposed to triggering agents. This abnormal increase triggers numerous biochemical activities including hyperkalemia and rhabdomyolysis from increased permeability of the muscle sarcoplasmic reticulum from low levels of ATP. This dysregulation of calcium channel in the skeletal muscle fibers results in persistent muscle contraction and rigidity [4].

For our patient, her family history was unfortunately vague and incomplete. There was a reported death on the paternal side of the family related to emergency surgery, but it was unclear if this was related to MH. It was not feasible for the team to attempt to get the previous anesthetic/surgical records of a distant relative. Our patient had two prior anesthetic exposure and is likely to have had exposure to one of the triggering agents in the past. Since she has many factors which put her at risk for MH, we believed that MH is the most probable cause of her fever.

6 How Does MH Cause Fever and Lead to Death?

Malignant hyperthermia is mediated by a dysregulation of the release of the calcium in the skeletal muscle typically on the RYR1 gene causing uncontrolled contraction and rigidity (see Fig. 1).

The uncontrolled muscle contraction leads to increased usage of oxygen and increased CO_2 production, heat production, muscle contractures due to increased glycolysis, uncoupling of oxidative phosphorylation, and activation of actin-myosin filaments [4].

The clinical picture usually presents as persistent tachycardia, rising end-tidal CO_2 production despite appropriate minute ventilation, hypertension, hypoxemia, combined metabolic and respiratory acidosis, hyperthermia, and muscle rigidity. If untreated, as the skeletal muscle continues to contract, both metabolic and respiratory acidosis progress with depletion of ATP stores leading to rhabdomyolysis. This leads to myocyte death resulting in hyperkalemia and myoglobin in the urine. The electrolyte disturbance of significant hyperkalemia (more than 6 mEQ) can lead to cardiac arrythmias. The rise in CPK levels in patients with MH will peak in 12–24 h after the MH episode to more than 20,000 I.U. Plasma and urine myoglobin can increase, and if not aggressively treated, myoglobinuria can lead to acute renal failure. The elevated temperature can lastly lead to disseminated intravascular coagulation (DIC) and death. Prompt treatment is needed to prevent this MH cascade. For our patient, since MH is high on our differential diagnosis list, treatment was initiated to prevent morbidity or mortality.

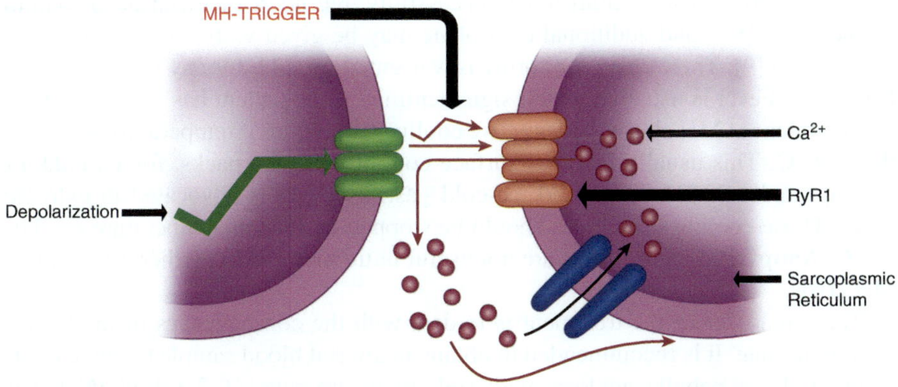

Fig. 1 MH trigger leads to dysregulation of RYR1 receptor leading to calcium release causing muscle contraction. Photo courtesy of Maya Santos

7 How Do You Treat MH?

Treatment of MH in the operating room begins with discontinuation of triggering agents. If a patient is still undergoing general anesthesia with inhalational anesthetic agents, this should be changed to a total intravenous anesthetic technique (TIVA) and strict avoidance of succinylcholine. Insertion of activated charcoal filters on both the expiratory and inspiratory limbs of the anesthesia circuit will help prevent further exposure. Under general anesthesia, the treatment also includes ventilation with 100% oxygen at high flows to flush the anesthesia circuit and hyperventilation to compensate for rising CO_2 from the hypermetabolic state.

Dantrolene (Ryanodex, Dantrium) is the primary treatment for treating MH. The dose is 2.5 mg/kg given every 5 min and repeated if signs and symptoms of MH are persisting. It may be given by continuous infusion 0.25 mg/kg/h until the patient is hemodynamically stable and the hypermetabolic state subsides. This usually presents as decreasing heart rate, decreasing temperature, and decrease in CO_2 production. There is no upper limit of dantrolene dose; however, if greater than 10 mg/kg is administered, an alternate diagnosis should be considered [4]. Dantrolene is a muscle relaxant which antagonizes the ryanodine receptor and slows the release of calcium in skeletal muscle. Dantrolene currently comes in two formulations. The older preparation is a 20 mg vial which dissolves in 60 cc of sterile water (slowly and poorly) and therefore very difficult to reconstitute in an emergency. The new preparation is in a concentrated form of 250 mg/5 cc of sterile water and therefore is easy to reconstitute. The newer formulation allows for ease of use and utilizes 1 vial only necessary for an average-sized adult. The potential side effects of dantrolene include weakness, dizziness, rash, phlebitis, and fatigue. If the patient is not intubated, care should be taken to watch for respiratory compromise and the need for respiratory support. The typical weakness seen with dantrolene is seen in the extremities. Dantrolene has reduced the mortality of MH from the high 70% in the 1970s to less than 5% in 2008 [11].

After dantrolene is administered successfully, recrudescence can occur within the next 24–48 h, and additional dantrolene may be given with a dose of 1 mg/kg every 4–6 h [9]. Therefore, monitoring is warranted for 24 h for any patient with an MH crisis. Fever is usually the first sign identified if the patient has recrudescence.

Treatment of MH also includes active cooling techniques if temperature is greater than 39 °C. This usually involves surface cooling with ice packs, forced cold air cooling, and cold IV fluids, and ice-cold gastric lavage is advocated in extreme cases. These cooling techniques should be stopped as soon as temperature reaches 38 °C. Antipyretic medications are not useful in treating the hyperthermia during a MH crisis.

The remainder of the treatment is to deal with the consequences of the hypermetabolic state. It is recommended to obtain an arterial blood sample to guide treatment of the metabolic acidosis with sodium bicarbonate (1–2 mEq/kg/dose) if acidosis is profound. The most common electrolyte abnormality is hyperkalemia. Hyperkalemia is usually treated with calcium (calcium chloride 10 mg/kg or calcium gluconate 10–50 mg/kg), sodium bicarbonate (1–2 meq/kg/dose), and glucose/insulin. And in severe cases of hyperkalemia, alternative treatment options include albuterol, dialysis, and ECMO. Ventricular arrythmias including ventricular bigeminy, V tachycardia, and fibrillation are also common. This may require treatment with antiarrhythmics like intravenous lidocaine infusion or amiodarone. In addition, MH can cause acute renal failure because of the myoglobin in the urine. Maintaining adequate urine output with fluids, mannitol (0.25 g/kg IV), and furosemide (1 mg/kg) and continuous monitoring in ICU are recommended.

For our patient, her clinical presentation in the PACU was highly suspicious of MH. Since MH has a high mortality and morbidity, prompt treatment is necessary. Since she was extubated, her treatment should include respiratory support with 100% nonrebreather mask, prompt treatment with dantrolene 2.5 mg/kg, and active cooling techniques. Careful observation of her respiratory status is warranted because of the respiratory acidosis and the effects of dantrolene as a muscle relaxant. If it becomes necessary, respiratory support with a breathing tube and ventilation may be needed. It would be necessary to start an additional peripheral IV for medication, A-line placement to monitor her degree of acidosis, and frequent laboratory testing which should include electrolytes like potassium, creatine kinase, and coagulation studies. She would need to be monitored in the intensive care unit for the next 24–48 to first stabilize her but also to watch for recrudescence. She may need additional dosages of dantrolene if the fever recurs. It is helpful to contact the Malignant Hyperthermia Association of the United States (MHAUS) during the treatment of a MH crisis especially if this occurs after hours in an emergency case to obtain support from MH expert on this disease [12].

8 Is There a Definitive Test to Confirm Diagnosis for MH?

The clinical presentation and supporting laboratory tests form the basis for diagnosis of a MH event. Researchers from the MHAUS (Malignant Hyperthermia Association of the United States) did develop a clinical grading scale to help in research and evaluate those patients who need more specific and sensitive diagnostic tests. The scale requires the provider to score the degree of five parameters: rigidity, muscle breakdown, respiratory acidosis, temperature, and cardiac involvement [13].

Since there is no "gold" standard test for MH, the best test for MH is in vitro contracture test (IVCT). This involves exposure of muscle tissue usually taken from the vastus muscle of the thigh under local anesthesia and propofol infusion to halothane and/or caffeine in vitro. In susceptible patients it produces an exaggerated muscle contracture. It is expensive and requires a surgical procedure under anesthesia (TIVA) and/or regional nerve block to obtain the tissue. This is done only in a few centers around the world. This test is the most sensitive and often done when the child is older than 5 years old [10]. A negative result rules out diagnosis of MH. But the test does have a high false-positive rate of 20%. This test cannot be done immediately after a MH crisis.

Genetic testing can also be used to look for mutation on specific chromosomes which are known to be related to MH. Genetic testing has less than 50% sensitivity.

There are three outcomes of genetic testing. The first is if a known mutation is identified, then the patient would be identified as MH susceptible. The second outcome could be that a DNA variation is identified with unknown significance. In those instances, patients would also need to be identified as MH susceptible. Lastly, the genetic results could have no known DNA mutations, but this does not rule out MH because only a small percentage of mutations are known. Genetic testing just like in vitro contracture test is quite expensive and completed in only specialized centers around the world [10].

For any patients who have had a MH crisis, any future surgeries/anesthetics should be performed with nontriggering agents with strict avoidance of inhalational anesthetic agents and succinylcholine. Barbiturate, opioids, propofol, benzodiazepines, nitrous oxide, anticholinergics, anticholinesterases, local anesthetics, and sympathomimetics may be used in children with MH. Parents and the child should be educated on the different aspects of this rare complex medical condition known as MH.

For our patient, her parents should go through genetic testing to identify which side of the family might have mutation related to MH. It is possible for genetic testing to be negative or inconclusive; and if it is feasible, an in vitro contracture test should be performed next. Our patient should be identified as MH susceptible for any future surgeries or anesthetics. A medical alert bracelet can be helpful to wear in case of emergencies. Any future anesthetics for her should strictly avoid inhalational agents and succinylcholine.

9 If This Was Not MH, Could This Be Aspiration of Secretion/Blood During Intubation/Extubation?

The fever could be a result of aspiration event leading to pneumonia or pneumonitis causing the fever in the immediate postoperative period. General anesthesia can leave patients susceptible to aspiration if they vomit during induction of anesthesia. Our nil per os (NPO) "nothing by mouth" guidelines help in minimizing this risk. NPO adherence takes careful preoperative instruction and communication with families. Many families are often worried about not allowing children access to nutrition and water for long periods of time. In some families, food is used as a motivation for good behavior. But the NPO guidelines help to alleviate much of the risk of aspiration. Careful clear communication with families is vital.

Other issues with our patient are the blood encountered during nasal intubation. This patient likely had adenoid hypertrophy. Studies have shown the incidence of adenoid hypertrophy for children and adolescence to be about 34%. Some studies report incidences up to 70% [14]. Typically, many anesthesiologists try to decrease the bleeding during a nasal intubation with the use of vasoconstrictors. Oxymetazoline 0.05% is the most used vasoconstrictor. But other vasoconstrictors, like cocaine or epinephrine, have been also described to be effective in decreasing bleeding [15]. Other techniques to decrease nasal intubation bleeding are use of gels to lubricate the nasal RAE tube, warming the intubation tube in warm saline to soften the tube, dilating the nares with nasal trumpets, and using a red-rubber catheter as a guide on the end of the nasal RAE tube to spread the adenoids as the tube passes the adenoids [16]. All these can decrease the amount of bleeding from the adenoids during nasal intubation.

In our patient, blood might have entered the trachea during the nasal intubation attempt. It is prudent to attempt to suction secretions and particularly blood out of the tracheal tree. Clotted blood can lead to severe obstruction and respiratory compromise. Removal of the blood with a saline lavage will greatly reduce this risk.

Since she was coughing in the recovery room, the question of aspiration was part of our differential diagnosis. If MH was not high on the differential diagnosis, it may be warranted to do a laboratory investigation looking for a leukocytosis and a chest film to look for an infiltration. The steady dramatic rise of body temperature immediately after surgery is uncommon after an aspiration event.

10 Could This Be Starting a Viral Illness in the Family? Should the Case Have Been Started Given the Child Had a Resolved Upper Respiratory Illness (URI) and a Sick Contact at Home?

In our patient, the onset of an URI in a child with known reactive airway should not be undertaken without careful assessment of risks and benefits. Most elective cases such as dental rehabilitation should be postponed especially if an intubation is necessary to accomplish the surgery. Research has shown that URI was associated with a higher risk of perioperative respiratory adverse reactions if the URI was less than 2 weeks before the procedure and if URI symptoms were present at the time of procedure [17].

Another review of several studies with focus on the safety of anesthesia in children with URI undergoing general anesthesia provided a proposal for a decision algorithm. The summary of the review of these pediatric studies concluded with safety guidelines that general anesthesia should be postponed for at least 2 weeks in children with symptomatic infections with fever, wheezing, and purulent secretions. This review also recommended anesthetic options for children with upper respiratory infection with a runny nose and cough to include preoperative inhalational therapy with albuterol, use of a face mask or laryngeal mask, intravenous induction with propofol and avoidance of desflurane, and endotracheal intubation whenever possible [18].

One of the most debated and discussed topics in pediatric anesthesia is the dilemma of a child with upper respiratory illness which started the evening before or the morning of surgery or whether to proceed with anesthesia/surgery or to postpone until the patient is without symptoms. It has been written and debated in many journal articles with pros and cons. Considering many children have six to eight URI per year on average [19], finding a window to schedule surgery may deprive the child of necessary surgical intervention and care. URIs increase the possibility of a perioperative respiratory event; but anesthesiologists are in better position to mitigate some of some those risks and manage some of the complications without associated morbidity [18].

Upper respiratory tract infections are usually virally mediated with rhinovirus making up 30–40% of those illnesses [19]. URIs are usually self-limiting but must be distinguished from more serious infections like pneumonia, bronchiolitis, croup, or streptococcal throat. Hyperactivity of the airways with URI is very common and can persist up to 6 weeks after the infection. The hyperactivity can lead to laryngospasm and bronchospasm which can complicate the anesthetic management.

The preoperative assessment of patients with URI needs to focus on symptoms such as fever, shortness of breath, energy level/lethargy, appetite, color of secretion, cough, sputum production, and wheezing. These symptoms can provide insight on the degree of disease and if the child is more at risk of respiratory sequelae after anesthesia. Children with mild symptoms often do well with anesthesia and surgery.

The risks and benefits of anesthesia and surgery must be carefully weighed in patients with URI. On occasion cancelation of surgery can lead to worsening of the disease process if surgery is postponed for the typical 4 weeks or resolution of URI. If the case is urgent, the anesthetic plan must be tailored to attempt to decrease the respiratory complication associated with URI, like suctioning of airway, use of laryngeal mask airway (LMA) for instrumenting the airway if appropriate, use of anticholinergics, or humidification.

Our patient had URI symptoms 4 weeks before and was currently asymptomatic even though she was exposed to a sick sibling at home. She was symptom-free for surgery, and it was the ideal time to have her anesthetic and surgery.

11 Is MH the Diagnosis for Rising Temperature in PACU?

She had the typical clinical presentation of malignant hyperthermia of developing dramatic increase in temperature after reaching PACU with persistent tachycardia, hyperventilation, and rigidity suggestive of an ongoing hypermetabolic syndrome. Intravenous administration of succinylcholine can result in masseter muscle contraction which can cause difficulty in opening the jaws for reintubation—a problem that was not seen in her. There was a definite triggering agent administered intramuscularly because of the lack of a functioning intravenous line. This choice of this route for drug administration was necessary and clinically significant since the IM dose of succinylcholine (mg/kg) administered is always much higher than if it was administered intravenously to treat laryngospasm. Hyperthermia is considered as a dramatic but frequently a late sign of MH, but the steady rate of increase can be as rapid as 1–2 ° every 5 min. If there is a delay in treating this rising temperature, it can lead hypercarbia, increase in oxygen consumption DIC, and multiple organ failure. Vigilant monitoring of temperature and aggressive measures to cool the patient down must be instituted as the treatment with dantrolene and other treatment modalities to correct the combined respiratory and metabolic acidosis [4].

Although we didn't have a quantitative measure of her CO_2, in PACU on arrival, she was tachypneic and trying to compensate for her metabolic acidosis. She had a steady rise in temperature in a short period of time after arrival which made the anesthesiologist suspect that MH was the possible diagnosis for this hyperthermia. It was evident that she was developing uncontrolled muscle contractures and limb rigidity as the second intravenous line was placed.

From her preoperative history, she had been exposed to triggering agents in the past. Her family history regarding MH was vague despite the history of a relative dying during emergency surgery under anesthesia. She was treated immediately with dantrolene 2.5 mg/kg every 5 min until her tachycardia decreased; her hyperthymia ceased to rise; and her rigidity became less. This required two doses of dantrolene. On her blood gas, pH is 7.15, PCO_2 55, pO_2 70, Na 135, K 5.3, and BE −10. She had both a metabolic and respiratory acidosis which were treated with sodium bicarbonate. After the second IV was placed, an arterial line and foley catheter were placed. She was treated with active cooling techniques which included surface ice packs and forced cool air. She fortunately did not have hyperkalemia. Her urine was sent for analysis for myoglobin and color was noted to be the classical cola urine appearance pointing to myoglobinuria which was later confirmed by the lab to be positive and significantly high. She was admitted to the intensive care unit for monitoring for 24 h. Her CPK rise was also significant reaching as high as 36,000 I.U. almost 8 h after the episode. She didn't have recrudescence during her stay in the hospital. She was discharged after 2 days with normal blood gases, electrolytes, and coagulation values. Her vital signs stabilized within 12 h, and she was afebrile and well hydrated with adequate urine output.

Education was given to both parents about the episode of MH with the help of an interpreter. The plan was for her family to have genetic testing soon. Depending on family genetic testing, a muscle biopsy may be warranted for her parents. Our patient will always be identified as malignant hyperthermia susceptible for the rest of her life and will benefit from having a medical alert bracelet to identify her as MH susceptible. An anesthesia alert about her MH susceptibility should be entered into her electronic data systems so that she will never be exposed to triggering agents. If she undergoes an anesthetic for future surgery, TIVA with propofol and opioids may be a choice with regional blocks with local anesthetics and nontriggering agents like nondepolarizing muscle relaxants if necessary to supplement the anesthetic. Prophylactic pretreatment with dantrolene is still controversial although its availability must be confirmed before the surgery starts.

12 Summary

It is fortunately rare to encounter MH in our daily clinical practice. However, it is vital for the anesthesiologists and perioperative caregivers to be aware of the development of MH, and so temperature monitoring should be undertaken in cases lasting longer than 30 min. MH is a hypermetabolic syndrome that can rapidly result in fatality if there is delay in diagnosis and treatment. When a child with occult MH susceptibility is exposed to triggering agents and develops signs persistent tachycardia, hyperventilation, hyperthermia, and muscle rigidity, aggressive measures should be taken to continuously monitor, treat, and reevaluate the ongoing hypermetabolic state with team effort to continue the treatment ultimately in an intensive care setting. A dramatic increase in temperature in the PACU should be investigated thoroughly to rule out onset of MH even if there are other differential diagnoses that could possibly be the etiology of a postoperative fever as in the patient described. The four "red herrings" or "false clues" for the postoperative fever in this patient are worth noting: a dental procedure where (1) the whole body is covered for the entire duration of surgery, (2) dental procedures with extraction of infected teeth after nasotracheal intubation causing bacteremia, (3) an ongoing viral infection, and (4) episode of aspiration of blood from the nose on anesthetic induction. Vigilance in monitoring and prompt treatment is vital in preventing morbidity and for improving safety in these children.

References

1. Lin WL, Li CH, Cherng CH. Body temperature management during pediatric full mouth rehabilitation surgery under general anesthesia. J Dent Sci. 2018;13(3):263–6. https://doi.org/10.1016/j.jds.2018.04.002. Epub 2018 Jun 7. PMID: 30895130; PMCID: PMC6388863
2. Ashley B, Spiegel DA, Cahill P, Talwar D, Baldwin KD. Post-operative fever in orthopaedic surgery: how effective is the 'fever workup?'. J Orthop Surg (Hong Kong). 2017;25(3):2309499017727953. https://doi.org/10.1177/2309499017727953.
3. Narayan M, Medinilla SP. Fever in the postoperative patient. Emerg Med Clin North Am. 2013;31(4):1045–58. https://doi.org/10.1016/j.emc.2013.07.011.
4. Rosenberg H, Pollock N, Schiemann A, Bulger T, Stowell K. Malignant hyperthermia: a review. Orphanet J Rare Dis. 2015;10:93. https://doi.org/10.1186/s13023-015-0310-1.
5. Desciak MC, Martin DE. Perioperative pulmonary embolism: diagnosis and anesthetic management. J Clin Anesth. 2011;23(2):153–65. https://doi.org/10.1016/j.jclinane.2010.06.011.
6. Onçağ O, Cökmez B, Aydemir S, Balcioğlu T. Investigation of bacteremia following nasotracheal intubation. Paediatr Anaesth. 2005;15(3):194–8. https://doi.org/10.1111/j.1460-9592.2005.01503.x.
7. Lockhart PB, Brennan MT, Kent ML, Norton HJ, Weinrib DA. Impact of amoxicillin prophylaxis on the incidence, nature, and duration of bacteremia in children after intubation and dental procedures. Circulation. 2004;109(23):2878–84. https://doi.org/10.1161/01.CIR.0000129303.90488.29. Epub 2004 Jun 1
8. Larach MG, Allen GC, Brandom BW, Lehman EB. Temperature changes are not late signs of malignant hyperthermia: a NAMH registry of MHAUS study. Anesthesiology. 2008;109:A374.
9. Kim K, Kriss RS, Tautz TJ. Malignant hyperthermia: a clinical review. Adv Anesth. 2019;37:35–51. https://doi.org/10.1016/j.aan.2019.08.003.
10. Ellinas H, Albrecht MA. Malignant hyperthermia update. Anesthesiol Clin. 2020;38(1):165–81. https://doi.org/10.1016/j.anclin.2019.10.010.
11. Larach MG, Brandom BW, Allen GC, Gronert GA, Lehman EB. Cardiac arrests and deaths associated with malignant hyperthermia in North America from 1987 to 2006: a report from the North American malignant hyperthermia registry of the malignant hyperthermia association of the United States. Anesthesiology. 2008;108(4):603–11. https://doi.org/10.1097/ALN.0b013e318167aee2.
12. Riazi S, Kraeva N, Hopkins PM. Updated guide for the management of malignant hyperthermia. Can J Anaesth. 2018;65(6):709–21.

13. Larach MG, Localio AR, Allen GC, Denborough MA, Ellis FR, Gronert GA, Kaplan RF, Muldoon SM, Nelson TE, Ording H. A clinical grading scale to predict malignant hyperthermia susceptibility. Anesthesiology. 1994;80(4):771–9. https://doi.org/10.1097/00000542-199404000-00008.
14. Pereira L, Monyror J, Almeida FT, Almeida FR, Guerra E, Flores-Mir C, Pachêco-Pereira C. Prevalence of adenoid hypertrophy: a systematic review and meta-analysis. Sleep Med Rev. 2018;38:101–12. https://doi.org/10.1016/j.smrv.2017.06.001. Epub 2017 Jun 14
15. Song J. A comparison of the effects of epinephrine and xylometazoline in decreasing nasal bleeding during nasotracheal intubation. J Dent Anesth Pain Med. 2017;17(4):281–7. https://doi.org/10.17245/jdapm.2017.17.4.281. Epub 2017 Dec 28. PMID: 29349350; PMCID: PMC5766085
16. Elwood T, Stillions DM, Woo DW, Bradford HM, Ramamoorthy C. Nasotracheal intubation: a randomized trial of two methods. Anesthesiology. 2002;96(1):51–3. https://doi.org/10.1097/00000542-200201000-00014.
17. Von Ungern-Sternberg BS, Boda K, Chambers NA, Rebmann C, Johnson C, Sly PD, Habre W. Risk assessment for respiratory complications in paediatric anaesthesia: a prospective cohort study. Lancet. 2010;376(9743):773–83. https://doi.org/10.1016/S0140-6736(10)61193-2.
18. Becke K. Anesthesia in children with a cold. Curr Opin Anaesthesiol. 2012;25(3):333–9. https://doi.org/10.1097/ACO.0b013e3283534e80.
19. Tait AR, Malviya S. Anesthesia for the child with an upper respiratory tract infection: still a dilemma? Anesth Analg. 2005;100(1):59–65. https://doi.org/10.1213/01.ANE.0000139653.53618.91.

Vomiting Blood After Routine T&A

Angela C. Lee

1 Stem Case

A 3-year-old, 10 kg, otherwise healthy, full-term boy underwent tonsillectomy and adenoidectomy for obstructive sleep apnea. A sleep study was not done. He snores every night, and his mother has noticed that he gasps and holds his breath. However, he starts breathing again on his own without his mother having to wake him up. He has a good appetite, but daycare staff have reported that he seems to be sleepier than other children. The child is scheduled to be observed overnight in the post-anesthesia care unit (PACU) as a 23-h stay due to his age, severity of symptoms, and parental preference.

Surgery was uneventful under general anesthesia, consisting of propofol, dexmedetomidine (1 mcg/kg), fentanyl (0.2 mcg/kg), acetaminophen (15 mg/kg), and sevoflurane (3%). He received dexamethasone and ondansetron, as well as 200 mL of Lactated Ringer's solution. You are called by the PACU nurse to assess this patient about 3 h after arrival. His nurse reports that he has vomited four times in the past hour, with vomitus becoming more bright red like fresh blood with each emesis. The child has consumed 4 ounces of apple juice and a popsicle. He is now awake and crying, with bright red blood visible on the lips and tongue. His parents are near him and appear anxious.

A. C. Lee (✉)
Division of Anesthesiology, Pain and Perioperative Medicine, Children's National Hospital, Washington, DC, USA
e-mail: alee@childrensnational.org

S. T. Verghese (ed.), *Anesthesia STAT! Acute Pediatric Emergencies in PACU*,
https://doi.org/10.1007/978-3-031-24396-7_22

1.1 How will you prepare this child for surgery? Do you keep the patient on his mothers lap?

As more medical providers approach this child's bedside to examine him, a 3-year-old child will inevitably become more anxious and frightened, leading to crying and increased bleeding. If the patient is kept on continuous monitoring with pulse oximetry and vital signs are stable, he should be allowed to remain on the parent's lap. However, the venous catheter should be checked for patency and further secured if needed. Furthermore, the parent and the PACU nurse should be instructed to stop feeding the child at this point. The anesthesiologist may help expedite the otolaryngologist's evaluation of the tonsillar pillar including a quick look with flashlight and inform the anesthesiologist-in-charge of a potential emergent return to the operating room (OR) to assure staffing and OR availability. A recent study at our tertiary care children's hospital found that in patients presenting with post-tonsillectomy hemorrhage (PTH), the longest mean time to OR occurred in the morning, 119.7 min (SD 101.5), versus all other periods of the day [1].

Tonsillectomy with or without adenoidectomy is one of the commonly performed surgeries in children. In the United States, it is estimated that over 500,000 cases took place in patients <15 years of age in 2006. Indications for tonsillectomy include recurrent throat infection and sleep disordered breathing [2]. Sleep disordered breathing is estimated to occur in 12% of children. Although in-laboratory polysomnography is the gold standard for the diagnosis of obstructive sleep apnea (OSA), this test is inconvenient and expensive. In fact, only about 10% of children undergo polysomnography prior to their adenotonsillectomy. Indications for polysomnography include complex medical conditions such as Down syndrome, craniofacial anomalies, sickle cell disease, obesity, etc. Tools such as questionnaires, clinical parameters (restless sleep, apneic pauses observed by caregivers, daytime sleepiness, and/or hyperactivity), and physical exam findings are more often used by otolaryngologists to determine the need for surgery [3]. Our patient's low-for-age weight (10 kg, <5th percentile for age), apneic pauses during sleep, and daytime somnolence indicate clinically significant sleep disordered breathing that has been affecting his growth and development. Anesthetic considerations for adenotonsillectomy with sleep disordered breathing as an indication include increased risk of ventilatory suppression from opioids. One study found almost double the level of respiratory suppression from opioids in these patients as compared to healthy controls. The American Society of Anesthesiologists has recommended reducing the amount of opioids by half in children and adults with OSA. This increased sensitivity to the respiratory depressive effects of opioids, as well as the increased attention brought to deaths in rapid metabolizers of codeine [3], has shifted the perioperative management of tonsillectomies toward reducing narcotics or avoiding them altogether in severe cases of OSA. Between 1969 and 2012, there were ten deaths and three overdoses in children treated with codeine reported to FDA's Adverse Event Reporting System. Eight of the 13 cases occurred in children after adenotonsillectomy. There is now a black box warning to the drug's label stating that codeine is contraindicated for treatment of pain in children after tonsillectomy or adenoidectomy.

Otolaryngologists have stopped prescribing codeine for postoperative pain after tonsillectomy. Anesthesiologists have been utilizing IV acetaminophen and dexmedetomidine to supplement inhalational agents as part of a balanced anesthetic technique. Other anesthetic considerations for tonsillectomy include its higher risk of postoperative nausea and vomiting compared to other pediatric surgeries, occurring in up to 70% of children [4].

Whether the procedure is performed on an outpatient or inpatient basis depends on patient age, comorbidities, and indication for the surgery. In 2019, the American Academy of Otolaryngology recommended inpatient admission and overnight observation after tonsillectomy for patients who are less than 3 years old or have severe OSA (apnea-hypopnea index ≥10 obstructive events/hr. and/or SaO_2 nadir <80%) [5]. Most patients generally tolerate tonsillectomy under general anesthesia without any complication, but occasionally patients present with PTH that requires surgical exploration and treatment. PTH that occurs in the first 24 h after surgery is considered primary and after 24 h, a secondary hemorrhage, with an estimated incidence of 0.6–0.7% for primary and 0.8–3.0% for secondary hemorrhage [1]. A fraction of these patients require revision surgery. An older study from the Hospital for Sick Children, Toronto, that examined 9409 healthy children ≤17 years old who were observed overnight after tonsillectomy, found the incidence of PTH to be 2.15% (202 patients), but those requiring a second anesthetic for hemostasis was only 0.06% (6 patients) [6]. Most PTH is secondary, after the fibrin clot has detached from the tonsillar fossae. Secondary PTH peaks between postoperative days 4 and 7 [7]. Factors that have been proposed to be associated with an increased risk of PTH have included surgeon inexperience, patient age, operating technique, and intraoperative blood loss [1, 8].

Our clinical scenario in the PACU is primary PTH and requires immediate attention. Although uncommon, PTH has potential to be life-threatening due to its brisk nature. Younger children less than 8 years of age have been shown to be more susceptible to severe PTH, that is, bleeding that leads to hemorrhagic shock, blood transfusion, ligature of the internal carotid artery, packing of the pharynx, tracheostomy, embolization, or resuscitation. With their lower total blood volume, PTH in younger children has the potential to become life-threatening earlier than the same amount of bleeding in an older child or adult [9]. With a blood volume of about 700 mL (70 mL/kg × 10 kg), 200 mL of blood loss, for instance, would be significant in a 10 kg toddler but not a 70 kg, 16-year-old.

At the end of tonsillectomy, the otolaryngologist typically passes an orogastric tube to evacuate any stomach contents, including residual swallowed blood. Blood vomited in PACU may be old blood from the surgery or may be active bleeding from the tonsillar pillars. Most of the blood from PTH is swallowed rather than spat out, and so an accurate estimate of blood loss is difficult. A patient who is vomiting blood after tonsillectomy requires immediate physical examination by the otolaryngologist. As the surgery team is being called to the bedside, the patient's disposition and fluid status should be assessed. Mental status appropriate for developmental age, vital sign trends, capillary refill time <2 s, and urine output, indicated by the number of wet diapers in this toddler, will assist in assessing his volume status. Hemodynamic compromise will occur when about 40% of the total blood volume has been lost. New, unexplained tachycardia and pallor may indicate that significant blood loss has already occurred before hypotension becomes apparent [4]. Prompt hydration with isotonic crystalloid solutions such as lactated Ringer's or normal saline is indicated to support hemodynamics. Complete blood count (CBC) and type and screen should be sent. A bedside point of care (POC) hemoglobin can provide rapid results to guide management while waiting for lab results. If bleeding is ongoing and profuse, particularly in the case of this young patient with a smaller total blood volume, crossmatch of red blood cell units as well as a coagulation profile should be considered early in the evaluation phase. For torrential PTH due to arterial bleeding, uncross matched emergency release red blood cells may be indicated. Rates of blood transfusion for PTH have been reported as low as 0% to as high as 0.7% for all age groups [10].

1.2 How will you manage loss of peripheral IV access?

The patient is being examined by an otolaryngology team, receiving 100 mL (10 mL/kg) of Lactated Ringer's bolus over 30 min while tubes for blood work are being prepared. At this point you notice that the peripheral intravenous (PIV) access has ceased to work, the child is crying, with bedside monitor alarms going off very loudly, and everyone around including the child's parents are appearing very distressed. You are called to bedside for an intravenous catheter placement. There are no obvious veins visible on this child's chubby extremities.

Reestablishment of intravenous access is of the highest priority. Children, particularly those under 3 years of age, have a thicker layer of subcutaneous fat and pose a challenge in peripheral IV cannulation [11]. In this child with difficult IV access and full stomach, sedation is not an option to facilitate IV access. Instead, speed is of the essence in this deteriorating clinical picture. Routine use of near infrared vein-viewing devices for peripheral IV access in children has not been shown to reduce time or number of attempts to successful cannulation [12]. However, such studies often do not account for inter-operator variability and individual facility with using the device and so should be considered if difficult intravenous access is anticipated depending on the operator's experience. Ultrasound guidance by the anesthesiologist most adept at using this to assist in PIV placement is an option as well, although studies on ultrasound-guided PIV placement on children with and without difficult PIV access have been mixed [13, 14]. If the patient must return to the operating room urgently and no IV access can be obtained, intraosseous access will be a faster and more feasible option than central venous access. Although most often used in the emergency room during resuscitation, intraosseous access devices are a part of the pediatric advanced life support algorithm and available in operating rooms for code situations. Maximum flow rates of up to 10 mL/min under gravity and > 20 mL/min under pressure from an infusion pump and 10 mL/min for blood transfusion have been reported via the intraosseous route [15].

The otolaryngology attending has diagnosed an area of brisk venous bleeding and posts the case as an emergency exploration to stop the tonsillar bleed. Peripheral IV access has been obtained in the saphenous vein after a single blind attempt. Point of care hemoglobin measures 10 g/dL on two readings. The child is still stable and alert on the mother's lap, with an emesis basin of bloody vomitus nearby. The patient has by now received 200 mL of Lactated Ringer's intraoperatively and 100 mL of Lactated Ringer's in the PACU, with 5% dextrose 0.45% sodium chloride solution also infusing at a maintenance rate of at 40 mL/h. Complete blood count and crossmatch are being sent. You return to the operating room to set up the anesthesia machine and necessary equipment for an urgent re-exploration for the bleeding site in OR.

2 What Are Some Special Considerations for Intraoperative Management?

Unless the PTH is a potentially catastrophic arterial bleed, induction of anesthesia should commence after fluid resuscitation to avoid hemodynamic instability at induction. Intravenous midazolam may be administered to achieve anxiolysis without sedation immediately before transporting the child to the operating room. Although inhalation induction of general anesthesia and intubation in the left lateral position for PTH have been described [16, 17], this technique has fallen in disuse and is not considered. Considerations at anesthesia induction for PTH include hemodynamic instability, hypoxemia, aspiration, and difficult intubation. A 2010 retrospective cohort study of PTH found that transient hypoxemia was the most common complication, with 9.9% of the 475 patients studied suffering hypoxemia although most occurred during emergence and extubation. In this same study, aspiration of blood into the glottis occurred in 0.8% of patients but was not associated with respiratory complications. At induction of anesthesia, bradycardia and hypotension were seen in 4.2% and 2.5% of patients, respectively [17].

Because of the potential for blood clots to obstruct the suction catheter, two suction systems should be set up. Anticipating and preparing for the presence of excessive blood in the posterior pharynx on laryngoscopy is essential to minimize time between anesthesia induction and intubation (see Fig. 1).

A secondary intubation technique should be readily available if intubation proves more difficult than the initial intubation for tonsillectomy. Cuffed endotracheal tubes of various sizes should also be prepared as interval airway swelling may necessitate a smaller endotracheal tube than was initially used for surgery.

The anesthesiologist should plan for rapid sequence intubation (RSI) with an induction agent (usually propofol) followed by succinylcholine, ideally after preoxygenation via face mask as the patient permits. Gentle bag mask ventilation with 1.0 FiO_2 at low pressures $\leq$12 cm H_2O without cricoid pressure after induction of

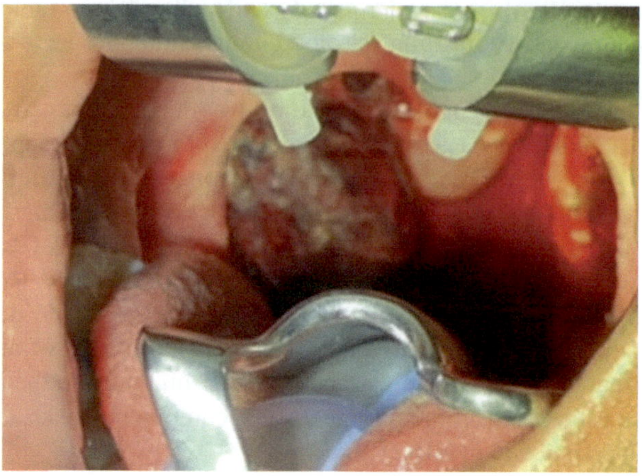

Fig. 1 Anatomic View. Copious blood in the pharynx due to PTH. Blood clot seen in patient's right tonsillar fossa (dark purplish-brown). Photograph printed with permission from Habib Zalzal, M.D.

general anesthesia, rather than the classical RSI technique with cricoid pressure and apnea modeled on adult anesthesia, may be considered in order to allow continued oxygenation, curb hypercarbia, and prevent atelectasis [18]. A 2019 retrospective audit of 110 surgical revisions in 103 children with PTH showed that compared to children who underwent classical RSI, patients who underwent modified RSI with gentle mask ventilation after anesthesia induction had less severe hypoxemia (defined as $SaO_2 < 80\%$), better view on laryngoscopy, and less hypertension at induction [19]. If the anesthesiologist does choose to use cricoid pressure at induction, gentle pressure of 10 Newtons (N) is recommended before general anesthesia is fully induced, increasing to 30 N after the patient loses consciousness. This is because a pressure of 20 N is painful in awake patients and can result in retching [20]. If the child is actively retching and vomiting, placing him in a slight left lateral position might help drain the blood to the dependent portion allowing the anesthesiologist to have a better visualization of the larynx during laryngoscopy after propofol and succinylcholine administration. In cases of active vomiting, cricoid pressure is contraindicated since it can result in esophageal rupture. Vomiting creates esophageal pressures in excess of 60 cm H_2O, and cricoid pressure would raise the intraesophageal pressure to dangerous levels in this situation [20].

More recently, apneic oxygenation administered via simple nasal cannula with low flow oxygen at a minimum of 0.2 L/kg/min up to 10 L/min [21] has been proposed as a change in routine practice at national meetings and in anesthesia literature to minimize desaturation during laryngoscopy in children. Due to their higher oxygen consumption and relative lower functional residual capacity, smaller children are uniquely more vulnerable to hypoxemia during laryngoscopy [22]. In our case, apneic oxygenation will provide a longer intubation window as conditions may be suboptimal due to airway swelling and secretions despite not being difficult to intubate previously. In this 10 kg patient, nasal cannula oxygen flow should be at least 2 L/min.

After induction and intubation with a cuffed 4.0 endotracheal tube and reduction of the inspired oxygen concentration to below 30% to minimize risk of airway fire, the operating room table is turned 90 °. The surgeon identifies one area of venous bleeding on the right tonsillar area and cauterizes it. The team waits an additional 10 min to look for signs of rebleeding and decides to pass an orogastric tube to evacuate swallowed blood. There are clots in the stomach, but most cannot be evacuated as the suction catheter keeps getting obstructed. Vital signs are stable.

3 What is the plan for emergence and recovery?

Barring major complications at induction such as aspiration, the vast majority of PTH patients are extubated at the end of the case. Patients should be extubated wide awake as they are still considered full-stomach candidates. Whether they can return to PACU for overnight observation or should go to the intensive care unit depends on the extent of blood loss and potential for hemodynamic instability. The presence of many clots suggests more swallowed blood than initially estimated. Obtaining a postoperative CBC and POC hemoglobin in the meantime is reasonable. Other diagnostic modalities to support the lab findings and supplement estimates of blood loss include POC gastric ultrasound as some studies have found good correlation between gastric antrum cross-sectional area and gastric volume, although these studies were done for gastric emptying time for food and drink rather than swallowed blood from bleeding in an emergency setting [23]. In any case, all PTH patients should be extubated awake.

4 Summary

Vomiting of blood in the PACU after tonsillectomy requires prompt assessment to evaluate for PTH. In a young patient with a smaller total blood volume, adequate medical treatment is essential to avoid major adverse sequelae. Our patient's PTH occurred in the PACU within the first 24 h after surgery, so was primary PTH by definition. Because it was not the torrential type of arterial bleeding that can quickly deteriorate into a life-threatening situation, there was time to assess the patient's volume status thoroughly and prepare for a controlled return to the OR. Patients who are discharged home and present later with secondary PTH should be questioned about aspirin or ibuprofen use in the interim. Although nonsteroidal anti-inflammatory medications such as ibuprofen and ketorolac have not been shown to increase bleeding, ketorolac is rarely administered intraoperatively for this surgery, while ibuprofen and acetaminophen are often prescribed as discharge medications [8]. While rare, PTH remains a potentially lethal complication of tonsillectomy. Particularly in practice settings other than large children's hospitals, simulation would be a valuable tool to review the anesthetic considerations for PTH and practice troubleshooting different case scenarios. These include difficult IV access, evaluation of volume status, difficult airway due to blood and airway swelling, and post-anesthesia disposition planning [24]. Simulation is a useful tool not only in training residents on PTH management but also as a continuing medical education exercise for attending anesthesiologists.

References

1. Michel M, Preciado D, Allen S, Behzadpour H, Pestieau S, Espinel A. Factors influencing time to operating room in children presenting with post-tonsillectomy hemorrhage. Int J Pediatr Otorhinolaryngol. 2021;141:110581. https://doi.org/10.1016/j.ijporl.2020.110581.
2. Subramanyam R, Varughese A, Willging JP, Sadhasivam S. Future of pediatric tonsillectomy and perioperative outcomes. Int J Pediatr Otorhinolaryngol. 2013;77(2):194–9. https://doi.org/10.1016/j.ijporl.2012.10.016.
3. Scalzitti NJ, Sarber KM. Diagnosis and perioperative management in pediatric sleep-disordered breathing. Paediatr Anaesth. 2018;28(11):940–6. https://doi.org/10.1111/pan.13506.
4. Lawson R. Anaesthesia for paediatric ENT surgery. Anaesth Intens Care Med. 2006;7(5):161–4.
5. Mitchell RB, Archer SM, Ishman SL, et al. Clinical practice guideline: tonsillectomy in children (update). Otolaryngol Head Neck Surg. 2019;160(1_suppl):S1–S42. https://doi.org/10.1177/0194599818801757.
6. Crysdale WS, Russel D. Complications of tonsillectomy and adenoidectomy in 9409 children observed overnight. CMAJ. 1986;135(10):1139–42.
7. McDougall RJ. Paediatric emergencies. Anaesthesia. 2013;68(Suppl 1):61–71. https://doi.org/10.1111/anae.12052.
8. Lee AC, Hache M. Pediatric anesthesia management for post-tonsillectomy bleed: current status and future directions. Int J Gen Med. 2022;15:63–9. https://doi.org/10.2147/IJGM.S312866.
9. Windfuhr JP, Schloendorff G, Baburi D, Kremer B. Serious post-tonsillectomy hemorrhage with and without lethal outcome in children and adolescents. Int J Pediatr Otorhinolaryngol. 2008;72(7):1029–40. https://doi.org/10.1016/j.ijporl.2008.03.009.
10. Windfuhr JP, Schloendorff G, Baburi D, Kremer B. Life-threatening posttonsillectomy hemorrhage. Laryngoscope. 2008;118(8):1389–94. https://doi.org/10.1097/MLG.0b013e3181734f7e.
11. Yen K, Riegert A, Gorelick MH. Derivation of the DIVA score: a clinical prediction rule for the identification of children with difficult intravenous access. Pediatr Emerg Care. 2008;24(3):143–7. https://doi.org/10.1097/PEC.0b013e3181666f32.
12. Rothbart A, Yu P, Muller-Lobeck L, Spies CD, Wernecke KD, Nachtigall I. Peripheral intravenous cannulation with support of infrared laser vein viewing system in a pre-operation setting in pediatric patients. BMC Res Notes. 2015;8:463. https://doi.org/10.1186/s13104-015-1431-2.
13. Munshey F, Parra DA, McDonnell C, Matava C. Ultrasound-guided techniques for peripheral intravenous placement in children with difficult venous access. Paediatr Anaesth. 2020;30(2):108–15. https://doi.org/10.1111/pan.13780.
14. Benkhadra M, Collignon M, Fournel I, et al. Ultrasound guidance allows faster peripheral IV cannulation in children under 3 years of age with difficult venous access: a prospective randomized study. Paediatr Anaesth. 2012;22(5):449–54. https://doi.org/10.1111/j.1460-9592.2012.03830.x.
15. Joseph G, Tobias JD. The use of intraosseous infusions in the operating room. J Clin Anesth. 2008;20(6):469–73. https://doi.org/10.1016/j.jclinane.2008.04.014.

16. Allen TH, Steven IM, Sweeney DB. The bleeding tonsil—anaesthesia for control of haemorrhage after tonsillectomy. Anaesth Intensive Care. 1973;1(6):517–20. https://doi.org/10.1177/0310057X7300100610.
17. Fields RG, Gencorelli FJ, Litman RS. Anesthetic management of the pediatric bleeding tonsil. Paediatr Anaesth. 2010;20(11):982–6. https://doi.org/10.1111/j.1460-9592.2010.03426.x.
18. Engelhardt T. Rapid sequence induction has no use in pediatric anesthesia. Paediatr Anaesth. 2015;25(1):5–8. https://doi.org/10.1111/pan.12544.
19. Kemper ME, Buehler PK, Schmitz A, Gysin C, Nicolai T, Weiss M. Classical versus controlled rapid sequence induction and intubation in children with bleeding tonsils (a retrospective audit). Acta Anaesthesiol Scand. 2020;64(1):41–7. https://doi.org/10.1111/aas.13473.
20. Landsman I. Cricoid pressure: indications and complications. Paediatr Anaesth. 2004;14(1):43–7. https://doi.org/10.1046/j.1460-9592.2003.01202.x.
21. Else SDN, Kovatsis PG. A narrative review of oxygenation during pediatric intubation and airway procedures. Anesth Analg. 2020;130(4):831–40. https://doi.org/10.1213/ANE.0000000000004403.
22. Sohn L, Hajduk J, Jagannathan N. Apneic oxygenation as a standard of care in children: how do we get there? Anesth Analg. 2020;130(4):828–30. https://doi.org/10.1213/ANE.0000000000004483.
23. Valla FV, Tume LN, Jotterand Chaparro C, et al. Gastric point-of-care ultrasound in acutely and critically ill children (POCUS-ped): a scoping review. Front Pediatr. 2022;10:921863. https://doi.org/10.3389/fped.2022.921863.
24. Breinholt CC, Obr CJ. General anesthesia for a posttonsillectomy and adenoidectomy bleed. MedEdPORTAL. 2016;12:10476. https://doi.org/10.15766/mep_2374-8265.10476.

O_2 Desaturation After Bariatric Surgery in a Teenager

Phayon U. Lee

A 17-year-old, 128-kilogram (Kg), 1.4-m-tall, Caucasian female arrived at the preoperative bay for her scheduled laparoscopic sleeve gastrectomy. Medical history included class 3 obesity, severe obstructive sleep apnea (OSA), mild asthma, prehypertension, hyperlipidemia, GERD, and nonalcoholic fatty liver disease.

Past surgical history was significant for tonsillectomy and adenoidectomy at age 6. The patient last had clear liquid at 10 pm the previous night.

Current medications included daily omeprazole, oral contraceptive pills (Loestrin), and albuterol prn. She mentioned that in addition she uses a CPAP machine at night. Previous anesthetic history was unremarkable, and the patient has no known drug allergies.

Physical examination of the patient revealed a wide neck circumference, Mallampati 3, but reassuring thyromental distance. In addition, she has large breasts and an obese abdomen. The respiratory exam showed distant breath sounds bilaterally, and her cardiac exam on auscultation revealed regular heart rate and rhythm. Additionally, the patient described that she did not walk much because of shortness of breath with activity and that she has been having difficulty lying flat. She regularly uses two pillows to prop her up at night when she goes to sleep. Preoperative ECG and ECHO were normal.

Her vital signs are as follows: blood pressure, 136/88 mmHg; heart rate, 80 beats per minute; respiratory rate, 25 breaths per minute; and spO_2, 96% on room air.

The patient agreed to a preoperative placement of IV although she was mildly anxious. With the use of a S-Caine patch™ to numb the skin, an intravenous catheter was placed on the dorsum of her hand as she was able to be kept calm through verbal reassurance [1]. She was brought to the operating room and positioned with

P. U. Lee (✉)
Children's National Hospital, The George Washington University School of Medicine, Washington, DC, USA
e-mail: Plee5@childrensnational.org

S. T. Verghese (ed.), *Anesthesia STAT! Acute Pediatric Emergencies in PACU*,
https://doi.org/10.1007/978-3-031-24396-7_23

a few blankets to prop her up. She was also placed in a slight reverse Trendelenburg position to assist with lung mechanics and to minimize passive regurgitation.

After monitors were placed, she was preoxygenated with 100% oxygen for about 4–5 min and anesthetic induction proceeded with 40 mg of intravenous lidocaine, 150 mg of propofol, and 25 μg of fentanyl. After the patient became apneic, an oral airway was placed, and patient was masked with 100% oxygen prior to the administration of succinylcholine. Intubation was accomplished with use of a CMAC, and endotracheal tube placement was confirmed with end-tidal carbon dioxide ($ETCO_2$) and bilateral auscultation of equal breath sounds. After inflating the cuff, the endotracheal tube was taped carefully with Tegaderm on either side of the mouth, and a temperature probe was placed in the mouth. The patient was paralyzed with rocuronium 50 mg after she showed clinical evidence of having recovered from succinylcholine and placed on pressure-controlled ventilation. A test dose of cefazolin of 50 mg was administered followed by the maximum recommended dose of cefazolin of 2 Gms prior to the surgical prep and clean for the planned laparoscopic gastric sleeve surgery (Fig. 1).

Sudden oxygen desaturation was seen immediately after insertion of an orogastric tube via the mouth into the stomach to aspirate gastric contents. This desaturation resolved after the ET tube that was inadvertently pushed in further into the trachea was pulled back to its original position. Placement of dilatational rubber bougies of increasing sizes often requested by the surgical team also can also cause the ET tube to move deeper into the trachea and cause sudden oxygen desaturation. The placement of temperature probe, orogastric tube, and dilatational rubber bougies can often push the tube tip into right main bronchus because of the patient's short neck and steep Trendelenburg position.

During the case, the patient again developed hypercarbia and decreased tidal volume after table position was changed to a sideway tilt combined with steep Trendelenburg position and when the insufflation of CO_2 commenced. After auscultation and determination that the tube tip was in the appropriate position above

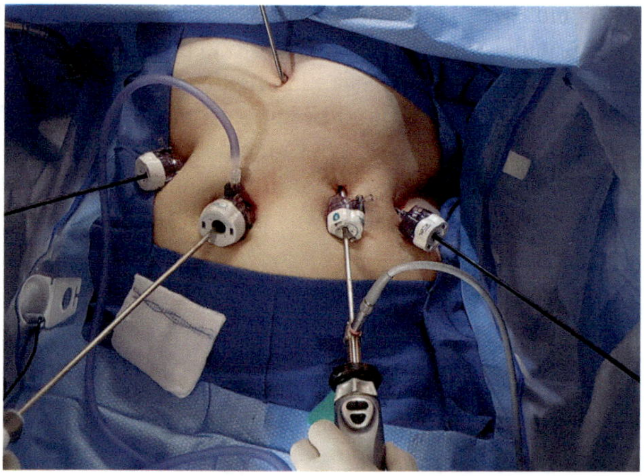

Fig. 1 Surgical setup for gastric sleeve surgery via laparoscopic approach. Photo courtesy of Dr. Evan P. Nadler

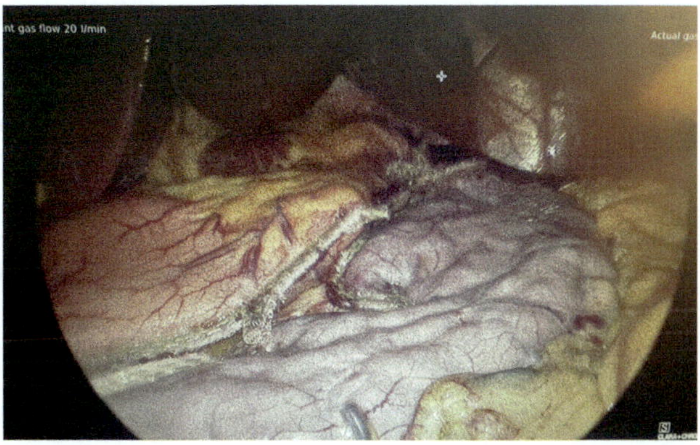

Fig. 2 Laparoscopic view after sleeve operation. Photo courtesy of Dr. Evan P Nadler

the carina, the inspired pressure was adjusted to improve the tidal volume to a volume of approximately 12–15 mL/kg and respiratory rate adjusted to reduce the $ETCO_2$. Maintenance anesthetic was accomplished with sevoflurane and pain management with multimodal analgesia: fentanyl 0.2 mcg/kg, iv acetaminophen, and iv ketorolac (Toradol) after the surgery was over and surgeon was satisfied with overall hemostasis (Fig. 2). Patient was given antiemetic prophylaxis with ondansetron and Decadron to prevent incidence of postoperative nausea and vomiting.

After completion of the gastric sleeve surgery, the plan was for awake extubation after complete muscle relaxant reversal with sugammadex. The need for awake extubation was discussed with patient and her parents during the preop interview that she might remember the presence of an endotracheal tube in her mouth for a brief period and that she may experience a mild sore throat which will be treated with blow by oxygen mist and if needed a nebulizing treatment of racemic epinephrine will be administered in PACU. The oropharynx was carefully suctioned, and a soft bite block was placed. During emergence, the patient had several episodes of coughing with increased peak airway pressures. The ETT was also suctioned with only minimal secretions. During this episode, the patient desaturated to 89%; auscultation revealed mildly coarse breath sounds that resolved with administration of albuterol. The patient was then successfully extubated in the semi-upright position after being fully awake. The patient was transferred to the hospital bed, and an attempt was made to have the head of the bed elevated and a few blankets rolled to form a firm shoulder roll prop which was placed behind the patient to help facilitate effective respirations. During transport to the post-anesthesia care unit, the patient was noted to have developed an obstructive pattern of breathing that was relieved by the chin lift and jaw thrust maneuver. Application of 100% oxygen by face mask connected to a Jackson-Rees circuit that was attached to a portable oxygen tank allowed the continuous assessment of adequate respiratory rate and volume.

On arrival to the PACU, the patient although breathing spontaneously was noted to slowly develop heavy snoring and somewhat difficult to arouse. The oxygen saturation was 96% even when continuing 100% oxygen by face mask. The patient was also repositioned to try and relieve her upper airway obstruction. An attempt was also made to place an oral airway; however, the patient was too awake for its placement. During the handoff process, the anesthesiologist emphasized to the PACU nurse the need to maintain the patient in an almost upright sitting position and about her sensitivity to narcotics and to place the patient on her home CPAP machine once it had been evaluated by the hospital biomed. Her vital signs were stable, and she appeared more responsive when the handoff was eventually over.

Approximately 25 min after the patient was dropped off at the PACU, anesthesia was called stat to the bedside for sudden onset of oxygen desaturation. On arrival, the patient was noted to be lying flat with the center of the bed sunken resulting in flexion of the patient's neck. The patient was also noted have any spontaneous respiratory effort, and no noticeable chest rise was seen, and chest auscultation revealed no breath sounds. The oxygen saturations were noted to be in the 70s. The patient was also difficult to arouse, and the patient was still not wearing the CPAP machine. As soon as the head was extended and firm jaw thrust was applied simultaneously by the anesthesiologist, it was followed by placement of an oral airway and controlled ventilation with 100% oxygen by face mask. There was a steady improvement of oxygen saturation, and after about 5 min, she was awake and maintained in a semi-sitting position with pillows and head of bed elevation. Her CPAP machine was placed without difficulty when she tolerated this well. For the rest of her stay in PACU, she was advised to remain in a semi-sitting state with supplemental oxygen via nasal cannula with the side port attached to the monitor to measure CO_2 in each breath. She had one to one nursing care and the orders to receive Tylenol and Motrin round the clock. She spent the rest of the day playing cards with her parents and sister and watching some movies on TV. Her saturation on room air was back to preoperative levels and she was instructed to take deep breaths and cough frequently and helped by the nurse to ambulate around the PACU corridors. She was discharged home the next day without any further problems with oxygen desaturation.

1 What Are the Differential Diagnoses for Postoperative Desaturation After Bariatric Surgery?

Patients who present for bariatric surgery secondary to clinically significant obesity are at increased risk of respiratory complications. Some common causes of desaturation in the PACU includes upper airway obstruction, including obstructive sleep apnea (OSA), laryngospasm, hypoventilation secondary to residual anesthetics/analgesics causing respiratory depression and or inadequate airway maintenance (secondary to reduced muscle tone/residual neuromuscular blockade), obesity hypoventilation syndrome (chronic hypoventilation), and atelectasis. Additionally, poor positioning compounding reduced thoracic compliance, mucus plug/secretions, and bronchospasm which may result in hypoxemia [2]. Pulmonary embolism should also be considered as a source of hypoxemia in this obese patient population postoperatively.

2 How Does Respiratory Mechanics Differ in an Obese Patient?

Obese patients have rapid desaturation during the period of apnea during laryngoscopy, and this is mainly because of a decrease in functional residual capacity reduction in expiratory reserve and decreased ventilation/perfusion (V/Q) ratio [3].

Prolonged pre-oxygenation in the "ramped-up" position is superior to the usual "sniff" position in morbidly obese patients to align oral, pharyngeal, and laryngeal axes and must be meticulously accomplished prior to laryngoscopy and intubation [4].

Video laryngoscopy should always be available and ready for use if there is a question about difficulty with direct laryngoscopy. Awake fiberoptic intubation is usually considered if the BMI is >50 kg/m^2 and/or a neck circumference is >42 cm.

After intubation, the tracheal tube position must be maintained at the correct depth, and ventilation must be optimized to maintain adequate oxygenation. Special ventilation techniques can improve oxygenation in morbidly obese patients undergoing anesthesia. Preoxygenation using a higher fraction of inspired oxygen with the patient at a 25 ° ramped-up position and rapid sequence intubation with succinyl choline to prevent air entry into the stomach with positive pressure ventilation by mask are suggested strategies in bariatric surgery. Laryngeal masks should be available as rescue devices and the difficult airway cart available in the OR.

Optimal ventilation strategies in obese patients include lung recruitment maneuvers up to 40 cm H_2O for 30–40 s, use of higher tidal volumes (10–12 cc/kg) and PEEP (7–10 cm H_2O), and complete muscle relaxation to maintain normocapnia [5].

During bariatric surgery, the need for creating a pneumoperitoneum and increase in abdominal pressure can affect the patient's respiratory mechanics [6]. The addition of carbon dioxide for abdominal cavity inflation can cause increased intra-abdominal pressure, systemic vascular resistance, and decreased venous return which causes lowering of cardiac output. Pneumothorax, air embolism, and mediastinal emphysema are some of the fatal complications of pneumoperitoneum.

Extubation is usually accomplished when the patient is fully reversed, wide awake, and following verbal commands. The patient is maintained with a 30–45 ° elevation of the upper torso and moved to the hospital bed with the help of Hover device. Patient is transported to the PACU with oxygen blow by in the same head-up position with a portable pulse oximeter attached to the finger for continuous monitoring of oxygen saturation.

General anesthesia commonly results in a reduced functional residual capacity (FRC) in normal individuals and results in atelectasis [7]. Being in the supine position also reduces the FRC by 20% secondary to compression atelectasis, and this is worsened in the obese patient. In the obese patient, the diaphragm is shifted upward, and the thorax becomes less compliant resulting in a restrictive ventilatory pattern and atelectasis [8]. Overall, the FRC, vital capacity (VC), and total lung capacity (TLC) are reduced in the obese population although closing capacity stays the same [9]. Any condition that worsens these volume relationships will result in potential small airway closure, V/Q mismatch, and hypoxemia. Because of this, patients must be monitored carefully in the PACU to minimize episodes of significant desaturation [7].

3 What Is the Prevalence of OSA in the Bariatric Population and What Role Did This Patient's OSA Play in Her Postoperative Desaturation?

Obstructive sleep apnea (OSA) is a disorder related to sleep and designated by prolonged or intermittent partial to complete upper airway obstruction during sleep. It affects 1.2–5.7% of children in the USA [10]. OSA was reported to have a prevalence of 13–59% in adolescents with severe obesity [11] and a prevalence of greater than 70% in a cohort of adults presenting for evaluation for bariatric surgery [12].

This patient had a known history of OSA, and CPAP machine was not appropriately applied during the postoperative period and may have contributed to the significant hypoxemia experienced in the PACU. One study by Gallagher et al. [2] (2010) found multiple episodes of desaturation with a nadir of 75% despite use of CPAP. Additionally, desaturation was seen in 100% of the patients in the first 24 h despite diagnosis and treatment for at least 6 weeks preoperatively. Therefore, based on these findings, it is unclear if the use of the CPAP machine would have prevented the desaturation episode in the PACU.

4 What Is Obesity Hypoventilation Syndrome and How Prevalent Is It in the Bariatric Population?

Obesity hypoventilation syndrome (OHS) is a sleep-related disorder defined by BMI $\geq$ 30 kg/m^2, sleep disordered breathing, and daytime hypercapnia. According to a study by Tran et al. [13] (2020), OHS is present in approximately two-thirds of patients being referred for bariatric surgery. They also determined that moderate to severe OSA was a significant predictor of OHS. Although it is possible that this patient may have had OHS contributing to her risk for respiratory complication, she was not formally evaluated for the syndrome and her daytime $PaCO_2$ was unknown.

Although, intuitively, hypoventilation may appear to be a significant contributor of postoperative desaturation, Gallagher et al. [2] (2010) found that it did not play a significant role in the cause of desaturation in their bariatric patient population. A study in adult patients with and without OSA who underwent laparoscopic bariatric surgery did not show a significant increase in the incidence of desaturations in patients with OSA [14].

5 What Role Does Opioid Administration Play in Postoperative Desaturation in Bariatric Patients and What Alternative Pain Management Strategy Could Have Been Employed in This Patient?

It is well known that one of the most feared side effects of opioid analgesics is respiratory depression. One potential cause of desaturation in the postoperative care unit in the obese population undergoing bariatric surgery is narcotic-induced decreased arousal. This decreased arousal was also seen with the use of PCA [2]. The presence of OSA and OHS also worsens the respiratory depressant effects of systemically administered opioids [15].

Enhanced recovery after surgery (ERAS) recommends the implementation of opioid-sparing analgesia [16] of which regional anesthesia is an important component [17]. It has been established that multimodal opioid-sparing analgesia is effective at controlling pain while also decreasing the narcotic use after bariatric surgery [18].

This patient was given a bolus of fentanyl postoperatively, and this most likely potentiated the decreased arousal resulting in increased obstruction and oxygen desaturation. The bariatric patient population benefits from multimodal analgesia that decreases the use of opioids. TAP blocks were employed in one study and was shown to be effective at improving pain management and decreasing the use of narcotics and essentially the respiratory depressant effects associated with narcotics use [19]. In addition to regional techniques for pain management, this patient may have benefited from use of non-opioids such as scheduled anti-inflammatories, for instance, acetaminophen was found to have opioid-sparing effect in a retrospective analysis [20]. Other infusions such as dexmedetomidine and ketamine that have opioid-sparing effects can also be considered. According to one study, preoperative administration of ketamine has been shown to reduce opioid consumption in postoperative bariatric patients along with the pain scores [21].

6 Could the Obstruction Have Been Secondary to Position?

Positioning of the patient in the supine position and flat may have potentially worsened the respiratory mechanics further resulting in desaturation. The supine position decreases the FRC, and this is worsened in the mild to moderate obese patient [22] respiratory mechanics.

7 Is It Possible for the Desaturation to Be Secondary to Atelectasis?

Atelectasis refers to the closure of small airway secondary to volume reduction. The extent of postoperative atelectasis depends on several factors such as type of surgical procedure, type of anesthesia, baseline pulmonary function, and position during surgery [23]. Obesity in bariatric patients increases the risk of postoperative atelectasis secondary to the reduced FRC [24]. Atelectasis may cause a V/Q mismatch and result in decreased compliance of the lung [22]. Atelectasis can increase morbidity and mortality. It was seen in one study to be the cause of 11% of postoperative respiratory failure and related death [25]. Not surprisingly, a study by Baltieri et al. [26] (2016) found atelectasis to be 37% prevalent in the bariatric surgery patient population even after exclusion of medical problems like OSA. In addition to the worsening and prolongation of atelectasis, laparoscopic surgery compounds this problem secondary to the reduced lung compliance with the institution of pneumoperitoneum [27].

Atelectasis is usually diagnosed after development of tachypnea and hypoxemia (from blood gas analysis) and is usually seen after discharge from the recovery area and can worsen and continue for up to 5 days [28].

The presence of atelectasis can result in severe hypoxemia secondary to decreased compliance of the lung tissue, V/Q mismatch, poor gas exchange, and an increase in pulmonary vascular resistance. The risk of infection is increased as the ability of antibiotics to penetrate the lung tissue in atelectatic areas is greatly reduced [29].

Preventing atelectasis in the postoperative period is therefore very important. Methods that can be implemented to reduce the risk after bariatric surgery includes lung recruitment maneuvers such as incentive spirometry, deep breathing exercise, coughing, CPAP and appropriate pain management with regional technique and patient-controlled analgesics over potent analgesics, early mobilization, and head-up position [30, 31].

8 Is Pulmonary Embolism a Potential Cause of the Postoperative Desaturation?

Pulmonary embolism (PE) is an uncommon cause of postoperative mortality. Patients undergoing treatment for obesity are at an increased risk for venous thromboembolism (VTE) and PE. This increased incidence of VTE is thought to be due to a combination of decreased venous return and stasis and the endocrine effect of adipose tissue resulting in a prothrombotic state [32, 33]. The signs and symptoms of PE can be obscure and mimic many other conditions; however, this diagnosis should be considered when a patient is experiencing hemodynamic instability and hypoxemia not responsive to oxygen therapy and airway maneuver [34].

9 What Were the Risk Factors for Postoperative Desaturation in This Bariatric Surgery Patient and How Could the Postoperative Outcome Have Been Optimized?

Postoperative pneumonia and respiratory failure are the most common non-wound complications after bariatric surgery [35]. Risk factors associated with the development of these respiratory complications include history of CHF and previous PCI, COPD, cigarette smoking [35], and increased age secondary to decreased oropharyngeal motor function, laryngopharyngeal sensitivity, and increased risk of atelectasis [36]. Additionally, history of stroke conferred a four times greater risk of postoperative pneumonia, and greater weight increased the risk of postoperative respiratory failure [35].

Our patient developed immediate/early postoperative respiratory complication and therefore postoperative pneumonia is less likely; however, it is very likely that her weight was a contributing factor to the development of the postoperative respiratory failure.

10 Could Residual Neuromuscular Blockade Be a Potential Cause of This Patient's Postoperative Desaturation?

She was administered neuromuscular blockade during the intraoperative period. It is possible that the reversal was not fully adequate and may have resulted in upper airway obstruction secondary to the decreased tone of the oropharyngeal tissue. Even though intermediate acting neuromuscular blocker was used and reversed pharmacologically for complete reversal, the complete recovery of muscle strength may not be accomplished fully prior to tracheal extubation [37]. Small degrees of residual neuromuscular blockade (TOF 0.7–0.9) can result in upper airway obstruction due to the decreased pharyngeal muscle tone; it also causes reduced hypoxic ventilatory response and airway reflexes and predisposes the patient to aspiration [38–40]. Another study by Kumar et al. [41] (2012) reported that residual neuromuscular blockade can decrease the forced vital capacity and peak expiratory flow in the immediate postoperative period. Sugammadex was used for reversal in this patient. Sugammadex is a selective relaxant-binding agent specifically developed for rapid reversal of nondepolarizing neuromuscular blockade induced by rocuronium. Its potential clinical benefits include fast and predictable reversal of any degree of block, increased patient safety, and reduced incidence of residual block on recovery when compared to neostigmine [42]. So inadequate reversal, though possible, may not have been the cause in our patient.

11 Could Bronchospasm or Laryngospasm Be Contributors to This Postoperative Desaturation? What Is the Treatment?

This patient has a history of asthma requiring rescue inhaler use and is morbidly obese, both of which are risk factors for developing perioperative respiratory adverse events. Due to this patient's history of asthma, she is at an increased risk of perioperative bronchospasm and laryngospasm and should have received preoperative bronchodilator to decrease the risk of perioperative respiratory adverse events. Von Ungern-Sternberg [43] reports that bronchial hyperreactivity has an exaggerated response to airway stimulation which leads to an increased risk of bronchospasm and desaturation.

Bronchospasm should be promptly treated with 100% oxygen and albuterol, and if this is insufficient, epinephrine, IV ketamine, or magnesium should be considered. Laryngospasm on the other hand should be treated with jaw thrust and continuous positive airway pressure (CPAP) with 100% oxygen; if these maneuvers are not breaking the laryngospasm, then propofol and/or succinylcholine should be administered [43].

12 What Was Determined to Be the Cause of the Desaturation in This Patient?

The desaturation in this patient may have been multifactorial; however, the major contributor was most likely the decreased respiratory drive and upper airway obstruction that resulted after the administration of opioid in the PACU. The level of decreased arousal was thought to be compounded by the presence of obesity and OSA. The patient did not have wheezing on auscultation in the PACU, and the patient did not show any signs straining during inspiratory or expiratory making bronchospasm and laryngospasm less likely.

13 Discussion

13.1 General Anesthesia for Morbidly Obese Teenagers for Gastric Sleeve Operation

Obesity is a very pressing public health issue in our country because of its prevalence in almost 600 million adults [44]. In adolescents the problem of obesity has been increasing steadily [45]. Bariatric surgery has been successful in select teenagers who cannot lose this excess weight by diet and exercise [46].

Bariatric surgery has become an effective surgical mode to reduce weight in obese teenagers in many pediatric hospitals in the USA. The last decade has seen an increase in obesity in adolescents in USA with at least 30% of them showing criteria for metabolic syndrome [47].

Body mass index (BMI) relates weight to the height of the patient and is the screening tool used for assessing obesity in patients. Dividing the weight of the patient in kilograms by the square of the height in meters is the method of calculating the BMI.

In children, the BMI can vary by age, gender, and maturity. Morbid obesity is defined as a BMI $\geq$ 120% of the 95th percentile for age and sex or a BMI $\geq$ 35 kg per m^2.

Currently, the guidelines for selection of teenagers for weight loss surgery include a (BMI) > 40 kg/m^2 with minor comorbidities or > _35kg/m^2 with comorbid disease state like diabetes mellitus, type 2 hypertension, and OSA with apnea-hypopnea index (AHI) > 15.

13.2 Types of Bariatric Surgery

The three different types of sleeve gastrectomy that are currently offered at our institution to these young patients are performed via a laparoscopic approach.

Roux-en-Y gastric bypass (RYGB), the vertical sleeve gastrectomy (VSG), and adjustable gastric banding (AGB) are the three main types of bariatric surgery with *VSG as the most popular procedure performed in our institution.*

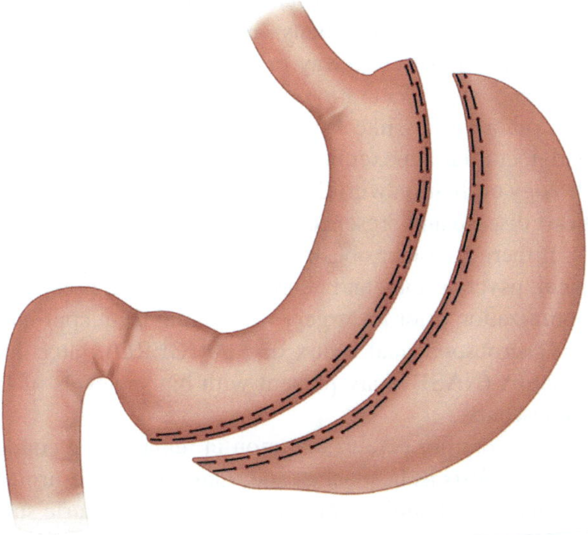

Fig. 3 Vertical sleeve gastrectomy

Due to their technical ease and lower complication rates, both laparoscopic sleeve gastrectomy and laparoscopic adjustable gastric banding have been popular alternatives to laparoscopic Roux-en-Y gastric bypass. However, AGB is not approved in children under the age of 18 and thus is not used in young teens [48].

Laparoscopic sleeve gastrectomy is currently the most performed bariatric procedure in the USA [49] (Fig. 3).

In adolescents, laparoscopic sleeve gastrectomy is an excellent option to provide excess weight loss and remission of comorbid conditions without long-term malabsorptive risks [50].

13.3 Preoperative Evaluation and Planning

A detailed preop evaluation of patients for bariatric surgery is essential for a smooth and safe perioperative course.

Comprehensive evaluation of comorbid conditions in the obese patient is vital for optimal preparation for the surgery.

Multidisciplinary preop clinics associated with bariatric surgery centers makes this in-person evaluation possible. In our institution, pediatric bariatric surgeon refers these patients to preoperative clinic supervised by the anesthesiologists and preop nurse practitioners for a complete preop evaluation which includes comprehensive history as well as physical evaluation with focus mainly on obesity-related diseases.

Perioperative morbidity is increased in obesity when a metabolic syndrome is clinically evident with hypertension, hyperinsulinemia, and high triglycerides.

History of snoring, obstructive sleep apnea diagnosis with polysomnography results with particular focus on apnea and hypopnea index (AHI) and HI, use of continuous positive airway pressure (CPAP) or bilevel positive pressure (BIPAP), baseline oxygen saturation on room air should be obtained during the evaluation.

Comorbidities like hypertension, hypercholesterolemia, and presence of OSA and nocturnal hypoxemia proven by sleep study should prompt one to obtain a cardiology evaluation with ECG and echocardiography to rule out early-onset ischemic heart disease and presence of pulmonary hypertension.

If there are other obesity-related comorbidities (diabetes, renal, hepatic involvement, psychosocial, and neurological), then a preop evaluation of these systems for optimization prior to surgery is essential from appropriate specialists.

Gastroesophageal reflux disease (GERD), fatty liver, and nonalcoholic steatohepatitis (NASH) may present with higher levels of liver enzymes in these obese adolescents.

Pseudotumor cerebri common in females is a condition associated with obesity and manifests as headaches and vomiting. A presurgical psychologic assessment is obtained in all adolescent patients prior to bariatric surgery in our institution.

A retrospective review of 167 patients undergoing laparoscopic sleeve gastrectomy with preexisting psychologic depression, anxiety, attention deficit, and binge-eating showed that their prescribed medications included selective serotonin reuptake inhibitors (SSRIs) and serotonin-norepinephrine reuptake inhibitors (SNRIs). Although this review did not see any significant drug interactions during anesthesia, it is important to obtain detailed account of medications that can interact with the anesthetic drugs. The combined use of potent anesthetic drugs in these patients on SSRIs and SNRIs can produce life-threatening symptoms of drug-drug interactions (DDIs) [51].

Physical evaluation of patient's body habitus, head, and neck to gauge the range of mouth opening, neck circumference and its mobility, and presence of large tongue, prominent teeth, and large tonsils by close examination will identify potential problems early to help prepare and plan for successful mask ventilation and ease of intubation and ventilation on the day of surgery.

Lab investigation should include a complete blood count, metabolic panel, coagulation and lipid profile, glycosylated hemoglobin, type and screen, electrocardiogram, transthoracic echocardiogram, baseline oxygen saturation, and polysomnography. Calculation of ideal body weight (IBW) should also be obtained for correct dosing of medications.

Morbidly obese patients have excess fatty tissue not only externally on the breast, neck, thoracic, and abdominal wall but also internally in the mouth, pharynx, and abdomen. This abundance of fatty tissue can make spontaneous ventilation during mild sedation, mask ventilation, and intubation during anesthesia induction extremely difficult. The increased size of abdominal contents due to visceral organomegaly can reduce the ability of the patient to breathe in the supine position. Trendelenburg can further decrease functional residual capacity and worsen the ventilation/perfusion (V/Q) mismatch. Elevation of patient's upper body head and neck and preoxygenation are mandatory during anesthetic induction. Rapid sequence or standard induction with intravenous hypnotics should be based on the ease of airway mask fit and evidence of an unobstructed airway. Irrespective of the choice of induction, airway manipulation should occur only when the depth of anesthesia is sufficient for laryngoscopy and intubation to avoid aspiration of stomach contents. Intubating laryngeal mask airway has been suggested as a rescue device in obese patients for failed ventilation and intubation. In the immediate postoperative period, frequent desaturation periods are reported in morbidly obese patients that can be treated with continuous positive pressure noninvasive ventilation and proper positioning [52].

Assessment of patient's neck circumference, Mallampati score, thyromental distance, and range of neck movement are all vital information required for plans to secure the airway successfully. Mallampati score is a simple evaluation which rates the visibility of the base of the uvula, faucial pillars, and soft palate to determine the difficulty with laryngoscopy and intubation. In a study of 100 morbidly obese patients, neither obesity nor body mass index predicted problems with tracheal intubation, but a high Mallampati score ($\geq$3) and large neck circumference $\geq$ 43 cm predicted an increase in the potential for difficult laryngoscopy and intubation [53]. In a close claimed US data about difficult intubation airway obstruction, Mallampati grades 3–4 and limited cervical extension were ranked as predictors of a difficult intubation [54].

Monitoring the obese patient and obtaining venous access during anesthesia may be difficult. Noninvasive blood pressure cuff monitoring at the brachial area is acceptable if the cuff encircles most of the upper arm circumference. The use of ultrasonography and transillumination may be helpful in obtaining venous access in these challenging individuals.

13.4 Drug Dosing

Drug dosing is an important area to pay close attention to during the perioperative period in the obese patient undergoing general anesthesia.

Standard dosing guidelines are not useful to the anesthesiologist to calculate the correct dose of medications in obese patients. Scalars such as total body weight (TBW), lean body weight (LBW), and ideal body weight (IBW) can be used for calculating the best dose based on the pharmacokinetics of each drug.

Obesity increases both fat and lean body mass, the latter being responsible for almost all of body's metabolic activity. Lean body mass (LBM) is the nonfat cell part of the body which includes intracellular connective tissue [55].

IBW does not include this increase in LBW. Since LBW is difficult to calculate, IBW is considered in its place. The method to calculate IBW in obese child is to multiply the BMI at the 50th percentile for the child's age by the square of the height in meters [56].

Multiple studies have looked at the effect of obesity on organs that are essential for the pharmacokinetics and pharmacodynamics of drugs. Providers of anesthesia should be knowledgeable about the physiological changes associated with obesity and the resultant changes in drug utilization and elimination that ensue [57].

When dosing obese patients, it is important to consider the changes in the size of elimination organs like liver and kidney and their function and composition as well as the specific properties of the drug administered (lipophilicity and elimination pathway) and use the correct body size metric: total body weight, lean body weight, and body surface area to calculate the appropriate dose required [58].

13.5 DVT Prophylaxis

Morbid obesity has been correlated to a higher risk of venous thromboembolism (VTE).

A history of deep vein thrombosis and pulmonary embolism must be obtained because of a strong correlation of high BMI with venous thromboembolism (VTE) with its complications. Both screening for VTE and use of pharmacologic as well as mechanical prophylaxis is currently utilized during bariatric surgery [59].

A dosing scheme of 40 mg vs. 60 mg enoxaparin stratified according to BMI (40 mg SC for a BMI < 50 kg/m^2) and 60 mg SC (for a BMI ≥ 50 kg/m^2) was effective in reaching prophylactic anti-FXa activity in 83% of adolescent patients [60].

13.6 Antibiotic Prophylaxis

Antibiotic prophylaxis is recommended for bariatric surgery although the surgical approach is closed via a laparoscope [61].

13.7 Postoperative Analgesia

A morbidly obese patient for bariatric surgery benefits from the use of multimodal analgesic approach with drugs combined to decrease opioid amount which can cause respiratory depression and hypoxemia. Pre-emptive analgesia can be effective in postoperative pain relief with regional blocks [62].

Transversus abdominal plane (TAP) block is a minimally invasive technique used for abdominal and gynecological surgeries and has been studied in obese patients with the help of ultrasound guidance (USG). The study results showed that USG-guided TAP block produced higher patient satisfaction scores, early ambulation, bowel function, decreased PONV, and early discharge readiness when compared to non-TAP group [63].

The effectiveness of accomplishing TAP block under direct vision with laparoscopic guidance instead of USG guidance before surgical closure has also been studied [64].

Another method of reducing analgesic requirement in the postoperative period is the use of intraperitoneal hydrocortisone with bupivacaine [65].

The use of intraoperative dexmedetomidine during bariatric surgery in the morbidly obese adolescent population can decrease the need for narcotics in the postoperative period [66].

The risk of anesthesia-related perioperative complications can be decreased in obese patients with strict adherence to safety protocols that have been developed to prevent the anticipated problems that can develop in them.

The following safety check list should be highlighted when anesthetizing morbidly obese patients for bariatric surgery.

14 Anesthetic Safety Checklist for Bariatric Surgery

1. *Patient positioning* for airway management—ramped-up position for intubation (external auditory meatus located at the level of anterior chest).
2. Availability of *difficult airway cart* and appropriately sized intubating LMA in case of airway rescue need) before induction.
3. Thorough *preoxygenation* prior to intubation with patient in the "ramped-up" position.
4. Careful *positioning of the ET tube* aiming to position the cuff just below the vocal cords.
5. Optimize *ventilation strategies*: recruitment maneuvers—(40 cm H_2O for 30–40 s) higher tidal volumes (12–15 cc/kg), PEEP (7–10 cm H_2O), and normocapnia.
6. Antibiotics intravenously before surgical incision.
7. Use of *pneumatic compressive devices* on both legs.
8. *DVT prophylaxis* induction using heparin (dose and method).
9. *Awake extubation and transport in semi-sitting position* with oxygen blow by.
10. *Early ambulation.*

15 Summary

The need to provide anesthesia for different types of surgical conditions in obese children and adolescent patients are continuously increasing and can be challenging if the pathophysiology of obesity is not clearly understood by all the members of the perioperative team. The deleterious changes in respiratory mechanics with obesity and anesthesia and the unique response to narcotic drugs and effect of adverse positioning are significant factors to be continuously monitored by all who are caring for obese patients during surgery and the immediate perioperative period for their optimal safety and comfort.

References

1. Sethna NF, Verghese ST, Hannallah RS, Solodiuk JC, Zurakowski D, Berde CB. A randomized controlled trial to evaluate S-Caine patch for reducing pain associated with vascular access in children. Anesthesiology. 2005;102(2):403–8. https://doi.org/10.1097/00000542-200502000-00025.
2. Gallagher SF, Haines KL, Osterlund LG, Mullen M, Downs JB. Postoperative hypoxemia: common, undetected, and unsuspected after bariatric surgery. J Surg Res. 2010;159(2):622–6. https://doi.org/10.1016/j.jss.2009.09.003.
3. Gabrielsen A-M, Lund MB, Kongerud J, Viken KE, Røislien J, Hjelmesæth J. The relationship between anthropometric measures, blood gases, and lung function in morbidly obese white subjects. Obes Surg. 2010;21(4):485–91. https://doi.org/10.1007/s11695-010-0306-9.
4. Collins JS, Lemmens HJM, Brodsky JB, Brock-Utne JG, Levitan RM. Laryngoscopy and morbid obesity: a comparison of the "sniff" and "ramped" positions. Obes Surg. 2004;14(9):1171–5. https://doi.org/10.1381/0960892042386869.
5. Grassi L, Kacmarek R, Berra L. Ventilatory mechanics in the patient with obesity. Anesthesiology. 2020;132(5):1246–56. https://doi.org/10.1097/aln.0000000000003.
6. Sprung J, Whalley DG, Falcone T, Warner DO, Hubmayr RD, Hammel J. The impact of morbid obesity, pneumoperitoneum, and posture on respiratory system mechanics and oxygenation during laparoscopy. Anesth Analg. 2002;94(5):1345–50. https://doi.org/10.1097/00000539-200205000-00056.
7. Pelosi P, Croci M, Ravagnan I, et al. The effects of body mass on lung volumes, respiratory mechanics, and gas exchange during general anesthesia. Anesth Analg. 1998;87(3):654–60. https://doi.org/10.1097/00000539-199809000-00031.
8. Paul DR, Hoyt JL, Boutros AR. Cardiovascular and respiratory changes in response to change of posture in the very obese. Anesthesiology. 1976;45(1):73–8. https://doi.org/10.1097/00000542-197607000-00013.
9. Jones RL, Nzekwu M-MU. The effects of body mass index on lung volumes. Chest. 2006;130(3):827–33. https://doi.org/10.1378/chest.130.3.827.
10. Marcus CL, Brooks LJ, Ward SD, et al. Diagnosis and management of childhood obstructive sleep apnea syndrome. Pediatrics. 2012;130(3) https://doi.org/10.1542/peds.2012-1672.
11. Verhulst SL, Van Gaal L, De Backer W, Desager K. The prevalence, anatomical correlates and treatment of sleep-disordered breathing in obese children and adolescents. Sleep Med Rev. 2008;12(5):339–46. https://doi.org/10.1016/j.smrv.2007.11.002.
12. Lopez PP, Stefan B, Schulman CI, Byers PM. Prevalence of sleep apnea in morbidly obese patients who presented for weight loss surgery evaluation: more evidence for routine screening for obstructive sleep apnea before weight loss surgery. Am Surg. 2008;74(9):834–8. https://doi.org/10.1177/000313480807400914.
13. Tran K, Wang L, Gharaibeh S, et al. Elucidating predictors of obesity hypoventilation syndrome in a large bariatric surgery cohort. Ann Am Thorac Soc. 2020;17(10):1279–88. https://doi.org/10.1513/annalsats.202002-135oc.
14. Ahmad S, Nagle A, McCarthy RJ, Fitzgerald PC, Sullivan JT, Prystowsky J. Postoperative hypoxemia in morbidly obese patients with and without obstructive sleep apnea undergoing laparoscopic bariatric surgery. Anesth Analg. 2008;107(1):138–43. https://doi.org/10.1213/ane.0b013e318174df8b.
15. Kositanurit W, Muntham D, Udomsawaengsup S, Chirakalwasan N. Prevalence and associated factors of obstructive sleep apnea in morbidly obese patients undergoing bariatric surgery. Sleep Breath. 2017;22(1):251–6. https://doi.org/10.1007/s11325-017-1500-y.
16. Thorell A, MacCormick AD, Awad S, et al. Guidelines for perioperative care in bariatric surgery: enhanced recovery after surgery (ERAS) society recommendations. World J Surg. 2016;40(9):2065–83. https://doi.org/10.1007/s00268-016-3492-3.

17. Kumar K, Kirksey MA, Duong S, Wu CL. A review of opioid-sparing modalities in perioperative pain management. Anesth Analg. 2017;125(5):1749–60. https://doi.org/10.1213/ane.0000000000002497.
18. Ziemann-Gimmel P, Hensel P, Koppman J, Marema R. Multimodal analgesia reduces narcotic requirements and antiemetic rescue medication in laparoscopic roux-en-Y gastric bypass surgery. Surg Obes Relat Dis. 2013;9(6):975–80. https://doi.org/10.1016/j.soard.2013.02.003.
19. Chenchen T, Shantanna H, Hong D, Oparin Y, Lee Y. Benefits of transversus abdominis plane block on postoperative analgesia after bariatric surgery: a systematic review and meta-analysis. Pain Physician. 2021;24(5):345–58. https://doi.org/10.36076/ppj.2021.24.345.
20. Song K, Melroy MJ, Whipple OC. Optimizing multimodal analgesia with intravenous acetaminophen and opioids in postoperative bariatric patients. Pharmacotherapy. 2014;34(S1) https://doi.org/10.1002/phar.1517.
21. Zeballos JL, Lirk P, Rathmell JP. Low-dose ketamine for acute pain management. Reg Anesth Pain Med. 2018;43(5):453–5. https://doi.org/10.1097/aap.0000000000000810.
22. Sebbane M, El Kamel M, Millot A, et al. Effect of weight loss on postural changes in pulmonary function in obese subjects: a longitudinal study. Respir Care. 2015;60(7):992–9. https://doi.org/10.4187/respcare.03668.
23. Degani-Costa LH, Faresin SM, dos Reis Falcão LF. Preoperative evaluation of the patient with pulmonary disease. Braz J Anesthesiol. 2014;64(1):22–34. https://doi.org/10.1016/j.bjane.2012.11.002.
24. Zammit C, Liddicoat H, Moonsie I, Makker H. Obesity and respiratory diseases. Int J Gen Med. 2010:335. https://doi.org/10.2147/ijgm.s11926.
25. Esquinas Rodriguez AM, Papadakos PJ, Carron M, Cosentini R, Chiumello D. Clinical review: helmet and non-invasive mechanical ventilation in critically ill patients. Crit Care. 2013;17(2):223. https://doi.org/10.1186/cc11875.
26. Baltieri L, Peixoto-Souza FS, Rasera-Junior I, Montebelo MI, Costa D, Pazzianotto-Forti EM. Analysis of the prevalence of atelectasis in patients undergoing bariatric surgery. Braz J Anesthesiol. 2016;66(6):577–82. https://doi.org/10.1016/j.bjane.2014.11.016.
27. Hu XY. Effective ventilation strategies for obese patients undergoing bariatric surgery: a literature review. AANA J. 2016;84(1):35–45.
28. Malbouisson LM, Humberto F, Rdos R, Carmona MJ, Auler JO Jr. Atelectasias durante anestesia: fisiopatologia e tratamento. Rev Bras Anestesiol. 2008;58(1):73–83. https://doi.org/10.1590/s0034-70942008000100011.
29. Rama-Maceiras P. Peri-operative atelectasis and alveolar recruitment manoeuvres. Arch Bronconeumol. 2010;46(6):317–24. https://doi.org/10.1016/s1579-2129(10)70074-4.
30. Sudré EC, de Batista PR, Castiglia YM. Longer immediate recovery time after anesthesia increases risk of respiratory complications after laparotomy for bariatric surgery: a randomized clinical trial and a cohort study. Obes Surg. 2015;25(11):2205–12. https://doi.org/10.1007/s11695-015-1855-8.
31. Karcz M, Papadakos PJ. Respiratory complications in the postanesthesia care unit: a review of pathophysiological mechanisms. Can J Respir Ther. 2013;49(4):21–9.
32. Ahima RS, Flier JS. Adipose tissue as an endocrine organ. Trends Endocrinol Metabol. 2000;11(8):327–32. https://doi.org/10.1016/s1043-2760(00)00301-5.
33. Melinek J, Livingston E, Cortina G, Fishbein MC. Autopsy findings following gastric bypass surgery for morbid obesity. Arch Pathol Lab Med. 2002;126(9):1091–5. https://doi.org/10.5858/2002-126-1091-affgbs.
34. Smith D, Murauski J. Pulmonary embolism in the postanesthesia care unit: a case study. J Perianesth Nurs. 2017;32(1):6–14. https://doi.org/10.1016/j.jopan.2015.12.016.
35. Gupta PK, Gupta H, Kaushik M, et al. Predictors of pulmonary complications after bariatric surgery. Surg Obes Relat Dis. 2012;8(5):574–81. https://doi.org/10.1016/j.soard.2011.04.227.
36. Evers BM, Townsend CM, Thompson JC. Organ physiology of aging. Surg Clin N Am. 1994;74(1):23–39. https://doi.org/10.1016/s0039-6109(16)46226-2.

37. Murphy GS, Szokol JW, Marymont JH, Franklin M, Avram MJ, Vender JS. Residual paralysis at the time of tracheal extubation. Anesth Analg. 2005;100(6):1840–5. https://doi.org/10.1213/01.ane.0000151159.55655.cb.
38. Sundman E, Witt H, Olsson R, Ekberg O, Kuylenstierna R, Eriksson LI. The incidence and mechanisms of pharyngeal and upper esophageal dysfunction in partially paralyzed humans. Anesthesiology. 2000;92(4):977–84. https://doi.org/10.1097/00000542-200004000-00014.
39. Eikermann M, Groeben H, Hüsing J, Peters J. Accelerometry of adductor pollicis muscle predicts recovery of neuromuscular blockade in anesthetized patients. Anesthesiology. 2003;98(6):1333–7. https://doi.org/10.1097/00000542-200306000-00006.
40. Eikermann M, Vogt FM, Herbstreit F, et al. The predisposition to inspiratory upper airway collapse during partial neuromuscular blockade. Am J Respir Crit Care Med. 2007;175(1):9–15. https://doi.org/10.1164/rccm.200512-1862oc.
41. Kumar GV, Nair AP, Murthy HS, Jalaja KR, Ramachandra K, Parameshwara G. Residual neuromuscular blockade affects postoperative pulmonary function. Anesthesiology. 2012;117(6):1234–44. https://doi.org/10.1097/aln.0b013e3182715b80.
42. Hristovska A-M, Duch P, Allingstrup M, Afshari A. Efficacy and safety of sugammadex versus neostigmine in reversing neuromuscular blockade in adults. Cochrane Database Syst Rev. 2017;2017(9) https://doi.org/10.1002/14651858.cd012763.
43. von Ungern-Sternberg BS. Respiratory complications in the pediatric postanesthesia care unit. Anesthesiol Clin. 2014;32(1):45–61. https://doi.org/10.1016/j.anclin.2013.10.004.
44. Obesity and Overweight. World Health Organization. https://www.who.int/news-room/fact-sheets/detail/obesity-and-overweight. Accessed 5 Aug 2022.
45. Ogden CL, Carroll MD, Kit BK, Flegal KM. Prevalence of childhood and adult obesity in the United States, 2011-2012. JAMA. 2014;311(8):806. https://doi.org/10.1001/jama.2014.732.
46. Tsai WS, Inge TH, Burd RS. Bariatric surgery in adolescents. Arch Pediatr Adolesc Med. 2007;161(3):217. https://doi.org/10.1001/archpedi.161.3.217.
47. Cook S, Weitzman M, Auinger P, Nguyen M, Dietz WH. Prevalence of a metabolic syndrome phenotype in adolescents. Arch Pediatr Adolesc Med. 2003;157(8):821. https://doi.org/10.1001/archpedi.157.8.821.
48. Griggs CL, Perez NP, Goldstone RN, et al. National trends in the use of metabolic and bariatric surgery among pediatric patients with severe obesity. JAMA Pediatr. 2018;172(12):1191. https://doi.org/10.1001/jamapediatrics.2018.3030.
49. Chung AY, Strassle PD, Schlottmann F, Patti MG, Duke MC, Farrell TM. Trends in utilization and relative complication rates of bariatric procedures. J Gastrointest Surg. 2019;23(7):1362–72. https://doi.org/10.1007/s11605-018-3951-2.
50. McGuire MM, Nadler EP, Qureshi FG. Laparoscopic vertical sleeve gastrectomy for adolescents with morbid obesity. Semin Pediatr Surg. 2014;23(1):21–3. https://doi.org/10.1053/j.sempedsurg.2013.10.021.
51. Williams EF, Vaughns JD, Mackey ER, Muret JC, Nadler EP, van den Anker JN. Implications of perioperative polypharmacy in adolescents undergoing bariatric surgery: a single-center experience. Obes Surg. 2020;30(7):2832–5. https://doi.org/10.1007/s11695-020-04456-w.
52. Kristensen MS. Airway management and morbid obesity. Eur J Anaesthesiol. 2010;27(11):923–7. https://doi.org/10.1097/eja.0b013e32833d91aa.
53. Brodsky JB, Lemmens HJ, Brock-Utne JG, Vierra M, Saidman LJ. Morbid obesity and tracheal intubation. Anesth Analg. 2002;94(3):732–6. https://doi.org/10.1097/00000539-200203000-00047.
54. Joffe AM, Aziz MF, Posner KL, Duggan LV, Mincer SL, Domino KB. Management of difficult tracheal intubation. Anesthesiology. 2019;131(4):818–29. https://doi.org/10.1097/aln.0000000000002815.
55. Han PY, Duffull SB, Kirkpatrick CM, Green B. Dosing in obesity: a simple solution to a big problem. Clin Pharmacol Therap. 2007;82(5):505–8. https://doi.org/10.1038/sj.clpt.6100381.
56. Holzman RS, Mancuso TJ, Polaner DM, Chatterjee D. A practical approach to pediatric anesthesia. 2nd ed. Philadelphia, PA: Wolters Kluwer; 2016. p. 806–20.

57. Smit C, De Hoogd S, Brüggemann RJM, Knibbe CA. Obesity and drug pharmacology: a review of the influence of obesity on pharmacokinetic and pharmacodynamic parameters. Expert Opin Drug Metab Toxicol. 2018;14(3):275–85. https://doi.org/10.1080/17425255.2018.1440287.
58. Gerhart JG, Balevic S, Sinha J, et al. Characterizing pharmacokinetics in children with obesity—physiological, drug, patient, and methodological considerations. Front Pharmacol. 2022:13. https://doi.org/10.3389/fphar.2022.818726.
59. Halvorson EE, Ervin SE, Russell TB, Skelton JA, Davis S, Spangler J. Association of obesity and pediatric venous thromboembolism. Hosp Pediatr. 2016;6(1):22–6. https://doi.org/10.1542/hpeds.2015-0039.
60. Vaughns JD, Ziesenitz VC, Williams EF, Nadler EP, Mikus G, van den Anker J. Prophylactic use of enoxaparin in adolescents during bariatric surgery—a prospective clinical study. Obes Surg. 2019;30(1):63–8. https://doi.org/10.1007/s11695-019-04135-5.
61. Soleimanpour H, Safari S, Sanaie S, Nazari M, Alavian SM. Anesthetic considerations in patients undergoing bariatric surgery: a review article. Anesthesiol Pain Med. 2017;7(4) https://doi.org/10.5812/aapm.57568.
62. Alvarez A, Singh PM, Sinha AC. Postoperative analgesia in morbid obesity. Obes Surg. 2014;24(4):652–9. https://doi.org/10.1007/s11695-014-1185-2.
63. Mittal T, Dey A, Siddhartha R, Nali A, Sharma B, Malik V. Efficacy of ultrasound-guided transversus abdominis plane (tap) block for postoperative analgesia in laparoscopic gastric sleeve resection: a randomized single blinded case control study. Surg Endosc. 2018;32(12):4985–9. https://doi.org/10.1007/s00464-018-6261-6.
64. Jalali SM, Bahri MH, Yazd SM, Karoobi M, Shababi N. Efficacy of laparoscopic transversus abdominis plane block on postoperative pain management and surgery side effects in laparoscopic bariatric surgeries. Langenbeck's Arch Surg. 2022;407(2):549–57. https://doi.org/10.1007/s00423-021-02400-9.
65. Amer GF, Hamed H, Salim MS, Hegazy MA. Effect of adding hydrocortisone to intraperitoneal bupivacaine in laparoscopic bariatric surgery. Anesth Essays Res. 2020;14(1):137. https://doi.org/10.4103/aer.aer_141_19.
66. Vaughns JD, Martin C, Nelson J, Nadler E, Quezado ZM. Dexmedetomidine as an adjuvant for perioperative pain management in adolescents undergoing bariatric surgery: an observational cohort study. J Pediatr Surg. 2017;52(11):1787–90. https://doi.org/10.1016/j.jpedsurg.2017.04.007. Epub 2017 Apr 19

Confusion and Sudden Onset of Left Sided Weakness in a Patient with Sickle Cell Disease (SCD) After Gall Bladder Surgery

Robert Scott Dingeman

Learning Objectives
By the end of this chapter, readers will be able to:

1. Describe the natural history and prevalence of SCD in children and its association with other disease states.
2. Summarize the most common perioperative risk factors for children with SCD undergoing elective surgeries.
3. Identify strategies to optimize perioperative preparation and conduct general anesthesia in the patient with SCD.
4. Differentiate between the most common postoperative complications in SCD patients and approaches to prevent their occurrence.
5. Formulate perioperative management plans for children with SCD that minimize postoperative morbidity and mortality.

1 Case Study Part I

A 9-year-old female presents to the preoperative clinic for evaluation prior to a laparoscopic cholecystectomy. The patient's mother accompanies her and states that her daughter has a history of sickle cell disease (SCD) and has had multiple vaso-occlusive crises (VOC) in the past requiring inpatient admissions for treatment but that she had not had any admissions or transfusions in the past 6 months prior to

R. S. Dingeman (✉)
The George Washington University School of Medicine and Health Sciences, Washington, DC, USA

Department of Anesthesiology, Pain and Perioperative Medicine, Children's National Hospital, Washington, DC, USA
e-mail: rdingeman@childrensnational.org

S. T. Verghese (ed.), *Anesthesia STAT! Acute Pediatric Emergencies in PACU*,
https://doi.org/10.1007/978-3-031-24396-7_24

surgery. The mother also says that her daughter had an adenotonsillectomy for OSA as a toddler but had no anesthetic complications and reports no known drug allergies. She denies any other significant past medical history or surgeries. She takes oral hydroxyurea and a multivitamin daily, but no other medications.

1.1 What Is Sickle Cell Disease (SCD)?

Hemoglobin (Hb), a protein located inside erythrocytes, is found in predominantly three forms. Hemoglobin A (also known as adult hemoglobin, A_1, or α2β2) is the most common making up 95–98% of hemoglobin and consists of two α and two β-globin chains. Hemoglobin A_2 ($\alpha_2\delta_2$) and fetal hemoglobin ($\alpha_2\gamma_2$) are less common, and other forms of hemoglobin, such as C, D, and E, are even more rare [1]. The α- and β-globin chains that make up HbA are produced by the genes known as HBA and HBB, respectively. Hemoglobin S (HbS), or sickle hemoglobin, occurs when a nucleotide, specifically glutamic acid, is substituted for valine at the sixth position on the HBB gene causing an abnormal version of the β-globin chain [1]. HbS proteins have the potential when oxygen is low to stick together inside erythrocytes forming long chains called polymers. Polymerization subsequentially produces conformational changes of erythrocytes altering their shape into sickles or crescent-like shapes resembling the harvesting tool (Fig. 1). When a child inherits the mutated allele from both parents, they are homozygous recessive for HbS and have sickle cell disease, also known as SCD or HbSS. Sickle cell trait (SCT), which generally bears no clinical significance, is a heterozygous and often benign state that occurs when a person inherits one normal hemoglobin and one abnormal β-globin gene, such as β-thalassemia (HbSβ), C (HbSC), or D-Punjab (HbSD) [2].

Although SCD is considered a genetic disorder, environmental factors in history may have triggered the first mutation of the gene [3]. The outbreak of plasmodium falciparum malaria in Africa, India, and the Middle East, secondary to deforestation

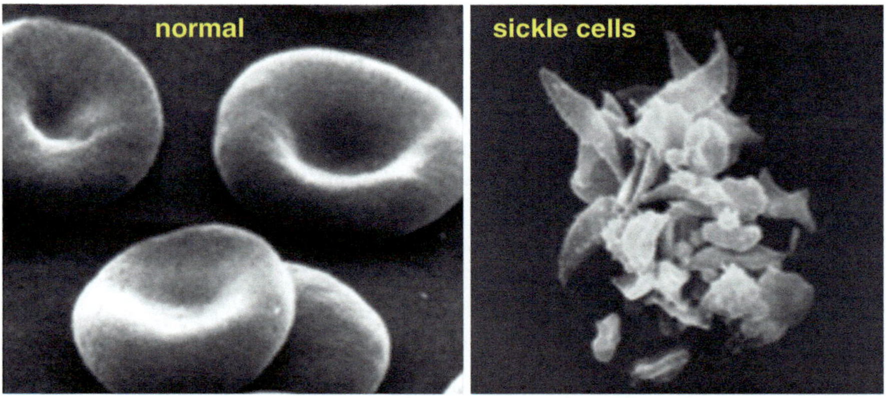

Fig. 1 Electron micrograph of red blood cells. (From Khurmi et al. [8])

and stagnant pools of water, coincides with the advent of the mutation. In the 1940s, J. B. S. Haladane observed that red blood cell disorders, such as SCD, were more common in areas where malaria was endemic and that individuals with these disorders did not contract malaria, and therefore he proposed the genetic link between the malaria endemic and the sickle cell gene (Haladane 1949) [3]. This theory may explain why SCD is more common among individuals of African descent.

SCD is diagnosed in nearly 275,000 children annually worldwide, and more than two million people throughout the world carry SCT [1, 4]. SCD is more common among African Americans with an incidence of 1 per 500 births and is estimated to affect between 70,000 and 100,000 Americans [5]. The life expectancy of Americans living with SCD is reduced to between 42 and 48 years due to complications of the disease, but improved newborn screening, vaccines, and antibiotic therapy, as well as other innovative treatments over the past two decades, have contributed to earlier diagnosis, better treatment options, and longer survival of individuals living with SCD [6, 7].

1.2 What Are the Most Common Clinical Presentations of SCD?

Individuals with SCD may not exhibit symptoms when their erythrocytes are behaving normally and are cylindrically shaped. Hypoxia may trigger polymerization of HbS and subsequent sickling of erythrocytes leading to an acute painful episode often referred to as a "sickle cell crisis" or vaso-occlusive crisis (VOC). Acidosis which decreases hemoglobin's affinity for oxygen may also cause sickling. Dehydration not only contributes to sickling by decreasing the osmolality of plasma which increases the concentration of HbS inside the erythrocyte but also decreases the volume and increases the viscosity of plasma resulting in slower blood flow through capillaries. Hypothermia triggers vasoconstriction limiting blood flow to organs which can also decrease the exchange of oxygen by the lungs worsening hypoxia and sickling. VOC symptoms and severity vary between individuals, but hemolytic anemia, infection, and organ damage can result from VOC [3].

Ninety percent of children have nonfunctioning spleens by the age of 6 due to multiple splenic microinfarcts secondary to VOC which leads to an increased risk of infection [2]. Acute chest syndrome (ACS) results when there is an area of poor ventilation within the lungs from an infection, such as RSV, causing a V/Q mismatch which leads to hypoxia, acidosis, and subsequent sickling which in turn leads to poor pulmonary perfusion and worsening hypoxia and further sickling [2]. ACS is more common in children between the ages of 2 and 4, and they often present with fever, respiratory symptoms, and chest pain [2]. The major clinical expressions of SCD are listed in Table 1. In addition to ACS, other serious life-threatening complications can occur, such as cerebrovascular accident, myocardial infarction, aplastic anemia, and acute renal failure. The most common permanent sequelae in patients with SCD are ischemic stroke and silent cerebral infarcts that can lead to cognitive impairment, disability, and death and occur in approximately 20% of

Table 1 Clinical expressions of sickle cell disease [7]

System	Clinical manifestations
Pulmonary	Acute chest syndrome, pulmonary hypertension, pulmonary infarction, asthma, airway hyperreactivity
Cardiac	Elevated cardiac output and cardiac enlargement, cardiac autonomic dysfunction, vasoocclusion of coronary arteries
Central nervous system	Ischemic stroke
Genitourinary	Renal failure, hematuria, renal tubular acidosis, priapism, nocturnal enuresis
Musculoskeletal	Dactylitis, osteomyelitis, bone infarction, osteopenia, osteoporosis, avascular necrosis
Hematological	Hemolytic anemia, acute a plastic anemia
Vascular	Leg ulcers
Immunological	Predisposed to infection due to functional asplenia and defective neutrophil responses, erythrocyte auto/alloimmunization, hemolytic transfusion reactions
Hepatobiliary	Increased risk of acute/chronic cholecystitis, bilirubin gallstones, chronic liver abnormalities, distended hepatic sinusoids, hepatomegaly
Eye	Sickle cell retinopathy
Spleen	Splenomegaly, splenic infarction leading to "autosplenectomy"
Other	*Pregnancy*: 30–50% preterm delivery, 20% low birth weight; increased rates of preeclampsia/eclampsia, intrauterine growth retardation, gestational hypertension, and Cesarean section, 20–50% higher mortality rate for mothers during pregnancy

patients with SCD by the age of 40 [9]. According to the US Cooperative Study of SCD, ischemic stroke is more likely to occur between the ages of 2 and 9 [10].

Hydroxyurea, the most prescribed medication for the treatment of SCD, reduces the incidence of VOC, ACS, and mortality [8]. The drug stimulates HbF formation, releases endogenous nitric oxide improving blood flow, and decreases the production of leukocytes and reticulocytes that cause inflammation [8]. Hydroxyurea and chronic transfusion therapy have been used to prevent ischemic stroke [10]. Symptomatic treatment for VOC continues to be hydration, supplemental oxygen with incentive spirometry, and aggressive pain management. Children under the age of 16 with severe complications from the disease may be eligible for a hematopoietic stem cell transplant [8].

1.3 What Are the Most Common Elective Surgeries in Children with SCD?

Children living with SCD may undergo inpatient and outpatient surgeries for similar reasons as children without SCD or for complications associated with their disease. The most common elective surgeries that children with SCD present to the operating room for are cholecystectomy, adenotonsillectomy, splenectomy, umbilical hernia repair, appendectomy, myringotomy, inguinal hernia repair, and hip replacement [2, 11]. Children with SCD may have high unconjugated bilirubin levels chronically leading to gallstones requiring gall bladder removal. In addition, more than two episodes of acute splenic sequestration may necessitate splenectomy. Avascular necrosis of the hip resulting from poor bone perfusion may require a total hip replacement for pain management and mobility [2].

1.4 What Other Disease States Are Associated With Sickle Cell Disease and May Affect Perioperative Outcomes?

Children with SCD are predisposed to vasculopathies. Moyamoya disease (MMD) is the presence of idiopathic internal carotid stenosis. Moyamoya is a Japanese word meaning "puff-of-smoke" which is how the stenotic arteries appear on cerebral angiogram (Fig. 2). When this stenosis occurs in the setting of SCD, it is called moyamoya syndrome [1]. Sickle cell-induced moyamoya syndrome (SCD-MMS) has been reported to occur in as many as 43% of all patients with SCD and occurs more commonly in SCD patients with abnormal transcranial Doppler (TCD) velocities [10]. Although TCD velocities can be used to screen SCD patients for cerebral vasculopathy, a cerebral angiogram or MRI should be done to confirm the diagnosis of SCD-MMS. SCD-MMS patients have greater than 12 times the risk of cerebral infarction making them high risk for neurologic complications especially perioperatively [10, 12, 13]. They also have three times the risk of having two or more cerebrovascular events during their lifetime when compared to SCD patients without MMS [13]. Hydroxyurea and chronic transfusion therapy have been used to prevent ischemic stroke in patients with SCD-MMS, but a systematic review of outcomes found that patients who underwent early indirect revascularization had lower rates of recurrent stroke and therefore suggest that early surgical intervention is safe and efficacious and may reduce the risk of future neurologic complications associated with SCD-MMS [10, 12, 13]. Patients undergoing revascularization surgery should have intraoperative EEG monitoring to assess cerebral blood flow [14].

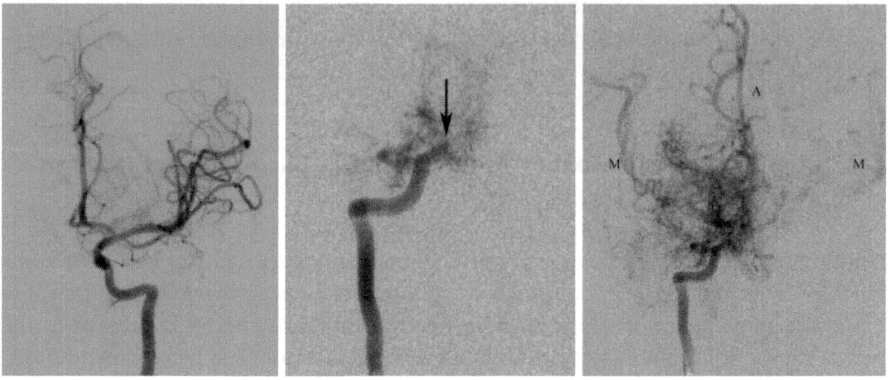

Image 1: Normal left internal carotid artery without stenosis.

Image 2: AP view of right internal carotid artery during early arterial phase with the characteristic "puff-of-smoke" collaterals

Image 3: AP view of right internal carotid artery during late arterial phase with the characteristic "puff-of-smoke" collaterals

Fig. 2 Angiographic findings of moyamoya [15]. AP views from a right internal carotid artery (ICA) angiogram during early and late arterial phases show occlusion of the terminal ICA (↓) with multiple moyamoya collaterals reconstituting the right middle cerebral (M) and anterior cerebral (A) territories. There is faint opacification of the left middle cerebral artery territory across a patent anterior communicating artery. (Images courtesy of Monica Pearl, M.D., Director of the Neurointerventional Radiology Program at Children's National Hospital)

1.5 Why Is This Patient Having an Elective Laparoscopic Cholecystectomy?

Prophylactic cholecystectomies help avoid emergency surgery for acute complications of SCD, such as cholecystitis, choledocholithiasis, and cholangitis, allowing for careful perioperative planning and optimization that decrease morbidity and mortality associated with sickle cell patients undergoing surgery [16]. In addition, elective laparoscopic cholecystectomies for asymptomatic cholelithiasis decrease hospital admissions for symptoms and complications associated with gall bladder disease [16]. Unlike the general population, over 50% of patients with SCD diagnosed with cholelithiasis develop complications within 3–5 years of their diagnosis compared to only 2–5% of the general population [16].

1.6 How Will You Preoperatively Assess Sickle Cell Patients and Plan for Surgery?

Since there are no published reports that preoperative screening for SCD decreases perioperative morbidity or mortality, routine preoperative screening for SCD is not recommended especially if neonatal screening is available locally [11]. If neonatal screening is not available, some researchers argue that preoperative screening for SCD in regions where malaria remains endemic should be considered although this may not be practical or affordable in resource-poor countries [11]. Most researchers agree that tailored perioperative care for children with SCD who are under 6 months of age presenting for surgery is unnecessary, since infants rarely manifest SCD-associated symptoms [14].

For those patients with SCD who are older than 6 months of age, a preoperative evaluation is recommended either in person or virtually to ensure the patient is medically optimized prior to surgery [17]. Additional goals of the preoperative evaluation are to estimate the risk associated with the surgery and create an individualized anesthetic plan that will minimize perioperative complications associated with SCD [17].

A thorough history and complete physical examination should be performed. A detailed history of pain and pain treatment strategies should be documented and may assist in perioperative pain management, especially in patients who have developed chronic pain, central desensitization, hyperalgesia syndrome, and opioid tolerance [11]. Many researchers recommend a detailed nervous system exam including TCD velocities, cerebral angiography, or MRI preoperatively to screen for SCD-MMS and other vasculopathies that may increase the risk of stroke [11]. An echocardiogram should be obtained for patients with a history of cardiac disease and obstructive sleep apnea. A complete blood count with differential should be obtained preoperatively, especially for those patients taking hydroxyurea which can cause neutropenia. Hemoglobin S percentage should be determined by electrophoresis or high-performance liquid chromatography prior to any medium- to high-risk surgery [11]. Since many SCD patients have had a prior blood transfusion and therefore mounted an immune response (i.e., alloimmunization), a type and crossmatch should be done prior to surgery even if intraoperative transfusion is unlikely. Other laboratory studies, such as renal and liver function tests and a chest radiograph, should be tailored to the patient's history and the procedure being performed.

Preoperative counseling to the patient and caregivers on how to avoid triggers of VOC, such as anxiety, stress, infection, and dehydration, should be included in the preoperative discussion [7, 17]. Many patients report that anxiety and stress, both physical and emotional, can precipitate VOC [7]. Anxiety can cause breath-holding and hypoxia triggering VOC. Patients with SCD should be scheduled as the first case of the day to reduce anxiety and minimize the risk of dehydration from prolonged fasting. Ambulatory surgery should be discouraged since patients must be monitored by experienced clinicians postoperatively for complications, although some argue that ambulatory surgery can be done safely if the patient is the first surgery of the day leaving plenty of time for postoperative monitoring [2, 11]. Children with SCD should be allowed to drink clear liquids up until the time of surgery or be admitted 1 day prior for IV fluid management to avoid dehydration [11]. A multidisciplinary team of specialists familiar with SCD that includes a hematologist, anesthesiologist, surgeon, blood bank specialist, and possible intensivist (if needed) should be available prior to admission [2, 11]. To avoid atelectasis, hypoxia, and other pulmonary complications that may lead to VOC, patients should be encouraged to perform incentive spirometry regularly both pre- and postoperatively [17].

Bicarbonate treatment to prevent acidosis has been suggested, but there is insufficient evidence [11]. Surgery should be postponed if the patient demonstrates signs of active, acute, or subacute infection [11].

1.7 Will You Transfuse a Sickle Cell Patient Prior to Surgery?

Preoperative transfusions remain controversial, and studies are limited and underpowered due to insufficient recruitment and loss to follow-up [4, 8, 11, 17, 19]. Nevertheless, several randomized controlled trials advocate for preoperative blood transfusions [8, 11, 17]. The largest cohort of SCD surgical patients to date from the 1990s reported lower rates of postoperative complications undergoing low-risk procedures in patients who received preoperative transfusions [17]. A multicenter randomized controlled trial from 2013 of patients over the age of 1 with red blood cell disorders presenting for low- to medium-risk surgery described a significantly higher rate of perioperative complications, especially ACS, in patients who were not transfused and reported no transfusion reactions [11, 19, 20]. Another analysis of 79 patients with SCD and abnormal TCD velocities found a higher rate of new MRI brain infarcts among patients who discontinued chronic transfusion therapy and therefore recommend transfusion therapy for SCD patients with a high risk of having cerebrovascular events [18, 19]. Another systematic review and meta-analysis of preoperative transfusion in patients with SCD found no difference in mortality or perioperative complications between patients who received preoperative exchange or simple transfusions and those who did not [4, 17]. Despite varying reports, preoperative transfusions of packed red blood cells up to a hemoglobin of 10 g dL^{-1} have become commonplace for all children undergoing low- to medium-risk surgery in the United States [2]. For children undergoing high-risk surgery, such as neurosurgery, cardiothoracic surgery, or major orthopedic surgery, or who are at high risk for perioperative complications due to previous stroke, ACS, or renal failure, exchange transfusions aiming for a hemoglobin of 10 g dL^{-1} and HbS < 30% are recommended [2, 18, 19].

2 Case Study Part II

The patient has arrived in the preoperative unit on the day of surgery. She has no peripheral IV.

2.1 How Will You Induce and Maintain Anesthesia, and What Intraoperative Management Strategies Benefit Patients with SCD?

All anesthesia techniques and standard medications can be used in SCD patients, if the primary goal of avoiding triggering erythrocytes to sickle is prioritized.

Oxygenation, hydration, normothermia, and analgesia should all be maintained to prevent VOC [11]. Preoperative anxiolysis may be required, since perioperative anxiety can lead to breath-holding, hypoxia, and sickling [8]. During the induction and emergence of anesthesia, obstruction and laryngospasm should be avoided or rapidly diagnosed and treated to minimize hypoxia. Hypoventilation and atelectasis should also be avoided, so controlled ventilation and the use of muscle relaxants may be preferred especially for laparoscopic procedures. To reduce the risk of infection postoperatively, prophylactic antibiotic administration is recommended for all procedures. The use of intraoperative tourniquets in sickle cell patients undergoing orthopedic surgery remains controversial, because there are no randomized controlled trials offering conclusive evidence. Some argue that tourniquets cause stasis, hypoxia, and acidosis which can trigger polymerization and sickling, but there are many reports of tourniquets being used in SCD patients without complications when vigilance is maintained. Overall, the benefits of less blood loss and therefore the avoidance of hypotension may outweigh the risk of the tourniquet triggering VOC [2, 3, 17]. Cell salvage is not recommended in sickle cell patients. Hypotension should be aggressively treated with intravenous fluids, vasopressors, and transfusions of red blood cells to a hemoglobin above 9–10 g dL^{-1}.

Since patients with SCD have an increased risk of perioperative stroke, cerebral oximetry or near-infrared spectroscopy (NIRS) may be a useful perioperative tool to assess brain oxygenation. Although studies have shown that children with SCD have lower cerebral oxygen saturation (% rSO_2) compared to normal individuals, there is no difference in NIRS spectra absorbance and therefore NIRS is a valid tool that may detect early perioperative changes in brain oxygenation in children with SCD [21].

Regional anesthesia can be safely used with or without general anesthesia for perioperative analgesia. Neuraxial anesthesia may provide superior analgesia and a sympathectomy causing vasodilation and improved blood flow, but hypotension and bradycardia should be avoided to decrease the risk of triggering VOC [8]. Transversus abdominis plane, erector spinae plane, quadratus lumborum, or rectus sheath single-shot blocks or catheters should be considered, especially for abdominal surgery such as cholecystectomy or splenectomy [2]. Multimodal analgesia that includes regional anesthesia techniques, NMDA antagonists such as ketamine, and α_2-agonist such as dexmedetomidine and clonidine are recommended to prevent hypoventilation associated with opioids but may also improve analgesia in patients with chronic pain from central sensitization and opioid-induced hyperalgesia. Acetaminophen and NSAIDs should be used with caution in patients with liver and renal disease.

If contrast is required for cardiac or neurologic procedures, hyperosmolar contrast media should be avoided since it may induce dehydration and subsequent polymerization and sickling. Isotonic contrast media should be used instead [17]. All contrast should be avoided in patients with renal disease.

The risk of a deep venous thromboembolism (DVT) is approximately 12% for SCD patients under the age of 40 years, so DVT prophylaxis with low-molecular weight heparin or low-dose unfractionated heparin is recommended [14, 17].

3 Case Study Part III

The patient is admitted to the post-anesthesia care unit (PACU) after surgery. The bedside nurse calls asking for someone to come evaluate the patient, because she appears confused with new-onset left-sided weakness.

3.1 What Are the Most Common Complications After Elective Surgery in Children with SCD?

There is a significant increase in cardiac, respiratory, and wound complications including pulmonary embolism, surgical site infection, and systemic infection in patients with a diagnosis of SCD as compared to the general population [22]. Vaso-occlusive episodes, ACS, and infection are the most common complications after surgery [23].

The most common symptom associated with vaso-occlusion is pain which can be severe and occurs more frequently in the long bones, back, chest, and abdomen [23]. Young children may present with dactylitis or pain in the hands and feet [23]. Pain management is key to postoperative care, and both long-acting and short-acting opioids should be considered. Alternatively, intravenous opioids may be administered by a patient-controlled analgesia (IV-PCA) pump with both continuous and demand features in patients expected to be admitted to the hospital after surgery [11]. There is a higher incidence of ACS after open abdominal surgery compared to laparoscopy, and therefore laparoscopic techniques are beneficial to patients with SCD [2].

All patients with SCD have a higher risk of postoperative stroke compared to the general population, but patients with abnormal TCD velocities and SCD-MMS are particularly susceptible to cerebrovascular events during and after surgery [2]. After splenectomy, thrombocytosis is common due to the unopposed effect of chronic bone marrow hyperactivity, and therefore SCD patients undergoing splenectomy have a higher risk of neurologic events as well [2, 24].

3.2 What Is Your Differential Diagnosis in the Patient With a New-Onset Neurologic Deficit?

The differential diagnosis for a patient with postoperative neurologic symptoms includes but is not limited to prolonged anesthesia, opioid overdose, seizure, metabolic encephalopathy, sepsis, hypotension, stroke, conversion disorder, emergence agitation/delirium, or a regional anesthesia complication. Ischemic stroke is more common in SCD patients than hemorrhagic stroke due to the sickling of erythrocytes, vasoconstriction, and hypercoagulability. Postoperative neurologic changes should be addressed straightaway, and ischemic stroke should be confirmed by computed tomography (CT) as soon as possible so that blood flow may be restored quickly to reduce the risk of long-term neurologic deficits [9]. If a stroke is suspected, consult neurology and neurosurgery immediately.

3.3 What Therapeutic Interventions Should Be Initiated for Neurologic Complications After Surgery?

If a transient ischemic attack or ischemic stroke is suspected or confirmed postoperatively, the American Society of Hematology (ASH) guideline panel recommends blood transfusion by simple modified exchange or apheresis immediately. If an exchange transfusion is not readily available within 2 h of the neurologic event and the patient's Hb is <8.5 g/dL, the ASH recommends immediate simple transfusions of packed red blood cells while the exchange transfusion or apheresis are being planned. Although intravenous (IV) tissue plasminogen activator (tPA) is recommended for adults within 4.5 h of neurologic symptoms consistent with acute ischemic stroke who show no evidence of intracranial hemorrhage on computed tomography (CT), IV tPA is not recommended for children <18 years of age with SCD [9]. The patient should be admitted to an intensive care or stroke unit as soon as possible.

3.4 What Other Interventions Should Be Considered Postoperatively for All Patients With SCD to Prevent Complications?

Since SCD patients are at increased risk of atelectasis, hypoxia, and other pulmonary complications that may lead to VOC and ACS, supplemental oxygen should be administered, and patients should be encouraged to perform incentive spirometry regularly postoperatively [5, 17]. All SCD patients should be monitored for fever and other signs of infection [14, 17]. Postoperative pain should be managed using a multimodal approach that balances the judicious use of analgesics to prevent splinting and breath-holding from pain as well as the risk of respiratory depression from opioids [2, 12]. Both long-acting and short-acting intravenous or oral opioids can be used for constant postoperative and breakthrough pain, respectively [17]. For patients who are expected to remain NPO postoperatively, an IV-PCA containing morphine or hydromorphone may be beneficial [5]. Urine output must be monitored, and a complete metabolic panel should be considered to assess for renal damage and electrolyte abnormalities. If necessary, an arterial blood gas and CXR, in addition to a physical examination, should be performed to diagnose ACS [2].

4 Case Study Part IV

The patient's postoperative neurologic symptoms in the PACU are consistent with a transient ischemic attack or ischemic stroke, and therefore she was transferred to the pediatric intensive care unit (PICU) immediately where she received an exchange transfusion that increased her hemoglobin to >10 g dl^{-1}. Neurosurgery and neurology were consulted, and an emergent CT of the brain showed no evidence of intracranial hemorrhage. She remained in the PICU overnight for frequent neurologic checks but did not receive tPA due to her age. Her symptoms resolved within 24 h, and she was eventually transferred to a regular floor on postoperative day two. She was discharged on postoperative day three without any permanent sequelae tolerating a regular diet. She and her family were instructed to follow up with neurosurgery for suspected SCD-MMS.

5 Summary and Conclusion

Children with SCD are at increased risk of morbidity and mortality during the perioperative period, and therefore careful preoperative assessment and planning are essential to reduce postoperative complications, such as ischemic stroke seen in this patient. SCD patients with abnormal TCD velocities are especially at risk for postoperative cerebrovascular events, and therefore all SCD patients should be screened preoperatively for SCD-MMS. Patients with SCD-MMS should consider early indirect revascularization surgery, which has been shown to be safe and efficacious in reducing the lifetime risk of cerebral infarcts and neurologic complications, prior to other elective surgeries. SCD-MMS patients having revascularization surgery should be monitored intraoperatively using EEG. Laparoscopic surgery, rather than open abdominal surgery, lowers the risk of postoperative ACS. Although preoperative transfusions remain controversial in SCD patients who do not have MMS, all SCD patients having major surgery should be transfused to a hemoglobin of 10 g dL^{-1} and a HbS < 30% to reduce the risk of perioperative complications. Perioperative reduction of hypoxia, hypothermia, hypotension, and acidosis reduces the likelihood of polymerization and sickling. Tourniquets can be used safely intraoperatively to reduce blood loss and minimize hypotension, but cell salvage is not recommended. Antibiotic and DVT prophylaxis are important to prevent infection and blood clots, respectively. Regional anesthesia can be done safely and may improve analgesia and blood flow to the surgical site reducing the risk of sickling. Pre- and postoperative incentive spirometry can reduce the incidence of ACS. NIRS may be a useful tool to detect changes in brain oxygenation and therefore reduce the risk of ischemic stroke perioperatively in patients with abnormal TCD velocities or SCD-MMS. All SCD patients should be monitored postoperatively and neurologic changes should be addressed and treated immediately to avoid long-term sequelae.

References

1. Scarlet S, Sweeting RS, Attaga KI, Redding-Lallinger RC, Meyer AA. An interdisciplinary perioperative management protocol for patients with sickle cell anemia: a single-surgeon experience. Am Surg. 2018;84:1120–2.
2. Akrimi S, Simiyu V. Anaesthetic management of children with sickle cell disease. BJA Educ. 2018;18(11):331–6.
3. Paradowski K. Pathophysiology and perioperative management of sickle cell disease. J Perioper Pract. 2015;25(6):101–4.
4. Alotaibi GS, Alsaleh K, Bolster L, McMurtry MS, Wu C. Preoperative transfusion in patients with sickle cell disease to prevent perioperative complications: a systematic review and meta-analysis. Hematology. 2014;19(8):463–71.
5. Howard J, Malfroy M, Llewelyn C, et al. The transfusion alternatives preoperatively in sickle cell disease (TAPS) study: a randomized, controlled, multicenter clinical trial. Lancet. 2013;381:930–8.
6. Cusano J, Curry EJ, Kingston KA, Klings E, Li X. Epidemiology and perioperative complications in patients with sickle cell disease after orthopedic surgery: 26 years' experience at a major academic center. J Am Acad Orthop Surg. 2019;27:e1043–51.
7. Stanley AC, Christian JM. Sickle cell disease and perioperative considerations: review and retrospective report. J Oral Maxillofac Surg. 2013;71:1027–33.
8. Khurmi N, Gorlin A, Misra L. Perioperative considerations for patients with sickle cell disease: a narrative review. Can J Anesth. 2017;64:860–9.
9. DeBaun MR, Jordan LC, King AA, Schatz J, Vichinsky E, Fox CK, McKinstry RC, Telfer P, Kraut MA, Daraz L, Kirkham FJ, Murad MH. American Society of Hematology 2020 guidelines for sickle cell disease: prevention, diagnosis, and treatment of cerebrovascular disease in children and adults. Blood Adv. 2020;4(8):1554–88.
10. Aguilar-Salinas P, Hayward K, Santos R, Agarwal V, Sauvageau E, Hanel RA, Aldana PR. Surgical revascularization for pediatric patients with sickle cell disease and moyamoya disease in the prevention of ischemic strokes: a single-center case series and a systematic review. World Neurosurg. 2019;123:435–442.e8.
11. Schyrr F, Dolci M, Nydegger M, Canellini G, Andreu-Ullrich H, Joseph JM, Diezi M, Cachat F, Rizzi M, Renella R. Perioperative care of children with sickle cell disease: a systematic review and clinical recommendations. Am J Hematol. 2020;95:78–96.
12. Newman S, Boulter JH, Malcolm JG, Pradilla I, Pradilla G. Outcomes in patients with moyamoya syndrome and sickle cell disease: a systematic review. World Neurosurg. 2020;135:165–70.
13. Yang W, Xu R, Porras JL, Takemoto CM, Khalid S, Garzon-Muvdi T, Caplan JM, Colby GP, Coon AL, Tamargo RJ, Huang J, Ahn ES. Effectiveness of surgical revascularization for stroke prevention in pediatric patients with sickle cell disease and moyamoya syndrome. J Neurosurg Pediatr. 2017;20(3):232–8.
14. Oyedeji CI, Welsby IJ. Optimizing management of sickle cell disease in patients undergoing surgery. Hematol Am Soc Hematol Educ Program. 2021;1:403–10.
15. Scott RM, Smith ER. Moyamoya disease and moyamoya syndrome. N Engl J Med. 2009;360:1226–37.
16. Muroni M, Loi V, Lionnet F, Girot R, Houry S. Prophylactic laparoscopic cholecystectomy in adult sickle cell disease patients with cholelithiasis: a prospective cohort study. Int J Surg. 2015;22:62–6.
17. Adjepong KO, Otegbeye F, Adjepong YA. Perioperative management of sickle cell disease. Mediterr J Hematol Infect Dis. 2018;10:e2018032.
18. Abboud MR, Yim E, Musallam KM, Adams RJ, STOP II Study Investigators. Discontinuing prophylactic transfusions increases the risk of silent brain infarction in children with sickle cell disease: data from STOP II. Blood. 2011;118(4):894–8.

19. Fortin PM, Hopewell S, Estcourt LJ. Red blood cell transfusion to treat or prevent complications in sickle cell disease: an overview of Cochrane reviews. Cochrane Database Syst Rev. 2018;8(8):CD012082.
20. Hyder O, Yaster M, Bateman BT, Firth PG. Surgical procedures and outcomes among children with sickle cell disease. Anesth Analg. 2013;117(5):1192–6.
21. Nahavandi M, Nichols JP, Hassan M, Gandjbakhche A, Kato GJ. Near-infrared spectra absorbance of blood from sickle cell patients and normal individuals. Hematology. 2009;14(1):46–8.
22. Enayatollahi MA, Novack TA, Maltenfort MG, Tabatabaee RM, Chen AF, Parvizi J. In-hospital morbidity and mortality following total joint arthroplasty in patients with hemoglobinopathies. J Arthroplasty. 2015;30(8):1308–12.
23. Brumm J, White RS, Arroyo NS, Gaber-Baylis LK, Gupta S, Turnball ZA, Mehta N. Sickle cell disease is associated with increased morbidity, resource utilization, and readmission after common abdominal surgeries: a multi-state analysis, 2007-2014. J Natl Med Assoc. 2020;112(2):198–208.
24. Snyder CW, Bludevich BM, Gonzalez R, Danielson PD, Chandler NM. Risk factors for complications after abdominal surgery in children with sickle cell disease. J Pediatr Surg. 2021;56:711–6.

Profound Bradycardia in a Child After Dexmedetomidine Treatment for Agitation on Induction and After Extubation: To Treat or Not to Treat?

Alberto A. Rivera Cintron and Susan T. Verghese

Learning Objectives

1. Describe clinical challenges in anesthetic induction in children with autism.
2. Types of sedatives for noninvasive studies in uncooperative children.
3. Discuss the type of drugs and routes utilized for premedication, induction, and sedation.
4. Expand on the hemodynamic side effects of DEX.

1 Stem Case

A young 4-year-old 20 kg boy with autism is scheduled for anesthesia for brain auditory evoked response (BAER) test for suspected hearing loss. He does not speak much and flaps his hands when agitated, and his vital signs are not obtained because he refuses placement of any monitors. He takes melatonin for sleep and lives at home with his siblings. He is nonverbal and uncooperative, makes no eye contact with any one, and is anxious around strangers. He remains in his street clothes refusing to wear the hospital gown or to take oral premedication. The mother is adamant that he does not get a premedication shot especially since he already had an unpleasant experience of getting an IM shot of ketamine before a brain MRI study earlier. At that time, he had woken up screaming and inconsolable and seemed afraid. His birth history and neonatal and infancy period are significant for delay in achieving physical milestones, speech delay, and failure to gain weight due to his poor eating habits.

A. A. Rivera Cintron · S. T. Verghese (✉)
Children's National Medical Center, Washington, DC, USA
e-mail: ariveracin@childrensnational.org; sverghes@childrensnational.org

S. T. Verghese (ed.), *Anesthesia STAT! Acute Pediatric Emergencies in PACU*,
https://doi.org/10.1007/978-3-031-24396-7_25

The anesthetic induction plans A and B, as well as maintenance of general anesthesia with an LMA, were discussed in detail with the mother who wished to be present with him for the anesthetic induction.

The plan A discussed was induction with a facemask in the procedure room with the patient on his mother's lap followed by an intravenous line prior to placement of an LMA. Plan B was to squirt DEX into the nostril since the mother did not want any intramuscular injections.

In the procedure room, he sat on his mother's lap, who was given specific instruction to hold his hands in hers to encircle him while the child life specialist showed him his favorite video. As soon as the mask flavored with chocolate (as per mom's request) carrying oxygen and 6% sevoflurane was gently placed over his face, he screamed and attempted to wiggle out of his mother's arms. Since his mother was also distressed and unable to hold him, the anesthesiologist had to abandon plan A and resort to plan B.

Plan B was to administer nasal DEX by squirting it from a small syringe into his nostril. The syringe had a blunt-tip laryngeal atomizer which was primed ready for administration with the appropriate dose, 3 mcg per kg (total 60 mcg). While he was playing his video game with the child life specialist who was able to distract him once again after a few minutes of crying, the premedication was rapidly and expertly squirted into one of his nostrils with the mother and nurse holding him and the anesthesiologist approaching him from behind. The speedily administered nasal dexmedetomidine caused the child to scream and struggle for some time, but this time the hold on him was firm and there was no danger of him falling or hurting himself or others. Since the mother had been warned in detail about this quick nasal drug administration technique in plan B, this stealthy approach from behind the patient did not take her by surprise and she was able to help. Although he continued to cry, it was evident after about 5–7 min that he was getting a bit drowsy. He was moved slowly with the mother's help to the stretcher, and the monitors were placed prior to securing an IV and airway for the procedure. The mother was then escorted out of the procedure room to the parent waiting room by the child life specialist. The anesthetic induction continued with oxygen and sevoflurane while an intravenous line was started on his hand and covered with Coban self-adhesive wrap to secure it for postoperative need.

An LMA was placed following administration of 30 mg of propofol and secured and his head was placed in the midline position. The audiologist proceeded placing appropriate electrodes on the scalp and each ear lobe to initiate the brain auditory evoked response test (Figs. 1 and 2).

Anesthesia was maintained by sevoflurane, oxygen, and air via the LMA with spontaneous ventilation, and he received 100 cc of lactated Ringer's solution during this procedure. The heart rate was high shortly after placement of monitors in the OR and came down to the range of 60–80 per minute, and his BP was 80/50 to 90/54 with normal spontaneous ventilation and 100% oxygen saturation.

At the end of the 30-min procedure, he was placed on his side or lateral (recovery) position, LMA was removed, and the intravenous line was disconnected from the IV fluids. The Coban-covered intravenous catheter was secured further and covered with a cotton sock, taped well to prevent him from pulling it out in PACU.

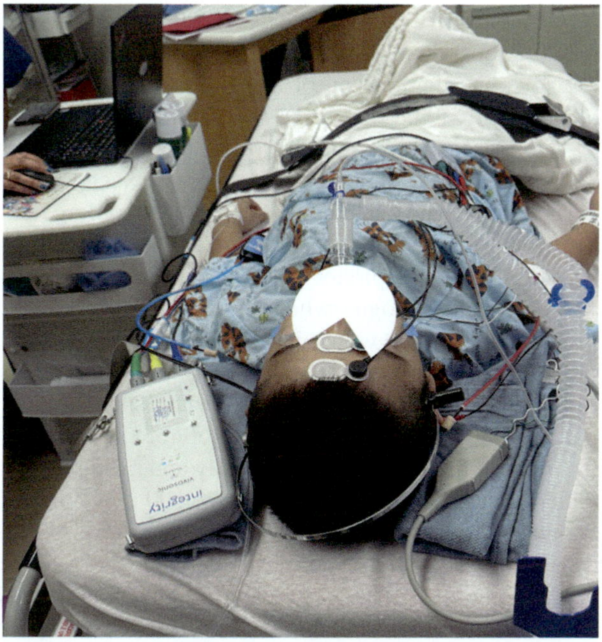

Fig. 1 Child anesthetized for BAER study

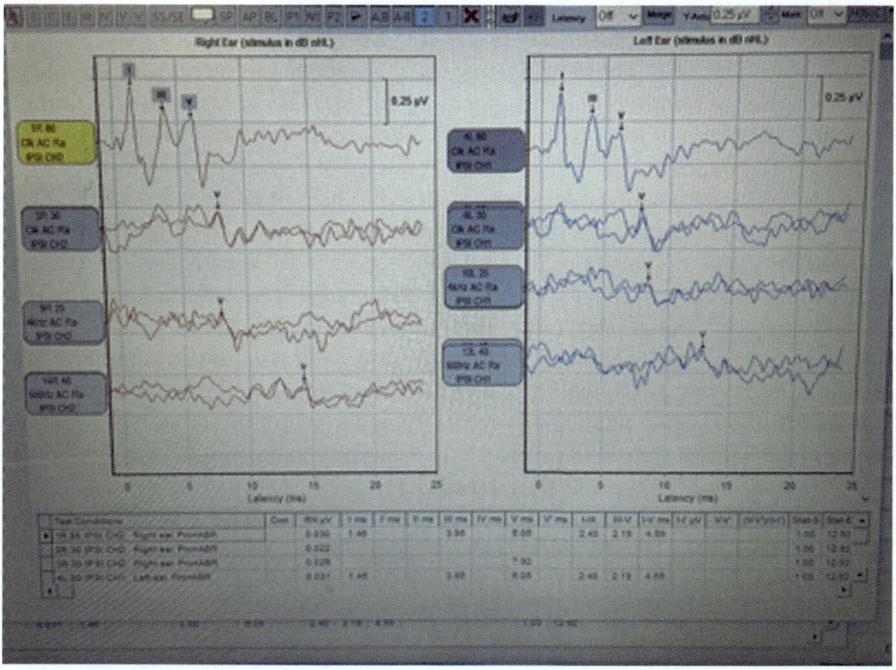

Fig. 2 ABR Results in a 4-year-old patient diagnosed with speech/language developmental delay. Testing completed as part of workup for autism. Auditory brainstem response (ABR) consistent with normal conductance of sound to the level of the brainstem (lateral lemniscus/inferior collisions) for 500–4000 Hz, bilaterally. Photo courtesy of Tracey Ambrose, AuD

On arrival in the PACU, he was taken to a side room with minimal noise, and the handoff report to PACU nurse included details about his phobias, ASD features, previous anesthetic, type of anesthetic induction, and need for his parents to be allowed early to be with him prior to emergence.

The parents were relieved to see their son lying on his side, with stable vital signs. His mother remarked that this was exactly how he was after the MRI but on awakening developed significant problems, pulling out iv catheter and monitors and screaming loudly. The heart rate on PACU admission was 80/min, blood pressure was 105/70, and respiratory rate was 20/min.

The anesthesiologist who was in PACU upon hearing this reminder from the mother about the previous anesthetic decided to give another dose of dexmedetomidine (0.5 mcg/kg to a total of 10 mcg) prophylactically (a "gilding-the-lily" situation), and that is when the unexpected hemodynamic response occurred. The patient's heart rate slowed down to 60/min and further lowered to 38–40/min with the monitor beginning to alarm loudly and raising the anxiety of all those around the patient. The decision to give 0.1 mg (100 mcg) of glycopyrrolate (5 mcg/kg body weight) intravenously to prevent further lowering of heart rate was made, and the drug was immediately administered. The heart rate increased to 130 min, and the next blood pressure showed an alarming increase to 180/100. The BP cuff was then tried in all four limbs and showed the BP to be persistently high. Intravenous propofol was administered in doses of 1–2 mg per kg (20–40 mg, in 10 mg increments) with the patient lying on his side and an oxygen mask placed close to his face. The patient was sedated, spontaneously breathing, 100% oxygen by face mask, and his oxygen saturation was consistently normal throughout this period of significant hemodynamic fluctuations. The exaggerated BP increase was eventually brought down to a high normal level with a few more boluses of intravenous propofol (total of 160 mg in 30 min).

When his hemodynamic status was assessed to be normal after an hour, he was moved to his mother's lap with the monitors still in place and the room lights dimmed for a smooth wake up. Eventually when he woke up, his mother held and rocked him. His father played his video, and the nurse watched the family from a short distance without approaching them or causing him any agitation.

The iv catheter was eventually removed an hour later with him crying during the process, and he was discharged 4 h later after monitoring for continuous hemodynamic stability. Despite the hemodynamic fluctuation after the treatment of bradycardia in the patient, the quality of wake up according to his mother was better than when he woke up after the anesthesia for his MRI.

The parents though anxious initially were able to be calmed down and they and the PACU nurse had several questions regarding the exaggerated BP increase with the treatment of bradycardia with intravenous glycopyrrolate.

Key Questions

1. *What happened to his HR and BP in PACU?*
2. *Could you have avoided this HR/BP problems by choosing another drug for anesthetic induction and maintenance?*
3. *What can be done differently in the future?*

2 Discussion

2.1 Autism and ASD

The number children with autism and autism spectrum disorders (ASD) has risen in the last two decades. CDC researchers reported that autism rates in the USA increased from 1 in 150 children in 2000 to 1 in 54 in 2016 and stands at 1 in 44 today. Autism or autism spectrum disorder refers to a range of neurological developmental disabilities characterized by challenges in children with social and communication skills, repetitive behaviors, delayed speech, and often inability to make eye contact. Children with autism have difficulty with loud noises, bright lights, and crowds and often like to be left alone since they lack any interest in interacting with others around them.

Anesthesia induction in children with autism and autism spectrum disorders can be labor intensive for the perioperative team because of the difficulty in assessing the child, the lack of cooperation, and the frequent need to resort to pharmacological means to calm the child to induce anesthesia. Most parents who know their children's lack of social skills can help with induction if they are given a clear understanding of what to expect. This might sometimes require isolating one parent to explain these details, while the other may be exclusively trying to control the distraught child from escaping from the room.

Understanding their child's need for a calm and safe induction of anesthesia, usually most parents call ahead to specify what the children will tolerate on arrival and what they will not. They may request a quiet room with a minimal number of health workers walking in and out of their child's room. Parents are encouraged during preop phone calls to bring anything that might calm their child: a favorite blanket or pillow, a stuffed animal toy or a squeezy toy, to be with the child on anesthetic induction. If the child would take oral premedication, midazolam can be administered to calm the child pharmacologically. In those children who will not take anything orally and will not let anyone come near them, intramuscular agents can be used by a stealth approach after explaining the process to the parent. IM ketamine is a suitable agent for IM induction, but the dose required is usually 3–4 mg/kg to achieve quick onset of sedation which could result in prolonged sleep after a minor procedure. IM DEX is being used with good success and may be the newer option in these children. The drug of choice for induction of anesthesia is currently DEX which can be administered either by the nasal route or by the intramuscular route.

2.2 Brain Evoked Auditory Response (BAER) Test

Encountering autistic children for a hearing test by using brain evoked auditory response (BAER) test is becoming more frequent in most surgical centers. The main problem of "questionable" hearing loss is because most autistic children behave apparently "deaf" to parents and family members by not responding to their name when called or to any other verbal commands. The ABR test in these children tends to be perfectly normal and therefore of a much shorter duration because most of them have normal hearing pathways. The apparent lack of response is often interpreted by family as potential sensorineural deafness because of their inability to process and respond to verbal commands. Once the induction is over, the anesthetic management is unremarkable and brief. Infants, children, and developmentally delayed or challenged children require anesthesia or deep sedation to remain motionless, for these very brief noninvasive procedures. The challenge for the anesthesia provider is how to assess the child, to plan and execute a smooth anesthetic induction, maintenance, and emergence, focusing on patient safety and parental satisfaction. This can be labor-intensive, involving several members of the perioperative team to keep the child calm and safe from the time of arrival till he is wake and reunited with his family without hurting himself or others.

3 Premedication or Preinduction Drugs

1. *What induction techniques are suitable in children with ASD?*
2. *What is the advantage of DEX over other sedative drugs?*
3. *What are the routes of administration of dexmedetomidine?*
4. *Are there studies to prove the effectiveness of DEX in children?*
5. *What are the unwanted side effects of dexmedetomidine?*
6. *Is pretreatment with anticholinergics necessary to prevent bradycardia?*
7. *Is dexmedetomidine approved to be used in children?*

The following discussion will focus on answering the above questions.

Dexmedetomidine is a potent highly selective alpha-2 adrenoreceptor agonist with anxiolytic, sedative, and analgesic effects. The sedative properties of dexmedetomidine (DEX) are desirable because the effects are very similar to natural sleep by its acts on the locus caeruleus, a nucleus in the pons of the brainstem involved with physiological response to stress and panic and a part of the reticular activating system.

Compared to sedatives like ketamine, DEX produces less secretions and does not have paradoxical reaction like midazolam. Intravenous route is commonly used, but intranasal administration of DEX is gaining popularity for anxiolysis and moderate sedation in children without intravenous lines.

Intranasal administration of DEX is less invasive than an intravenous route, and if parents have been warned and prepared about that route of administration, it can be useful in calming children as a preinduction agent. DEX is an effective sedative drug for noninvasive procedures like BAER, CT, MRI, nuclear medicine scans, ECHO, and EEG studies. DEX has minimal effect on respiratory depression in healthy children especially when a nasal route is utilized.

A prospective observational study was undertaken to evaluate the use of nasal DEX in children 6 months to 18 years with an ASA status I or II, undergoing noninvasive procedures such as radiological studies, electroencephalography, echocardiography, and BAER. The researchers reported that a dose of 3mcg/kg of DEX administered nasally as a sole agent or in combination with nasal midazolam had a very high success rate of sedation in 92% of patients [1]. Previous studies have shown that DEX produces bradycardia and hypotension in patients, and secondary to its effects on the α_2-adrenoreceptor, DEX can also decrease cardiac output, as clonidine does.

Another double-blind study compared nasal DEX (3mcg/kg) to nasal midazolam (0.3 mg) in 162 children undergoing CT scans and found more decreases in HR and BP with DEX group but more decreases in oxygen saturation with midazolam group. They concluded that DEX 3mcg/kg is superior to midazolam in faster-onset sedation satisfaction by parents and physicians and with fewer side effects [2].

Comparison of sedative effects of oral midazolam 0.5 mg/kg to nasal DEX 2.5 mcg/kg in 59 children aged 1–6 years similarly showed children in the DEX group having better Ramsay Sedation Scores during their CT scans compared to the midazolam group [3].

In 100 children aged 2–12 years, with ASA status I and II undergoing elective surgery, the onset time and duration of sedation of DEX were found to be 25 and 85 min, respectively. The overall satisfactory sedation at the time of intravenous cannulation attempt in children was only 62% perhaps due to the lower nasal DEX dose (1 mcg/kg) used [4].

Nasal delivery of DEX is achieved using an atomizer or drops from a syringe.

Mucosal atomization devices help efficient delivery of atomized solution to the nasal mucosa which is absorbed rapidly and taken up into the systemic circulation. A comparative study of these two nasal delivery methods, namely, atomizer and syringe, showed similar effectiveness [5].

Intramuscular route of delivering DEX (mean: 2.4–2.9 mcg/kg) was reported to be successful in producing sedation with mean time to achieve sedation of 13 min, in 65 children undergoing CT and MRI [6].

Randomized double blind controlled trials comparing the use of nasal DEX (3mcg/kg) to other sedatives like oral chloral hydrate (50 mg/kg) specifically for auditory brain response (ABR) showed the distinct advantages of DEX. A higher incidence of testing completion with a single dose with shorter time to desired sedation level and return to baseline activity on the same day were seen in those receiving DEX compared to oral chloral hydrate [7, 8].

Another study compared the sedative effects of oral chloral hydrate 50 mg/kg with intranasal DEX (3 mcg/kg) with buccal midazolam (0.1 mg/kg) for ABR testing. Intranasal DEX and buccal midazolam group had higher sedation success as well as deeper level of anesthesia compared to the oral chloral hydrate group with similar discharge times [9].

A systematic review of literature on the use and effect of intranasal DEX in children for ABR testing was undertaken by a study group in Italy. They reviewed all six articles published between 2016 and 2021 on the use of DEX in ABR testing, and the results were published early this year. The results showed high sedation effectiveness and success with DEX in all but one study. The dose used was 3 mcg/kg and the comparative groups in three studies used oral chloral hydrate [10].

Another systematic review meta-analysis based on the Cochrane Review methods included 1168 participants in 13 randomized controlled studies and evaluated the effect of intranasal DEX as a premedication in children. DEX provided satisfactory sedation at parent separation than other premedication agents requiring less rescue analgesics. In addition, DEX produced less nasal irritation and postoperative nausea and vomiting compared to other premedication drugs [11].

A retrospective data collection on 17,948 children in a tertiary hospital in China reported that combining DEX and ketamine administered nasally was effective with a success rate of 93% for sedation and low rate of adverse events during diagnostic studies [12].

Many studies with DEX have shown transient hypertension, bradycardia, and hypotension secondary to its peripheral vasoconstriction and sympatholytic properties. DEX activates the central pre- and post-alpha 2 receptors in the locus caeruleus and produces hypnosis and unconsciousness. The size of the body, hepatic function, plasma albumin, and cardiac output have significant effect on the pharmacokinetics of DEX [13].

Incidence of bradycardia with the use of DEX in children has been an area of interest to many researchers. Meta-analyses of 21 studies evaluated 2835 patients for this phenomenon of bradycardia after the use of DEX. They found that the incidence of bradycardia in dexmedetomidine-treated pediatric patients was 3%. In the meta-regression analyses, the patient's age, body weight, and DEX dose were not significantly associated with the incidence of bradycardia. The minimum heart rate observed during treatment with DEX however was positively associated with the patient's baseline heart rate [14].

DEX has tremendous usefulness as a sedative agent for anesthesia induction whether it is administered intravenously, intramuscularly, or intranasally. Selection of types of cases, concomitant drugs, and total dosage used is important to avoid the incidence of bradycardia and other hemodynamic adverse events. The incidence of bradycardia and the risk factors for bradycardia after intranasal administration were studied in 9984 children who underwent noninvasive studies. The overall incidence of bradycardia after sedation with intranasal DEX was 2.3% with normal blood pressure with male children showing a 1.48-fold higher risk. Children who received additional doses of DEX had more incidences of bradycardia compared to those who had a single dose. Simple wake up was effective in managing the bradycardia [15].

A case report of vasovagal syncope and severe bradycardia after the administration of intranasal DEX for sedation in an 11-year-old girl undergoing voiding cystourethrogram highlights the importance of continuing EKG monitoring in these patients for a longer period even if consciousness and vital signs are back to pre-sedation levels [16].

The effect of DEX on cardiac conduction tissue in children undergoing electrophysiological studies showed significant depression of both sinus and AV node function. This was evidenced by prolongation of the sinus cycle length, sinus node recovery time as well as AV nodal effective refractory period, Wenckebach cycle length, and ventriculo-atrial block cycle length. Arial excitability was decreased by DEX by increasing the atrial refractory period.

Despite the absence of spontaneous AV nodal block, the researchers cautioned the use of DEX in children at risk for bradycardia or AV nodal dysfunction [17, 18].

A case report of profound bradycardia with the use of DEX as a sedative infusion in the pediatric ICU in a 5-week-old infant on a ventilator with the diagnosis of AV canal and acute RSV should serve as a warning to avoid its use in infants on digoxin [19].

A review paper by Mason and Lerman in 2011 summarized the knowledge of DEX gleaned from many studies and concluded that DEX is an effective sedative, analgesic, and anxiolytic in children, maintaining the airway with minimal respiratory depression and decreasing shivering postoperatively. However, varying degrees of bradycardia, hypotension, and hypertension can still be evidenced depending on the age of the child and the dose administered. Recovery from DEX, which has a 2-h elimination half-life, may be protracted compared to the other sedatives. Appropriate monitoring and prompt interventions can maintain the continual safe use of DEX children without adverse cardiovascular complications [20].

In a 2013 study published by Mason and her colleagues, the effect of DEX on children undergoing nuclear medicine scans was evaluated. DEX was administered as an intravenous bolus of 2 mcg/kg over 10 min followed by a continuous infusion of 1 mcg/kg/h, in 669 patients with 99.7% success. Hypotension, hypertension, and bradycardia (defined as deviations of more than 20% from age-adjusted awake norms) occurred in 58.7%, 2.1%, and 4.3% of patients, respectively. Both hypotension and bradycardia were related to age, with older children tending to experience more hypotension and bradycardia but not requiring any pharmacologic therapy [21].

Another study by the same group reviewed the database on 3522 children undergoing radiological imaging (MRI) to determine the incidence and the predictors of hypertension. The children who received high-dose DEX sedation showed a hemodynamic change in the form of hypertension. 4.9% of patients had hypertension with a higher incidence in the younger group (0–3 years) when compared to older children (3–18 years) and those who received more than one bolus. The conclusion of this study was that hypertension is most likely to occur in infants during continuous infusion and after receiving an additional bolus of DEX [22].

When high doses of DEX are used, bradycardia can be severe. However, there is a need for caution before using an anticholinergic drug to counter this low heart rate. An anticholinergic like glycopyrrolate (5 mcg/kg) can increase the low heart rate and cause an exaggerated increase in arterial blood pressure. An interesting case report on three cases where the authors saw this unusual effect is worth remembering when one encounters profound bradycardia in children receiving high-dose DEX infusion [23].

Currently, there are no guidelines to pilot one to treat or even pretreat a drop-in heart rate by using an anticholinergic, when DEX is administered. In a retrospective descriptive study, a group of researchers reviewed the records of 163 children receiving DEX infusion during the MRI studies followed by administration of an anticholinergic. The mean age was 94.5 months and 32% had the diagnosis of Down syndrome. During the scan, the heart rate and systolic blood pressure decreased when no anticholinergics were given. Heart rate decreased by 26.6% in the non-pretreated patients compared to only 16.7% in the treated group. However, the systolic blood pressure increased significantly in the anticholinergic treated group compared to the untreated group (20.2% vs. 10.4%, respectively; $P = 0.02$). The maximal systolic blood pressure increased significantly, compared with baseline, in the anticholinergic group in comparison with the non-anticholinergic group. In children with Down syndrome, this blood pressure increase was even more exaggerated, 36 times greater when anticholinergic was given compared to the blood pressure in children who did not receive the anticholinergic. The conclusion of this study is that prophylactic administration of anticholinergic shows no advantage other than a transient clinically insignificant increase in heart rate but may precipitate an exaggerated increase in systolic blood pressure in patients treated with anticholinergic [24].

Despite the lack of approved pediatric labeling, DEX has been used almost daily in clinical practice in pediatric anesthesia and sedation services. Its bioavailability by nasal, IM, IV, and even subcutaneous routes make DEX very valuable in children with no intravenous access [25].

An international study to evaluate the prescription practices of DEX by pediatric anesthesiologists was undertaken by an online survey, and the results were published in 2021. Data from 791 responses (17% of 5171 invitees) were analyzed and showed that DEX was prescribed by 70% of those who responded.

Members of the pediatric specialty societies and their usage of DEX are shown within as percentages: Europe, (ESPA-53%), New Zealand and Australia (SPANZA-69%), Great Britain and Ireland (APAGBI-34%), and the USA (SPA-96%).

The marked difference in the use of DEX is probably reflective of lack of education or experience with DEX and because of lack of approved pediatric labeling. The current worldwide practice in the use of DEX in anesthesia and sedation will hopefully continue to improve in the future [26].

4 Conclusion

Dexmedetomidine is an extremely valuable drug in the anesthesiologist armamentarium. DEX is unique in being able to be administered by different routes for induction of anesthesia. In children undergoing pain-free noninvasive sedation procedures, the use of this drug is unique. It is versatile and superior to other premedication drugs because of the quality of sedation it provides described as being similar to natural sleep. To continue the safety record of this off-label drug, it is important for those who prescribe this drug to be thoroughly knowledgeable about its mode of action and side effects and to choose the right patient and the right dose to achieve the desired sedation goal.

References

1. Behrle N, Birisci E, Anderson J, Schroeder S, Dalabih A. Intranasal dexmedetomidine as a sedative for pediatric procedural sedation. J Pediatr Pharmacol Ther. 2017;22(1):4–8. https://doi.org/10.5863/1551-6776-22.1.4. PMID: 28337075; PMCID: PMC5341530
2. Azizkhani R, Heydari F, Ghazavi M, Riahinezhad M, Habibzadeh M, Bigdeli A, Golshani K, Majidinejad S, Mohammadbeigi A. Comparing sedative effect of dexmedetomidine versus midazolam for sedation of children while undergoing computerized tomography imaging. J Pediatr Neurosci. 2020;15(3):245–51. https://doi.org/10.4103/jpn.JPN_107_19. Epub 2020 Nov 6. PMID: 33531939; PMCID: PMC7847110
3. Ghai B, Jain K, Saxena AK, Bhatia N, Sodhi KS. Comparison of oral midazolam with intranasal dexmedetomidine premedication for children undergoing CT imaging: a randomized, double-blind, and controlled study. Paediatr Anaesth. 2017;27(1):37–44. https://doi.org/10.1111/pan.13010. Epub 2016 Oct 13. PMID: 27734549
4. Yuen VM, Hui TW, Irwin MG, Yao TJ, Wong GL, Yuen MK. Optimal timing for the administration of intranasal dexmedetomidine for premedication in children. Anaesthesia. 2010;65(9):922–9. https://doi.org/10.1111/j.1365-2044.2010.06453.x. PMID: 20645951
5. Li BL, Zhang N, Huang JX, Qiu QQ, Tian H, Ni J, Song XR, Yuen VM, Irwin MG. A comparison of intranasal dexmedetomidine for sedation in children administered either by atomizer or by drops. Anaesthesia. 2016;71(5):522–8. https://doi.org/10.1111/anae.13407. Epub 2016 Mar 3. PMID: 26936022
6. Mason KP, Lubisch NB, Robinson F, Roskos R. Intramuscular dexmedetomidine sedation for pediatric MRI and CT. AJR Am J Roentgenol. 2011;197(3):720–5.
7. Reynolds J, Rogers A, Medellin E, Guzman JA, Watcha MF. A prospective, randomized, double-blind trial of intranasal dexmedetomidine and oral chloral hydrate for sedated auditory brainstem response (ABR) testing. Paediatr Anaesth. 2016;26(3):286–93. https://doi.org/10.1111/pan.12854. PMID: 26814038
8. Delvi MB. Is intranasal dexmedetomidine superior to oral chloral hydrate for procedural sedation in children: a systematic review. Saudi J Anaesth. 2022;16(1):82–5. https://doi.org/10.4103/sja.sja_489_21. Epub 2022 Jan 4. PMID: 35261594; PMCID: PMC8846254
9. Li BL, Yuen VM, Zhou JL, Zhang N, Huang JX, Tian H, Song XR. A randomized controlled trial of oral chloral hydrate vs intranasal dexmedetomidine plus buccal midazolam for auditory brainstem response testing in children. Paediatr Anaesth. 2018;28(11):1022–8. https://doi.org/10.1111/pan.13498. Epub 2018 Oct 3.PMID: 30281180.
10. Marra P, Di Stadio A, Colacurcio V, Scarpa A, La Mantia I, Salzano FA, De Luca P. Sedation with intranasal dexmedetomidine in the pediatric population for auditory brainstem response testing: review of the existing literature. Healthcare (Basel). 2022;10(2):287. https://doi.org/10.3390/healthcare10020287. PMID: 35206901; PMCID: PMC8872591
11. Jun JH, Kim KN, Kim JY, Song SM. The effects of intranasal dexmedetomidine premedication in children: a systematic review and meta-analysis. Can J Anaesth. 2017;64(9):947–61. English. https://doi.org/10.1007/s12630-017-0917-x. Epub 2017 Jun 21. PMID: 28639236.
12. Yang F, Liu Y, Yu Q, Li S, Zhang J, Sun M, Liu L, Lei Y, Tian Q, Liu H, Tu S. Analysis of 17 948 pediatric patients undergoing procedural sedation with a combination of intranasal dexmedetomidine and ketamine. Paediatr Anaesth. 2019;29(1):85–91. https://doi.org/10.1111/pan.13526. Epub 2018 Nov 28. PMID: 30484930

13. Weerink MAS, Struys MMRF, Hannivoort LN, Barends CRM, Absalom AR, Colin P. Clinical pharmacokinetics and pharmacodynamics of dexmedetomidine. Clin Pharmacokinet. 2017;56(8):893–913. https://doi.org/10.1007/s40262-017-0507-7. PMID: 28105598; PMCID: PMC5511603
14. Gong M, Man Y, Fu Q. Incidence of bradycardia in pediatric patients receiving dexmedetomidine anesthesia: a meta-analysis. Int J Clin Pharm. 2017;39(1):139–47. https://doi.org/10.1007/s11096-016-0411-5. Epub 2016 Dec 31. PMID: 28040841
15. Lei H, Chao L, Miao T, Ya Jun L, Shen Ling L, Yan Ying P, Xiao Han P, Yun Bo X, Xin T. Incidence and risk factors of bradycardia in pediatric patients undergoing intranasal dexmedetomidine sedation. Acta Anaesthesiol Scand. 2020;64(4):464–71. https://doi.org/10.1111/aas.13509. Epub 2019 Dec 2. PMID: 31736052
16. Patel VJ, Ahmed SS, Nitu ME, Rigby MR. Vasovagal syncope and severe bradycardia following intranasal dexmedetomidine for pediatric procedural sedation. Paediatr Anaesth. 2014;24(4):446–8. https://doi.org/10.1111/pan.12368. Epub 2014 Feb 26. PMID: 24571687
17. Hammer GB, Drover DR, Cao H, Jackson E, Williams GD, Ramamoorthy C, Van Hare GF, Niksch A, Dubin AM. The effects of dexmedetomidine on cardiac electrophysiology in children. Anesth Analg. 2008;106(1):79–83, table of contents. https://doi.org/10.1213/01.ane.0000297421.92857.4e. PMID: 18165557.
18. Ergul Y, Unsal S, Ozyilmaz I, Ozturk E, Carus H, Guzeltas A. Electrocardiographic and electrophysiologic effects of dexmedetomidine on children. Pacing Clin Electrophysiol. 2015;38(6):682–7. https://doi.org/10.1111/pace.12623. Epub 2015 Apr 11. PMID: 25753681
19. Berkenbosch JW, Tobias JD. Development of bradycardia during sedation with dexmedetomidine in an infant currently receiving digoxin. Pediatr Crit Care Med. 2003;4(2):203–5.
20. Mason KP, Lerman J. Review article: dexmedetomidine in children: current knowledge and future applications. Anesth Analg. 2011;113(5):1129–42. https://doi.org/10.1213/ANE.0b013e31822b8629. Epub 2011 Aug 4. PMID: 21821507
21. Mason KP, Robinson F, Fontaine P, Prescilla R. Dexmedetomidine offers an option for safe and effective sedation for nuclear medicine imaging in children. Radiology. 2013;267(3):911–7.
22. Mason KP, Zurakowski D, Zgleszewski S, Prescilla R, Fontaine PJ, Dinardo JA. Incidence and predictors of hypertension during high dose dexmedetomidine sedation for pediatric MRI. Paediatr Anaesth. 2010;20(6):516–23. https://doi.org/10.1111/j.1460-9592.2010.03299.x. Epub 2010 Apr 14. PMID: 20412458
23. Mason KP, Zgleszewski S, Forman RE, Stark C, DiNardo JA. An exaggerated hypertensive response to glycopyrrolate therapy for bradycardia associated with high dose dexmedetomidine. Anesth Analg. 2009;108(3):906–8. https://doi.org/10.1213/ane.0b013e3181948a6f.
24. Subramanyam R, Cudilo EM, Hossain MM, McAuliffe J, Wu J, Patino M, Gunter J, Mahmoud M. To pretreat or not to pretreat: prophylactic anticholinergic administration before dexmedetomidine in pediatric imaging. Anesth Analg. 2015;121(2):479–85.
25. Mahmoud M, Barbi E, Mason KP. Dexmedetomidine: what's new for pediatrics? A narrative review. J Clin Med. 2020;9(9):2724. https://doi.org/10.3390/jcm9092724. PMID: 32846947; PMCID: PMC7565844
26. van Hoorn CE, Flint RB, Skowno J, Davies P, Engelhardt T, Lalwani K, Olutoye O, Ista E, de Graaff JC. Off-label use of dexmedetomidine in paediatric anaesthesiology: an international survey of 791 (paediatric) anaesthesiologists. Eur J Clin Pharmacol. 2021;77(4):625–35. https://doi.org/10.1007/s00228-020-03028-2. Evpub 2020 Oct 29. PMID: 33119787; PMCID: PMC7935836

Index

S. T. Verghese (ed.), *Anesthesia STAT! Acute Pediatric Emergencies in PACU*, https://doi.org/10.1007/978-3-031-24396-7

GPSR Compliance

The European Union's (EU) General Product Safety Regulation (GPSR) is a set of rules that requires consumer products to be safe and our obligations to ensure this.

If you have any concerns about our products, you can contact us on ProductSafety@springernature.com

In case Publisher is established outside the EU, the EU authorized representative is:

Springer Nature Customer Service Center GmbH
Europaplatz 3
69115 Heidelberg, Germany

Batch number: 10726135

Printed by Printforce, the Netherlands